Cardiac Assist Devices

Edited by

Daniel J. Goldstein, MD
Clinical Instructor in Cardiothoracic Surgery
Department of Surgery
Division of Cardiothoracic Surgery
Columbia Presbyterian Medical Center
New York, NY

and

Mehmet C. Oz, MD, MBA
Irving Assistant Professor of Surgery
Department of Surgery
Division of Cardiothoracic Surgery
Columbia Presbyterian Medical Center
New York, NY

Futura Publishing Company, Inc.
Armonk, NY

Library of Congress Cataloging-in-Publication Data

Cardiac assist devices / edited by Daniel J. Goldstein and Mehmet Oz.
    p. ; cm.
    ISBN 0-87993-449-2 (alk. paper)
    1. Cardiovascular instruments, Implanted. 2. Blood—Circulation, Artificial. 3.
    Heart—Surgery—Instruments. I. Goldstein, Daniel J., MD. II. Oz, Mehmet, 1960–
    [DNLM: 1. Heart-Assist Devices. 2. Intraoperative Care. WG 169.5 C267 1999]
    RD598.3.C37 1999
    617.4'10592—dc21

                                                                    99-048126

Copyright © 2000
Futura Publishing Company, Inc.

Published by
Futura Publishing Company
135 Bedford Road
Armonk, New York 10504

LC#: 99-048126
ISBN#: 0-87993-449-2

We dedicate this book to our wives,
Stephanie and Lisa,
for their endless patience, support,
love, and understanding

Foreword

The pandemic of congestive heart failure affects 1% of the western world and has become the source of increasing consternation for governments that are obliged to provide expensive treatments, sometimes with limited benefits, for patients who are often terminal.

I became a student of surgical options for this disease first as a heart and lung transplant surgeon, then as a principal investigator for a left ventricular assist device. I have continued to follow the impressive developments in the field ever since, now as a US senator responsible for funding our federal investment in biomedical research. In addition to the obvious, these options also provide a remarkable case study of how an entire treatment strategy can continue to evolve in an arena once felt to be mature—reminding us that our self-perceived limitations are often fictitious and can be overcome by creatively pursuing new frontiers with a healthy optimism.

The current trials evaluating long-term use of mechanical support in lieu of medical management, unimaginable even a decade ago, would never have come to fruition without such optimism and our aggressive use of pumps to salvage dying patients as a bridge to transplantation.

In *Cardiac Assist Devices*, editors Goldstein and Oz have not only summarized the developments in this rapidly evolving field, but have placed the current progress in an appropriate perspective. While early innovations in heart support during the middle part of the last century were designed by individuals who worked with relative independence, our own national policy makers came to appreciate the epidemiological impact of heart disease. Formal federal encouragement, through organizations such as the National Institutes of Health, has helped promote multidisciplinary approaches to the design of mechanical cardiac assist devices, and these research endeavors spawned numerous initiatives by small companies that have subsequently evolved into a thriving industry. In effect, the alliance of biomedical science, federal support, and industry has culminated in the creation of clinically viable heart pumps. A similar paradigm dominates developments in many other health-related fields as well.

By reviewing the history of mechanical pumps and exploring the fragile relationship between humans and machine through an overview of the biochemical and immune response changes associated with the use of artificial organs in living organisms, the book's contributors, many of whom are colleagues from my 20 years in medicine, help the reader understand how the fertile fields of innovation that today characterize the industry were sown.

Finally, experts in the field evaluate which pumps should be used in specific situations, make predictions for future developments, and, most importantly, review the nuances of creating successful programs. The lessons learned from this last topic alone are applicable to most of the substantive endeavors occurring in biomedicine as we approach the new millennium.

The heart specialists, the healthcare professionals, the policy makers—all will delight in reading this treatise. But the real beneficiary, shadowing the contributions discussed in each chapter, is the patient with heart disease, who will live a more fulfilling life because of the dedicated work of his fellow man.

Bill Frist, MD
US Senator

Preface

In 1896, Stephen Paget prophetically surmised that "surgery of the heart had probably reached the limits set by Nature to all surgery and that no new method and no new discovery could overcome the natural difficulties that attended a wound of the heart." Moreover, sentiments at the turn of the century regarding the heart as the "seat of the soul" and the "wellspring of life itself" pervaded poetry, philosophy, and the social sciences and rendered the heart a surgically untouchable organ. This *fin de siecle* skepticism permeated society, extending to another critical event in modern history occurring at this time—the introduction of the automobile. As a mechanical alternative to the long-lived and time-honored horse drawn carriage, it drew harsh criticism for being an unfulfillable, high-technological scam. Fortunately, Paget's foreboding vision proved erroneous, with both heart surgery and the motorcar rapidly becoming cultural icons, a fixture of our daily lives and a ubiquitous presence in our society.

Ambivalence (if not frank dubiousness) again beset heart surgery when Americans of the 1980s saw that the artificial heart, a product of cutting edge technology, did not provide the expected panacea. They saw Barney Clark wobbling on national television and witnessed his death (and those of most artificial heart recipients) without the quality of life promised by this space age technology. Despite these failures, mechanical hearts are increasingly being used to support patients with end-stage heart disease, and are swiftly entering the lexicon and armamentarium of cardiothoracic surgeons worldwide.

Certain similarities exist between the automotive and the mechanical support industries. In the most basic sense, the major function of both the car and the ventricular assist device (VAD) is to assist (a person or blood) in circulation. Both the car and the VAD can be mass-produced for wide distribution and are available for those who can afford the price. And importantly, both technologies provide users with a certain degree of freedom and independence.

Both cardiac surgery and the automotive industry have benefited from advances made in other fields, such as battery cells, which contributed to modern engine design and to the recent development of portable wearable VADs. Equally important, the development of both the car and the VAD have sparked advances in other fields. The widespread use of fossil fuel in cars (and subsequent bio-environmental pollution) has created a sub-industry dedicated to finding cleaner alternatives, while the application of textured-surface left VADs (LVADs) has engendered an entire field of immunology focused on gaining an understanding of the interaction between biomaterials and the immune system.

Both industries place a high premium on the safety of their technology. The automotive industry has developed anti-lock brakes, air-bags and steel reinforcement cages, while the VAD industry has manufactured pumps that are emboli-free and have multiple back-up mechanisms should equipment failure occur. Yet, unlike the car, and because VADs are so clearly linked to death when they fail, we hold them to much higher performance standards. Finally, both VAD and car companies have to design their devices to meet the needs and desires of their customers. The modern VAD industry, however, has only been in existence for two decades and, as a result, current VAD technology should be considered to be in its infancy. Most likely, one day we will view current devices the same way we now view Henry Ford's Model T.

The pursuit of long-term devices as a solution for heart failure, one of the leading killers of humans, must be accompanied by a rational understanding of how these advances will take place. We will only advance the technology by pushing it to failure and modifying the devices as we learn from their shortcomings. In a way, failure must be viewed as the road to progress. In this book, we seek to advance the knowledge of the readership by approaching the study of VADs from this vantage point.

Why a Book about Cardiac Assist Devices?

At first, the concept of writing a book about a seemingly narrow subject with an even narrower audience appears inconsequential. In the editors' minds, the book's *raison d'être* extends far beyond the needs of today's heart surgeon. It is our strong belief that while the book is mainly aimed at cardiologists, circulatory physiologists, critical care specialists, anesthesiologists, cardiac surgeons, and other healthcare professionals taking care of patients with end-stage heart disease, the content should apply to all healthcare providers, as this technology will undoubtedly touch all of our lives. Moreover, the development of the field of mechanical circulatory support represents the paradigm upon which many future medical industries will be built.

Furthermore, the topic discussed in the book pertains to an evolving technology aimed at treating one of the greatest and most expensive public health problems, congestive heart failure. Indeed, heart failure afflicts close to one percent of the adult population in the United States, is a contributing factor in over 250,000 deaths annually, is the primary diagnosis for more than 900,000 hospitalizations per year, and commands total treatment costs that approach $38 billion annually or nearly 4% of total healthcare costs. And despite the availability of heart transplantation as the preferred surgical treatment for end-stage heart disease, this mode of therapy is limited and clearly insufficient to meet the increasing demands for donor organs. The most recent figures available suggest that only 1 in 24 patients who could benefit from heart transplantation actually receives a donor organ, underscoring the crucial need for alternatives to cardiac allotransplantation.

Cardiac Assist Devices is organized into three different sections encompassing 30 chapters written by recognized leading investigators actively involved in their respective fields. The editors painstakingly surveyed colleagues and the literature to identify authors who 1) have extensive and current clinical experience with the topic; 2) have contributed vastly to the literature on the subject; and/or 3) have been closely involved in the development of a particular idea or device that has contributed to our understanding of circulatory assistance.

The first major section, entitled "General Aspects of Mechanical Support," presents an overview of the field of mechanical circulatory support with emphasis on the perioperative care of these fragile patients. Dr. Frazier, a pioneer in the field, and colleagues from the Texas Heart Institute, provide a historical perspective on mechanical support. Dr. Farrar, who has substantially advanced our understanding of ventricular interactions, contributes a chapter on the physiology of ventricular assistance.

Dr. Benjamin Sun, from the Pennsylvania State University, an institution with a long recognized history of significant contributions to the field of mechanical support, takes the reader through the algorithms used in selecting the best suited device for a given patient. With an unsurpassable clinical experience, Dr. Tom Karl from the Royal Children's Hospital in Australia presents an authoritative review of the limited options available for neonates, infants, and children who require mechanical support. The cardiothoracic anesthesia team from Columbia Presbyterian Medical Center, armed with experience in more than 170 cases involving implantable LVADs, succinctly presents the salient aspects necessary for a successful anesthetic approach to this complex patient population.

The ensuing four chapters comprise the perioperative management of the Achilles' heels of LVAD surgery, namely, bleeding, right heart failure, arrhythmias, and vasodilatory shock. Dr. Van Meter, from one of the leading implant centers in the country, addresses the etiology, complications, and management of perioperative bleeding, the most common complication plaguing LVAD surgery. Drs. Chen and Rose, recognized authors in the field, provide what is perhaps the most thorough review of the pathogenesis and management of right heart failure following LVAD placement, an entity responsible for most of the early mortality following this operation. A subject that has undeservedly received very little attention in the field is that of arrhythmias in the setting of LVAD placement. Based on their extensive institutional experience, Drs. Coromilas and Williams from Columbia Presbyterian examine the limited literature on the subject and provide important insights into the management of the frequent malignant ventricular arrhythmias that can affect this patient population. Finally, Drs. Argenziano and Landry discuss vasodilatory shock, a clinical entity that has received increasing attention in the literature, and review the successful use of vasopressin, a novel approach first proposed by the authors.

The topic of myocardial recovery is perhaps one of the most hotly debated and controversial in the field of LVAD support. With their contribution, Dr. Mueller and colleagues from the University of Berlin discuss their forefront efforts aimed at documenting myocardial recovery during LVAD support and predicting successful and long-lasting device explantation. Drs. Mancini and Beniaminovitz, medical leaders of one of the most active transplantation programs in the country, apply their tremendous experience with end-stage heart failure to review the effects of chronic LVAD support on submaximal and maximal exercise physiology.

A successful bridge to transplantation requires more than a skilled surgeon and caring cardiologist. An aggressive period of nutritional support and rehabilitation in the outpatient setting ensures that this process occurs and that the patient experiences an optimal quality of life. The nursing, rehabilitation, and psychiatric teams at Columbia Presbyterian exhaustively discuss the topics of outpatient support, rehabilitation, and quality of life.

In the current era of constrained healthcare resources, the increasing application of an expensive therapy such as LVAD support must be guided by trials that evaluate the benefits and costs of this emerging technology. Dr. Moskowitz and colleagues from the International Center for Outcomes Research examine the data on the economic impact of this technology, and advance the concept of cost effectiveness as a means of measuring the success of LVAD technology.

As pointed out earlier, investigation of the effects of biomaterials on the immune system and circulating blood elements has given rise to the field of LVAD immunobiology. The leader in this field, Dr. Silviu Itescu, examines in great detail the host—LVAD interaction and unveils a fascinating immunosuppressive effect reminiscent of systemic immunodeficient states such as AIDS and lupus erythematosus.

Part II, entitled "Available Devices," focuses on an individual characterization of the currently available and most widely used extracorporeal and intracorporeal ventricular assist devices. Each of the nine chapters is written by a leading investigator(s) who has extensive clinical and research experience with the device. Each chapter follows a similar format that comprises 1) a description of the device; 2) implantation technique; 3) limitations of the device; 4) results and outcomes; and 5) future directions.

In the final section of the book, entitled "Future Devices," the editors have searched for the most promising devices currently undergoing preclinical evaluation, and have asked their developers to describe the device and insinuate a plausible timeline for the clinical availability of their devices.

We hope that the readership will understand the practical aspects of device selection, implantation, and management, and learn of advances made during the evolution of this field that may impact on their daily practice. Perhaps more importantly, readers will develop insights into how high technology in modern medicine evolves—an observation that will color their view of this and other developments. The readership should be reminded of these lessons the next time they step into their cases, turn on their TVs, or send an E-mail over the web. As is usually the case, advances in medicine are paralleling changes in our society. Enjoy our "user's manual."

Contributing Authors

Hendrik-Jan Ankersmit, MD Post-doctorate Fellow in Cardiothoracic Surgery, Department of Surgery, Columbia Presbyterian Medical Center, New York, NY

Francisco Arabia, MD Department of Surgery, Section of Cardiovascular and Thoracic Surgery, University of Arizona Health Science Center, Tucson, AZ

Michael Argenziano, MD Fellow in Cardiothoracic Surgery, Department of Surgery, Division of Cardiothoracic Surgery, Columbia Presbyterian Medical Center, New York, NY

John H. Artrip, MD Cardiothoracic Research Fellow, Department of Surgery, Columbia Presbyterian Medical Center, New York, NY

Ainat Beniaminovitz, MD Assistant Professor of Medicine, Department of Medicine, Division of Cardiology, Columbia Presbyterian Medical Center, New York, NY

Lori A. Buck, MS, PT, CCS Department of Physical Therapy, Columbia Presbyterian Medical Center, New York, NY

Daniel Burkhoff, MD, PhD Associate Professor of Medicine, Department of Medicine, Division of Circulatory Physiology, Columbia Presbyterian Medical Center, New York, NY

Katharine A. Catanese, MSN Department of Surgery, Division of Cardiothoracic Surgery, Columbia Presbyterian Medical Center, New York, NY

Jonathan M. Chen, MD Department of Surgery, Columbia Presbyterian Medical Center, New York, NY

Jack Copeland, MD Professor and Chief, Department of Surgery, Section of Cardiovascular and Thoracic Surgery, University of Arizona Health Science Center, Tucson, AZ

James Coromilas, MD Associate Professor of Medicine, Division of Cardiology, Columbia Presbyterian Medical Center, New York, NY

Jack J. Curtis, MD Professor of Surgery, Chief, Cardiothoracic Surgery, Department of Surgery, University of Missouri-Columbia, Columbia, MO

Michael E. DeBakey, MD Chancellor Emeritus, Department of Surgery, Baylor College of Medicine, Houston, TX

Joseph J. DeRose, Jr., MD   Fellow in Cardiothoracic Surgery, Department of Surgery, Division of Cardiothoracic Surgery, Columbia Presbyterian Medical Center, New York, NY

Marc L. Dickstein, MD   Assistant Professor of Anesthesiology, Department of Anesthesiology, Columbia Presbyterian Medical Center, New York, NY

David J. Farrar, PhD   Vice President of Research and Development, Thoratec Laboratories Corporation, Pleasonton, CA; Department of Cardiac Surgery, California Pacific Medical Center, San Francisco, CA

O.H. Frazier, MD   Chief, Division of Cardiovascular and Thoracic Surgery, Professor of Surgery, Department of Surgery, The University of Texas-Houston Medical School; Chief, Cardiopulmonary Transplantation, St. Luke's Episcopal Hospital, Texas Heart Institute, Houston, TX

John M. Fuqua, Jr.   Medical Device Consultant, Cullen Cardiovascular Research Laboratory, Texas Heart Institute, Houston, TX

Annetine C. Gelijns, PhD   International Center for Health Outcomes and Innovation Research, Department of Surgery, College of Physicians and Surgeons, Joseph L. Mailman School of Public Health, Columbia University, New York, NY

Daniel J. Goldstein, MD   Clinical Instructor in Cardiothoracic Surgery, Department of Surgery, Division of Cardiothoracic Surgery, Columbia Presbyterian Medical Center, New York, NY

Mark J.S. Heath, MD   Assistant Professor of Anesthesiology, Department of Anesthesiology, Columbia Presbyterian Medical Center, New York, NY

David N. Helman, MD   Department of Surgery, Division of General Surgery, Massachusetts General Hospital, Boston, MA

Paul J. Hendry, MD   Associate Professor, Cardiovascular Devices Division, University of Ottawa Heart Institute, Ontario, Canada

Roland Hetzer, MD, PhD   Professor of Surgery, Humboldt University, Berlin; Chairman and Chief Surgeon, Department of Thoracic and Cardiovascular Surgery, Deutsches Herzzentrum Berlin, Berlin, Germany

Stephen B. Horton, MD   Clinical Perfusionist, Royal Children's Hospital, Melbourne, Australia

Suellen Irwin, RN   Department of Surgery, Baylor College of Medicine, Houston, TX

Silviu Itescu, MD   Assistant Professor of Surgical Sciences, Director of Transplant Immunology, Department of Surgery, Columbia Presbyterian Medical Center, New York, NY

Robert K. Jarvik, MD   Jarvik Heart Incorporated, New York, NY

Richard J. Kaplon, MD   Fellow in Cardiothoracic Surgery, Department of Thoracic and Cardiovascular Surgery, Cleveland Clinic Foundation, Cleveland, OH

Tom R. Karl, MD   Director, Victorian Pediatric Surgical Unit, Royal Children's Hospital, Melbourne, Australia

Friedrich Kaufmann   Engineer, Department of Thoracic and Cardiovascular Surgery, Deutsches Herzzentrum Berlin, Berlin, Germany

Wilbert J. Keon, MD   Professor and Chairman, Division of Cardiac Surgery, University of Ottawa Heart Institute, Ontario, Canada

G. Kimble Jett, MD   Chief, Cardiothoracic Surgery, Providence Seattle Medical Center, Seattle, WA

Robert L. Kormos, MD   Associate Professor of Surgery, Director of Artificial Heart Program, University of Pittsburgh Medical Center, Pittsburgh, PA

Donald W. Landry, MD, PhD   Department of Medicine, Division of Nephrology, Columbia Presbyterian Medical Center, New York, NY

Robert R. Lazzara, MD   Director, Minimally Invasive Surgery, Cardiovascular Surgery, Providence Seattle Medical Center, Seattle, WA

Ronald G. Levitan, BS   International Center for Health Outcomes and Innovation Research, Columbia University, New York, NY

Matthias Loebe, MD, PhD   Head, Assist Device Program, Senior Surgeon, Department of Thoracic and Cardiovascular Surgery, Deutsches Herzzentrum Berlin, Berlin, Germany

Douglas P. Lohmann, M.Eng.   Coordinator of Circulatory Support, Department of Cardiothoracic Surgery, Wake Forest University School of Medicine, Winston-Salem, NC

Donna Mancini, MD   Associate Professor of Medicine, Medical Director of Cardiac Transplantation, Department of Medicine, Division of Cardiology, Columbia Presbyterian Medical Center, New York, NY

Roy G. Masters, MD   Associate Professor of Surgery, Program Director, Cardiac Surgery, University of Ottawa Heart Institute, Ontario, Canada

Sanjay M. Mehta, MD   Fellow in Cardiothoracic Surgery, Division of Cardiothoracic Surgery, Penn State Geisinger Health System, The Pennsylvania State University, Hershey, PA

Berend Mets, MB, ChB, FRCA, PhD   Associate Professor of Clinical Anesthesiology, Department of Anesthesiology, Columbia Presbyterian Medical Center, New York, NY

David L.S. Morales, MD   Department of Surgery, Columbia Presbyterian Medical Center, New York, NY

Deborah Morley, PhD   Director, Regulatory and Clinical Affairs, MicroMed Technology, Inc.; Department of Surgery, Baylor College of Medicine, Houston, TX

Theresa M. Morrone, MS, PT, CCS   Department of Physical Therapy, Columbia Presbyterian Medical Center, New York, NY

Alan J. Moskowitz, MD   International Center for Health Outcomes and Innovation Research, Departments of Surgery and Medicine, College of Physicians and Surgeons, Joseph L. Mailman School of Public Health, Columbia University, New York, NY

Johannes Mueller, MD   CEO, Mediport Corporation; Department of Thoracic and Cardiovascular Surgery, Deutsches Herzzentrum Berlin, Berlin, Germany

Tofy Mussivand, PhD   Professor of Surgery and Engineering, Chair, Cardiovascular Devices Division, University of Ottawa Heart Institute, Ontario, Canada

Paul Nolan, PhD   Department of Surgery, Section of Cardiovascular and Thoracic Surgery, University of Arizona Health Science Center, Tucson, AZ

George P. Noon, MD   Professor of Surgery, Department of Surgery, Baylor College of Medicine, Houston, TX

Timothy E. Oaks, MD   Assistant Professor, Cardiothoracic Surgery, Director, Thoracic Transplantation, Department of Cardiothoracic Surgery, Wake Forest University School of Medicine, Winston-Salem, NC

Mehmet C. Oz, MD, MBA   Irving Assistant Professor of Surgery, Department of Surgery, Division of Cardiothoracic Surgery, Columbia Presbyterian Medical Center, New York, NY

Walter E. Pae, Jr., MD   Professor of Surgery, Director, Cardiac Transplantation, Division of Cardiothoracic Surgery, Penn State Geisinger Health System, The Pennsylvania State University, Hershey, PA

D. Glenn Pennington, MD   Howard Holt Bradshaw Professor of Surgery and Chair, Department of Cardiothoracic Surgery, Wake Forest University School of Medicine, Winston-Salem, NC

Peer M. Portner, PhD   Chairman, Novacor Division, Baxter Healthcare Corporation, Oakland, CA; Consulting Professor, Cardiothoracic Surgery, Stanford University School of Medicine, Stanford, CA

Narayanan Ramasamy, PhD   Director of Scientific Affairs, Novacor Division, Baxter Healthcare Corporation, Oakland, CA

Eric A. Rose, MD   Rose and Morris Milstein Johnson & Johnson Professor, Chairman, Department of Surgery, Division of Cardiothoracic Surgery, Columbia Presbyterian Medical Center, New York, NY

Peter A. Shapiro, MD   Associate Professor of Clinical Psychiatry, Department of Psychiatry, Columbia Presbyterian Medical Center, New York, NY

Nicholas G. Smedira, MD   Department of Thoracic and Cardiovascular Surgery, Cleveland Clinic Foundation, Cleveland, OH

Richard Smith, MSEE   Department of Surgery, Section of Cardiovascular and Thoracic Surgery, University of Arizona Health Science Center, Tucson, AZ

Benjamin C. Sun, MD   Assistant Professor of Surgery, Section of Cardiothoracic and Vascular Surgery, Penn State Geisinger Health System, Milton S. Hershey Medical Center, Hershey, PA

Anita Tierney, MPH   International Center for Health Outcomes and Innovation Research, Columbia University, New York, NY

Clifford H. Van Meter, Jr., MD   Chief, Division of Cardiothoracic Surgery and Transplantation, Ochsner Clinic, New Orleans, LA

Rita L. Vargo, MSN, RN   Senior Clinical Consultant, Novacor Division, Baxter Healthcare Corporation, Oakland, CA

Gus J. Vlahakes, MD   Associate Professor of Surgery, Harvard Medical School; Visiting Surgeon, Division of Cardiac Surgery, Massachusetts General Hospital, Boston, MA

Colette Wagner-Mann, DVM, PhD   Research Assistant Professor, Department of Surgery, University of Missouri-Columbia, Columbia, MO

Deborah L. Williams, MPH   International Center for Health Outcomes and Innovation Research, Departments of Surgery and Medicine, Columbia Presbyterian Medical Center, New York, NY

Mathew Williams, MD   Department of Surgery, University of California at Los Angeles, Los Angeles, CA

Joshua Zivin, PhD   International Center for Health Outcomes and Innovation Research, Joseph L. Mailman School of Public Health, Columbia University, New York, NY

Contents

Foreword v
  Bill Frist, MD
Preface vii
Contributing Authors xi

Part I
General Aspects of Mechanical Support

1. Clinical Left Heart Assist Devices: A Historical Perspective
   O.H. Frazier, MD, John M. Fuqua, Jr., and David N. Helman, MD 3

2. Physiology of Ventricular Interactions During Ventricular Assistance
   David J. Farrar, PhD 15

3. Device Selection
   Benjamin C. Sun, MD 27

4. Options for Mechanical Support in Pediatric Patients
   Tom R. Karl, MD and Stephen B. Horton, MD 37

5. Anesthetic Considerations During Left Ventricular Assist Device
   Implantation
   Marc L. Dickstein, MD, Berend Mets, MB, ChB, FRCA, PhD,
   and Mark J.S. Heath, MD 63

6. Perioperative Management of Bleeding
   Clifford H. Van Meter, Jr., MD 75

7. Management of Perioperative Right-Sided Circulatory Failure
   Jonathan M. Chen, MD and Eric A. Rose, MD 83

8. Perioperative Management of Arrhythmias in Recipients of Left
   Ventricular Assist Devices
   Mathew Williams, MD and James Coromilas, MD 103

9. Management of Vasodilatory Hypotension After Left Ventricular
   Assist Device Placement
   Michael Argenziano, MD and Donald W. Landry, MD, PhD 111

10. Left Ventricular Recovery During Left Ventricular Assist Device
Support
Johannes Mueller, MD and Roland Hetzer, MD, PhD   121

11. Exercise Performance in Patients with Left Ventricular Assist Devices
Donna Mancini, MD and Ainat Beniaminovitz, MD   137

12. Outpatient Left Ventricular Assist Therapy
Katharine A. Catanese, MSN and David L.S. Morales, MD   153

13. Rehabilitation of the Ventricular Assist Device Recipient
Theresa M. Morrone, MS, PT, CCS and Lori A. Buck, MS, PT, CCS   167

14. Quality of Life Issues Associated with the Use of Left Ventricular
Assist Devices
Peter A. Shapiro, MD   177

15. Economic Considerations of Left Ventricular Assist Device
Implantation
Alan J. Moskowitz, MD, Deborah L. Williams, MPH,
Anita Tierney, MPH, Ronald G. Levitan, BS, Joshua Zivin, PhD, and
Annetine C. Gelijns, PhD   183

16. Immunobiology of Left Ventricular Assist Devices
Hendrik-Jan Ankersmit, MD and Silviu Itescu, MD   193

Part II. Available Devices:
A. Extracorporeal Devices

17. Extracorporeal Support: Centrifugal Pumps
Jack J. Curtis, MD and Colette Wagner-Mann, DVM, PhD   215

18. Extracorporeal Support: The ABIOMED BVS 5000
G. Kimble Jett, MD and Robert R. Lazzara, MD   235

19. Extracorporeal Support: The Thoratec Device
D. Glenn Pennington, MD, Timothy E. Oaks, MD,
and Douglas P. Lohmann, M.Eng.   251

20. Extracorporeal Membrane Oxygenation in Adults
Richard J. Kaplon, MD and Nicholas G. Smedira, MD   263

21. Extracorporeal Support: The Berlin Heart
Matthias Loebe, MD, PhD, Friedrich Kaufmann,
and Roland Hetzer, MD, PhD   275

Part II. Available Devices:
B. Intracorporeal Devices

22. Intracorporeal Support: The Intra-aortic Balloon Pump
David N. Helman, MD and Gus J. Vlahakes, MD   291

23. Intracorporeal Support: Thermo Cardiosystems Ventricular Assist
Devices
Daniel J. Goldstein, MD   307

24. Intracorporeal Support: The Novacor Left Ventricular Assist System
Narayanan Ramasamy, PhD , Rita L. Vargo, MSN, RN,
Robert L. Kormos, MD, and Peer M. Portner, PhD   323

25. Intracorporeal Support: The CardioWest Total Artificial Heart
Jack Copeland, MD, Francisco Arabia, MD, Richard Smith, MSEE,
and Paul Nolan, PhD   341

Part III. Future Devices

26. Axial Flow Pumps
Joseph J. DeRose, Jr., MD and Robert K. Jarvik, MD   359

27. The DeBakey Ventricular Assist Device
George P. Noon, MD, Deborah Morley, PhD, Suellen Irwin, RN,
and Michael E. DeBakey, MD   375

28. Epicardial Compression Mechanical Devices
John H. Artrip, MD and Daniel Burkhoff, MD, PhD   387

29. The Pennsylvania State University Totally Implantable Left Ventricular
Assist Device and Total Artificial Heart
Sanjay M. Mehta, MD and Walter E. Pae, Jr., MD   403

30. The HeartSaver VAD: A Fully Implantable Ventricular Assist Device
for Long-Term Support
Tofy Mussivand, PhD, Paul J. Hendry, MD, Roy G. Masters, MD,
and Wilbert J. Keon, MD   417

Appendix   431

Index   435

Part I

General Aspects of Mechanical Support

Chapter 1

Clinical Left Heart Assist Devices:

A Historical Perspective

*O.H. Frazier, MD, John M. Fuqua, Jr., and
David N. Helman, MD*

Introduction

Heart disease kills as many persons as nearly all other causes of death combined. Chronic, progressive, end-stage heart failure results in untold suffering and economic hardship both for individuals and for society. To combat end-stage heart failure, various ventricular assist devices (VADs) have been developed with the goal of treating and rehabilitating patients with severe circulatory compromise by providing escalating levels of circulatory support. Today, however, because of the portability of current systems, these patients may return to their homes and even to their jobs while awaiting transplantation.[1] In this introductory chapter, we present a historical overview of the evolution of mechanical assist devices.

The Modern Era of Mechanical Circulatory Support

The modern era of mechanical circulatory support began in 1953 with the work of Gibbon,[2] the first surgeon to use cardiopulmonary bypass (CPB) successfully in a clinical setting. His CPB machine performed the work of the heart and lungs, providing a quiet, bloodless field for open heart surgery. As their experience grew, the pioneers of open heart surgery realized that some patients required 1 to 2 hours of additional support before they could be successfully weaned from CPB after cardiac surgery. Patients who could not be weaned died. Thus, surgeons were convinced that a more prolonged form of cardiac support was needed, as pulmonary function was usually adequate in these patients. The short-term support of CPB was beneficial

From Goldstein DJ and Oz MC (eds). *Cardiac Assist Devices*. Armonk, NY: Futura Publishing Co., Inc.; ©2000.

but proved damaging to end-organ function and to other formed blood elements. CPB (with the bubble oxygenator) also had a practical limit of 4 to 6 hours. A less physiologically damaging, longer term device (days to weeks) was needed that might allow the heart to rest long enough for intrinsic reparative processes to occur.[3]

In 1965, Spencer and colleagues[4] described a series of four patients with postcardiotomy heart failure who had been supported by postcardiotomy femoral-femoral CPB. One of these patients survived and was discharged from the hospital. To provide a device for more prolonged treatment of left ventricular failure, Hall and colleagues[5] developed an intrathoracic left ventricular bypass pump. This artificial left ventricle was placed in the left thorax and was connected between the left atrium and the descending thoracic aorta (Fig. 1). The device consisted of an inner blood chamber surrounded by an outer air chamber, which was fabricated from a Dacron® reinforced silicone rubber material molded to the appropriate size and shape and then heat set in an autoclave. When pulses of compressed air were supplied to the air chamber, the inner blood chamber collapsed and expelled blood from the lumen. Ball valves at the inlet and outlet allowed for unidirectional flow. An external pneumatic controller that was triggered by the R wave of the electrocardiogram powered the pump. After successful testing in animals, this implantable left VAD (LVAD) was first used in a human on July 18, 1963[5] in a patient who had developed cardiogenic shock after undergoing aortic valve replacement. Although the pump worked well, the patient had suffered a neurologic injury before the implantation, that did not improve despite adequate circulatory support. Mechanical support was discontinued after 4 days. In 1966, a subsequent version of the DeBakey blood pump was successfully implanted in a patient following double valve replacement (Fig. 2).[6] This device, which was placed extracorporeally and connected between the left atrium and the axillary artery, could be removed without opening the chest. In this case, the patient

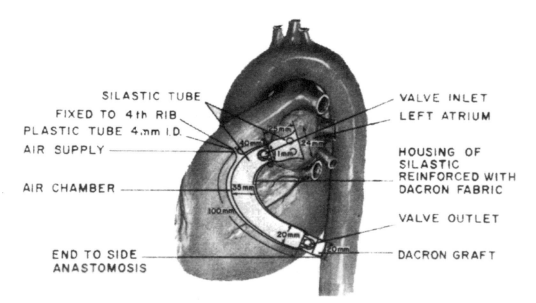

Figure 1. Intrathoracic circulatory device developed in 1963 by DeBakey for left ventricular bypass.

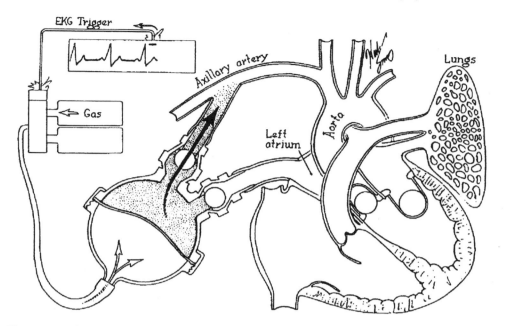

Figure 2. Left ventricular bypass pump, used successfully by DeBakey in 1966 to support a patient after double valve replacement.

was supported by the LVAD for 10 days at flows up to 1200 mL/min. The patient survived and was discharged, making this the first successful use of an LVAD for postcardiotomy heart failure.

National Programs

The National Heart Institute (now called the National Heart, Lung, and Blood Institute, or NHLBI) became actively involved in the support of heart assist system research after the formation of the Artificial Heart Program in 1964. Through grants and contracts, this program supported applied research studies at multiple centers. In 1966, a systems analysis approach was adopted to allow integration and optimization of resources from clinical centers, basic science research institutes, and the medical device industry. The program's technical objectives were originally directed toward the development of component parts for circulatory support systems. In 1970, the Artificial Heart Program became the Medical Devices Applications Branch of the (renamed) National Heart and Lung Institute (NHLI). The long-term objectives of this program were to develop: 1) emergency cardiac assist systems that could treat acute circulatory insufficiency; 2) temporary cardiac assist systems that could support the circulation for days to months, until the patient's clinical condition could be reversed or stabilized; 3) permanent heart assist systems that could provide circulatory support for the remainder of a patient's life; and 4) totally implantable artificial hearts that could replace irreparably damaged natural hearts. This effort was stimulated by the LVAD conference of 1972, which was sponsored by the NHLI and

Table 1

The Early LVAD Program

Institution/Investigator	Device	Description	Current Device and Institution
Avco-Everett Research Labs/Param I. Singh David M. Lederman Everett, MA	AVCO LVAD	Sac-type LVAD	ABIOMED BVS 5000 ABIOMED Inc.
Andros, Inc./Peer M. Portner Berkeley, CA	Andros model 11A solenoid actuated LVAS system	Dual pusher-plate diaphragm-type pump	Novacor LVAD Baxter Healthcare
Texas Heart Institute/ John C. Norman Houston, TX and Thermo Electron/ Victor L. Poirier Waltham, MA	THI-E type LVAD	Pusher-plate diaphragm-type pump	HeartMate LVAD Thermo Cardiosystems Inc.
Thoratec Labs/ J. Donald Hill Berkeley, CA	Thoratec Model VI-C LVAD	Pusher-plate diaphragm-type pump	Thoratec VAD Thoratec Labs

which emphasized the development of long-term (permanent) LVADs. In 1977, two requests for proposals were issued by John Watson, newly appointed director of the Devices and Technology Branch of the NHLBI: one for the development of "Left Heart Assist Blood Pumps"[7] and the other for the "Development of Electrical Energy Converters to Power and Control Left Heart Assist Devices."[8] These proposals were followed in 1980 by another, for the "Development of an Implantable Integrated Electrically Powered Left Heart Assist Systems,"[9] designed to provide circulatory support for more than 2 years. These proposals laid the foundation upon which the entire field has evolved.[10] The initial awardees of these requests for proposal developed the left ventricular assist systems that have been used in more than 4000 patients throughout the world (Table 1).

The Texas Heart Institute Program

The first implantation of the total artificial heart as a bridge to transplant[11] was the impetus for the formation of the Cardiovascular Surgical Research Laboratories of the Texas Heart Institute in 1972. Early investigators in the laboratories, headed by John Norman, collaborated with engineers at the Thermo Electron Research and Development Center (Waltham, MA) to design and test prototype nuclear-fueled mechanical circulatory support systems intended for permanent implantation. These systems consisted of an LVAD and a miniature nuclear-fueled, abdominally positioned thermal engine that provided power to the LVAD.[12] Concurrently, a separate but complementary research program was conducted in the laboratories, to develop a pneumatic abdominal LVAD (ALVAD) for the temporary treatment of cardiogenic shock.[13] This abdominally positioned blood pump was interposed between the apex of the left ventricle and the infrarenal abdominal aorta.[14] An external pneumatic

Table 2

Early Bridge-to-Transplantation Procedures at the Texas Heart Institute

Patient	Diagnosis	Date	Procedure	Duration
1. 47 yo man	CAD, LVA	4/4/69	TAH	64 hrs
		4/7/69	Transplantation	32 hrs
2. 21 yo man	SBE, MR, AR	2/9/78	LVAD	5 days
	Stone heart	2/14/78	Transplantation	14 days
3. 36 yo man	CAD	7/23/81	TAH	54 hours
		7/25/81	Transplantation	7 days

CAD = coronary artery disease; LVA = left ventricular aneurysm; TAH = total artificial heart; SBE = subacute bacterial endocarditis; MR = mitral regurgitation; AR = aortic regurgitation; LVAD = left ventricular assist device.

console provided programmed pulses of air to the ALVAD through a percutaneous drive line.[15] The ALVAD had a stroke volume of approximately 80 mL and could provide outputs of 9 L/min. Inlet and outlet disc valves provided unidirectional blood flow.

The first use of the LVAD as a bridge to transplant occurred in 1978, when a 23-year-old patient undergoing double valve replacement developed irreversible stone heart syndrome postoperatively. Despite severely impaired right ventricular function, the patient was supported for 7 days with univentricular support by the ALVAD.[16] A second artificial heart (Akutsu) was implanted at the Institute as a bridge to transplant in 1981.[17] Although the three devices used as bridges performed satisfactorily (Table 2), the patients died of infectious complications after transplantation. These complications were related to the aggressive use of the pan-immunosuppressant azathioprine (Imuran, Glaxo Wellcome Inc., Research Triangle Park, NC) in the patients already at high risk for infection—a result of general contamination from the procedures needed to implant the circulatory support devices.

Experiments were also performed in the laboratories to investigate the interactions between the biologic heart and circulatory support devices. The Institute's researchers studied the physiologic effects of the ALVAD on left ventricular work, cardiac output, myocardial blood flow, and myocardial oxygen consumption.[18] These studies showed that the ALVAD could reduce all indices of myocardial work yet increase systemic perfusion and coronary blood flow. Initial clinical trials of the ALVAD began in 1976.[19] Meanwhile, LVAD research had continued at other centers.

Bridge to Transplant

In the early 1980s, the more effective immunosuppressant cyclosporine (Sandimmune, Sandoz Pharmaceutical Corporation, East Hanover, NJ) was fortuitously discovered. With this discovery, transplant centers that had discontinued their programs again began to accept patients. Donor hearts remained scarce, and many patients died while awaiting transplant. To decrease the number of deaths, the left ventricular assist systems that had been developed as long-term support devices through the NHLBI program were approved as investigational devices by the United States Food and Drug Administration (FDA) to bridge such patients to transplant. In 1985, Portner and coworkers[20] at Stanford reported the first successful use of the Novacor LVAD (Baxter Healthcare Corp., Oakland, CA), an implantable, electromagnetic, solenoid-powered device, as a bridge to transplantation. At the Texas Heart Institute, we reported the first clinical trials of the Thermo Cardiosystems pneumatic (IP) HeartMate LVAD (Thermo Cardiosystems Inc., Woburn, MA), an implantable, pusher-plate blood pump used for long-term support in bridge-to-transplant procedures,[21] the Nimbus Hemopump (Nimbus Medical Inc., Rancho Cordova, CA), a miniature axial-flow pump for short-term temporary use,[22] and the TCI vented electric (VE) HeartMate LVAD, an implantable, untethered, electrically powered LVAD for long-term use.[23,24] The HeartMate was the first to be approved by the FDA for general clinical use. When patients with this device were compared to patients in a control group, the HeartMate recipients showed a significant clinical benefit (quality of life and survival).[21] Costs of caring for these patients were also significantly reduced.

Today, several extracorporeal blood pumps are routinely used for temporary left and/or right ventricular support in patients with reversible (usually postcardiotomy) heart failure.[25,26] These devices include the centrifugal Biopump[25] developed by Bio-Medicus (Medtronic Inc., Minneapolis, MN), the ABIOMED BVS 5000[26] (ABIOMED Inc., Danvers, MA), and the Thoratec VAD[27] (Thoratec Laboratories Corp., Berkeley, CA). Whereas the Biopump can be used for only a few days, the other blood pumps can provide circulatory support for a period of weeks to months.

At present, four LVADs are approved by the FDA for use as bridges to transplantation: 1) the Novacor implantable LVAD (Fig. 3); 2) the HeartMate pneumatic IP-LVAD; 3) the HeartMate VE-LVAD (Fig. 4); and 4) the Thoratec extracorporeal VAD (Fig. 5). The implantable LVADs have accounted for more than 2300 bridges to transplant. These devices are discussed separately elsewhere in this volume.

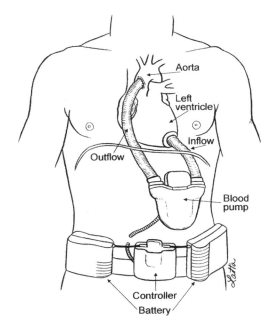

Figure 3. Novacor implantable left ventricular assist device.

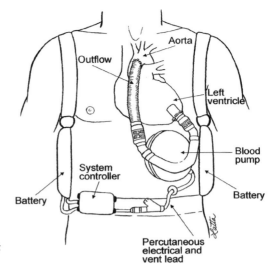

Figure 4. HeartMate implantable VE left ventricular assist device.

The successful clinical use of the Hemopump in 1988[22] validated the applicability of implantable, high-speed (25,000 rpm) axial flow pumps. Studies of these pumps also showed that nonpulsatile (or continuous) flow was well tolerated by the mammalian circulation. Continuous flow pumps have several advantages: they can be made much smaller than pulsatile pumps, they can function without a compliance chamber, and they offer the attractive possibility of total implantability. In 1994, a proposal ("Innovative Ventricular Assist Systems") was issued for the development of innovative LVAD technologies.[28] Six contracts were awarded: Transicoil/Jarvik

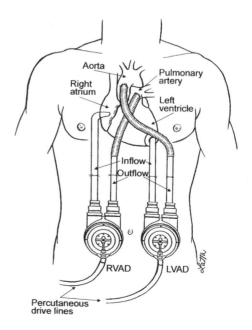

Figure 5. Thoratec extracorporeal ventricular assist device.

Heart/ Texas Heart Institute; Nimbus/Thermo Cardiosystems Inc./University of Pittsburgh; ABIOMED/Columbia University; Arrow/Penn State University; Whalen Biomedical/University of Utah; and Cleveland Clinic/Ohio State University.

Long-Term Support

Clinical applications for these devices have continued to expand. In 1991, another milestone was reached: the first patient with an LVAD (the portable VE HeartMate) was allowed to leave the hospital to await transplantation at home.[29] Shortly thereafter, another patient with a VE HeartMate was discharged and returned to his usual employment to await transplantation (Fig. 6).

Since the 1960s, experience gained from use of the LVAD as a bridge to recovery from acute postcardiotomy heart failure has stimulated further studies of patients with chronic heart failure. We first documented recovery from chronic heart failure with long-term LVAD support in a patient who died of a stroke after 505 days of support.[30] Subsequently, others documented myocardial recovery that occurred between the time the assist device was implanted (the time of maximal heart failure)

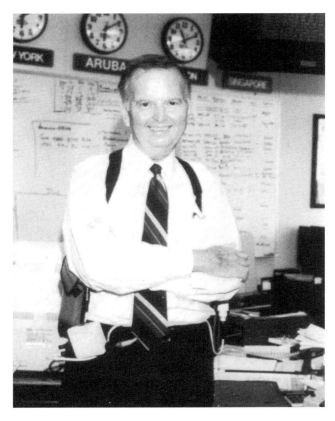

Figure 6. Patient with a VE-HeartMate LVAD returns to work as he awaits his heart transplant operation.

to the time it was removed (transplantation).[31] Thus, heart transplantation offers an unparalleled opportunity to study the effects of prolonged cardiac rest on myocardial function by allowing investigators to compare myocardial tissue samples harvested at the time of maximal heart failure during LVAD implantation with samples taken from the heart at the time of transplantation. As a result of these studies, we have learned that long-term LVAD support results in improvements in gross and histologic anatomy, physiology (as documented by pump-off studies before transplantation), and cellular function, including calcium transport[32] and glucose utilization.[33] This experience has led to successful removal of LVADs, followed by long-term survival in patients with chronic heart failure—an experience now termed "bridge to recovery" in Europe and in the United States. If this approach can evolve into a structured program that will allow prospective identification of patients who may benefit from long-term LVAD support, the need for heart transplants may be reduced, particularly in young patients with idiopathic cardiomyopathies.

The successful experience with long-term support in bridge-to-transplant patients led to the initiation of the multicenter clinical trial called REMATCH (Randomized Evaluation of Mechanical Assistance for the Treatment of Congestive Heart failure).[34] This study is designed to test the clinical benefit of long-term LVAD implantation as end therapy rather than as a bridge to transplantation, the original goal of the 1980 proposal.[9]

Summary

The formation of the Artificial Heart Program in 1964 and the subsequent evolution of the LVAD have had a major impact on the care of patients with terminal heart failure. Important milestones in this field are summarized in Table 3. These successes were made possible by the long-term committed support of NHLBI (1977 to present), under the Devices and Technology Branch directed by John Watson. The demonstration of clinical benefit when patients who received LVADs were compared

Table 3

Landmark Events in the Development of Left Ventricular Assist Devices

Investigator/Author	Year	Event
Hall[5]	1963	First clinical implantation of a LVAD
DeBakey[6]	1966	First successful clinical use of a LVAD
Norman[19]	1970s	Use of temporary LVADs for postcardiotomy failure
Norman[16]	1978	First use of a LVAD as a bridge to transplantation
Oyer[20]	1984	First use of an implantable long-term device as a bridge to transplantation
Frazier[30]	1991	First use of an untethered implantable LVAD as outpatient support
REMATCH Investigators[34]	1996–present	Initiation of prospective multicenter trial of LVAD versus medical therapy
Various authors	1996–present	Demonstration of ventricular recovery and successful LVAD removal

LVAD = left ventricular assist device.

with a nonrandomized, concurrent control group contributed to a wider use of this lifesaving technology. Today, the future of implantable long-term LVADs seems more promising than ever before.

Although heart transplantation has become a fairly routine procedure, the supply of donor hearts will continue to fall far short of the demand, creating a definite need for long-term mechanical circulatory support.[35] As smaller, more effective cardiac assist devices become available, this should increase the number of patients who can benefit from permanent circulatory support. The fact that myocardial function can improve enough with chronic ventricular unloading to allow removal of the device may further broaden the use of this technology.

References

1. Frazier OH. Long-term mechanical circulatory support. In Edmunds LH Jr. (ed): *Cardiac Surgery in the Adult*, ed 1. New York: McGraw-Hill; 1997:1477–1490.
2. Gibbon JH Jr. Application of a mechanical heart and lung apparatus in cardiac surgery. *Minn Med* 1954;37:171–185.
3. Liotta D, Hall CW, Henly WS, et al. Prolonged assisted circulation during and after cardiac or aortic surgery. *Am J Cardiol* 1963;12:399–405.
4. Spencer FC, Eiseman B, Trinkle JK, Rodd NP. Assisted circulation for cardiac failure following intracardiac surgery with cardiorespiratory bypass. *J Thorac Cardiovasc Surg* 1965;49: 56–73.
5. Hall CW, Liotta D, Henly WS, et al. Development of artificial intrathoracic circulatory pumps. *Am J Surg* 1964;108:685–692.
6. DeBakey ME. Left ventricular bypass pump for cardiac assistance. Clinical experience. *Am J Cardiol* 1971;27:3–11.
7. Department of Health and Human Services. National Institutes of Health. National Heart, Lung, and Blood Institute. Request for proposal. Left Heart Assist Blood Pumps. Bethesda, MD: 1977.
8. Department of Health and Human Services. National Institutes of Health. National Heart, Lung, and Blood Institute. Request for proposal. Development of Electrical Energy Converters to Power and Control Left Heart Assist Devices. Bethesda, MD: 1977.
9. Department of Health and Human Services. National Institutes of Health. National Heart, Lung, and Blood Institute. Request for proposal. Development of an Implantable Integrated Electrically Powered Left Heart Assist System. Bethesda, MD: 1980.
10. Fuqua JM Jr, Igo SR, Hibbs CW, et al. Development and evaluation of electrically actuated abdominal left ventricular assist systems for long-term use. *J Thorac Cardiovasc Surg* 1981; 81:718–726.
11. Cooley DA, Liotta D, Hallman GL, et al. Orthotopic cardiac prosthesis for two-staged cardiac replacement. *Am J Cardiol* 1969;24:723–730.
12. Norman JC, Harmison LT, Huffman FN. Nuclear-fueled circulatory support systems. *Arch Surg* 1972;105:645–647.
13. Norman JC, Whalen RL, Daley BDT, et al. An implantable left ventricular assist device (LVAD). *Clin Res* 1972;20:855. Abstract.
14. Fuqua JM, Igo SR, Edmonds CH, et al. Evaluations of left ventricular apex orientation in patients with congestive cardiomyopathy: Implications for long-term left ventricular assist devices. *Clin Res* 1978;26:6. Abstract.
15. Fuqua JM, Hibbs CW, Gernes DB, et al. A pneumatic control console for clinical left ventricular assist device operation. *Proceedings, 13th Annual Meeting, Association for the Advancement of Medical Instrumentation*. March 28-April 1, 1978:100.
16. Norman JC, Brook MI, Cooley DA, et al. Total support of the circulation of a patient with post-cardiotomy stone-heart syndrome by a partial artificial heart (ALVAD) for 5 days followed by heart and kidney transplantation. *Lancet* 1978;1:1125–1127.

17. Cooley DA, Akutsu T, Norman JC, et al. Total artificial heart in two-staged cardiac transplantation. *Tex Heart Inst J* 1981;8:305–319.
18. Robinson WJ, Migliore JJ, Arthur J, et al. An abdominal left ventricular assist device: Experimental physiologic analyses, II. *Trans Am Soc Artif Intern Organs* 1973;19:229–234.
19. Norman JC, Fuqua JM, Hibbs CW, et al. An intracorporeal (abdominal) left ventricular assist device: Initial clinical trials. *Arch Surg* 1977;112:1442–1451.
20. Portner PM, Oyer PE, McGregor CGA, et al. First human use of an electrically powered implantable ventricular assist system. *Artif Organs* 1985;9:36. Abstract.
21. Frazier OH, Rose EA, Macmanus Q, et al. Multicenter clinical evaluation of the HeartMate 1000 IP left ventricular assist device. *Ann Thorac Surg* 1992;53:1080–1090.
22. Frazier OH, Wampler RK, Duncan JM, et al. First human use of the Hemopump, a catheter-mounted ventricular assist device. *Ann Thorac Surg* 1990; 49:299–304.
23. Frazier OH. Chronic left ventricular support with a vented electric assist device. *Ann Thorac Surg* 1993;55:273–275.
24. Golding LR, Jacobs G, Groves LK, et al. Clinical results of mechanical support of the failing left ventricle. *J Thorac Cardiovasc Surg* 1982;83:597–601.
25. Magovern GJ, Park SB, Maher TD. Use of a centrifugal pump without anticoagulants for postoperative left ventricular assist. *World J Surg* 1985;9:25–36.
26. Guyton RA, Schonberger JP, Everts PA, et al. Postcardiotomy shock: Clinical evaluation of the BVS 5000 Biventricular Support System. *Ann Thorac Surg* 1993;56:346–356.
27. Farrar D, Hill JD, Pennington DG, et al. Preoperative and postoperative comparison of patients with univentricular and biventricular support with the Thoratec ventricular assist device as a bridge to cardiac transplantation. *J Thorac Cardiovasc Surg* 1997;113:202–209.
28. Department of Health and Human Services. National Institutes of Health. National Heart, Lung, and Blood Institute. Request for proposal. Innovative Ventricular Assist Systems. Bethesda, MD: 1994.
29. Frazier OH. First use of an untethered, vented electric left ventricular assist device for long-term support. *Circulation* 1994;89:2908–2914.
30. Frazier OH, Benedict CR, Radovancevic B, et al. Improved left ventricular function after chronic left ventricular unloading. *Ann Thorac Surg* 1996;62:675–682.
31. Hennig LM, Mueller J, Spiegelsberger S, et al. Long-term circulatory support as a bridge to transplantation, for recovery from cardiomyopathy, and for permanent replacement. *Eur J Cardiothorac Surg* 1997;11:S18-S24.
32. Bick RJ, Poindexter BJ, Buja LM, et al. Improved sarcoplasmic reticulum function after mechanical left ventricular unloading. *Cardiovasc Pathobiol* 1998;2:159–166.
33. Torre-Amione G, Stetson SJ, Youker KA, et al. Decreased expression of tumor necrosis factor α in failing human myocardium after mechanical circulatory support: A potential mechanism for cardiac recovery. *Circulation* 1999;100:1189–1193.
34. Rose EA, Moskowitz A, Packer M, et al. Randomized evaluation of mechanical assistance for the treatment of congestive heart failure: Rationale, design and endpoints. *Ann Thorac Surg* 1999;67:723–730.
35. Goldstein DJ, Oz MC, Rose EA. Implantable left ventricular assist devices. *N Engl J Med* 1998;339:1522–1533.

Chapter 2

Physiology of Ventricular Interactions During VentricularAssistance

David J. Farrar, PhD

Introduction

Due to the close anatomic coupling between the right and left hearts, the volume and pressure of one ventricle can affect the volume, pressure, and performance of the contralateral ventricle.[1–10] Various terms have been used to describe these phenomena, including ventricular interference, cross-talk, interdependence, and ventricular interaction. Ventricular assist devices can cause dramatic changes in ventricular volumes and hemodynamic conditions, and therefore substantial direct and indirect changes to the contralateral ventricle due to ventricular interactions.

The purpose of this chapter is to review the effects of left ventricular assist device (LVAD) support on the determinants of right ventricular function. Since the right ventricle is closely coupled to the left ventricle, it can be affected by various factors that can be altered with an LVAD, such as venous return, coronary artery perfusion pressure, septal motion, and pulmonary vascular pressures. Depending on the extent of cardiac and pulmonary disease and also on chosen cannulation sites and flow rates, these changes can be either beneficial or detrimental to the determinants of right ventricular function as described by preload, afterload, and contractility.[1]

There are two basic ways in which the right and left ventricles interact (Fig. 1): hemodynamic interactions (also referred to as indirect interactions), and mechanical interactions (also referred to as direct or anatomic interactions).[1,4,5] The former occur because the right and left hearts are connected in series and therefore the output of one ventricle becomes the input of the other. Mechanical interactions are due to the close anatomic coupling between the right and left ventricle via the shared interventricular septum, common muscle fibers in the free walls, and the pericardium. Ventricular assist devices can affect either or both of these interactions with resulting changes in ventricular function.[1,9,10]

From Goldstein DJ and Oz MC (eds). *Cardiac Assist Devices*. Armonk, NY: Futura Publishing Co., Inc.; ©2000.

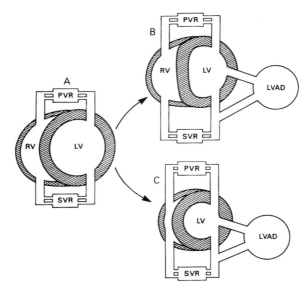

FIGURE 1. Hemodynamic ventricular interactions are due to the right (RV) and left (LV) ventricles being in series, connected by the systemic (SVR) and pulmonary (PVR) vascular resistance; mechanical interactions are due to the anatomic coupling provided by the shared interventricular septum and common muscle fibers of the RV and LV (A). A left ventricular assist device (LVAD) in parallel with the LV (B and C) can increase RV venous return and reduce RV afterload by shifting blood volume from the pulmonary to the systemic vascular systems. An LVAD that unloads the LV (B) can produce a leftward septal shift by reducing the transseptal pressure gradient, potentially improving RV filling but decreasing the systolic LV contribution to RV contraction. If the pulmonary arterial and RV pressures are also reduced during LVAD support, then both ventricles can become dimensionally unloaded (C). Reproduced, with permission, from Reference 14.

Hemodynamic Interactions

Cardiac Output and Venous Return

The main goal of using an LVAD in a patient with advanced heart failure is to increase blood flow to the end organs. Due to the in-series nature of the right and left hearts, any increase in flow to the systemic circulation from the LVAD will result in an increase in venous return to the right ventricle (Fig. 1). For successful return of flow to the left heart (and to the LVAD), the right ventricle must be capable of increasing its cardiac output to at least the amount being pumped by the LVAD. In human subjects with heart failure there is, on average, an approximate doubling of flow (from preoperative values) with institution of LVAD support. Indeed, in 74 patients who underwent insertion of a Thoratec LVAD (Thoratec Laboratories Corp., Berkeley, CA) as a bridge to transplant, average blood flow increased from a preoperative cardiac index of 1.6 ± 0.6 to 2.8 ± 0.5 L/min/m^2 under resting conditions after 30 days of isolated LVAD support.[11] In patients with isolated LVADs, the right ventricle must thus be capable of also pumping at least 2.8 L/min/m^2. In 139 patients receiving biventricular assist devices or biVADs,[11] average LVAD blood flow increased from a preoperative cardiac index of 1.4 ± 0.8 to 3.0 ± 0.5 L/min/m^2, under resting conditions after 30 days. Thus, in patients with biVADs the sum of blood flow from the right ventricular assist device (RVAD) and the output from the natural right ventricle must be at least 3.0 L/min/m^2. Therefore, the first basic principle of hemodynamic ventricular interactions in the setting of LVAD support as it relates to right ventricular function is that there is increased venous return to and increased cardiac output from the right ventricle.

The in-series concept explains how an LVAD can unmask preexisting right ventricular dysfunction by attempting to increase venous return beyond the capability of the right ventricle (see Chapter 7). Right ventricular dysfunction may only become clinically apparent after the left side is assisted.

Pulmonary Circulation

In patients with congestive heart failure, there can be substantial passive pulmonary hypertension secondary to elevated left atrial and pulmonary venous pressures. This results in a significant increase in right ventricular afterload. Since right ventricular function is significantly afterload-dependent, this pulmonary congestion can depress right ventricular function, even in patients with normal pulmonary vascular resistance (PVR). LVAD support has the ability to produce dramatic improvements in right ventricular afterload due to reversal of passive pulmonary hypertension. This is a direct result of the reductions in left heart filling pressures as the LVAD pumps blood from the pulmonary venous circulation to the systemic circulation. Thus, in the presence of high right ventricular afterload, LVAD placement often improves right heart function by reducing left atrial pressure and enhancing transpulmonary blood flow. Thus, the second basic principle of the effect of an LVAD on right ventricular function via ventricular interactions is that pulmonary artery pressures and right ventricular afterload will normally fall due to decreased left atrial pressure and relief from passive pulmonary hypertension.

This improvement is most apparent in patients with acute passively elevated pulmonary artery pressures but with relatively normal transpulmonary pressure gradient and PVR. In patients with fixed elevated PVR (eg, chronic obstructive pulmonary disease) this benefit may not become apparent, and pulmonary pressures in fact may rise with increased flow through this fixed resistance.

Right ventricular afterload can be described by pulmonary artery input resistance (R_{in}) (sometimes called total pulmonary resistance), which is calculated as mean pulmonary artery pressure divided by cardiac output. We first noticed the potential beneficial effects of left ventricular unloading on right ventricular afterload in an animal model[12] and in a clinical model of left ventricular bypass.[13,14] In patients undergoing routine coronary artery bypass grafting, left ventricular unloading resulted in a 57% reduction in R_{in} with markedly improved right ventricular function. Experimental studies yielded similar but less dramatic reductions in R_{in} (15%) during left ventricular unloading.[12] Clinical studies in LVAD recipients have documented 30% to 40% reductions in mean pulmonary artery pressure,[13,15–19] which accounted for the significant improvements in right ventricular cardiac output during bridging to cardiac transplantation.

The beneficial effect of LVAD support on right ventricular afterload as mani-

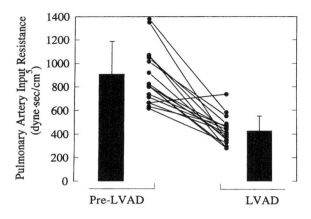

FIGURE 2. Pulmonary artery input resistance, as a measure of right ventricular afterload, was significantly reduced in patients supported with Thoratec left ventricular assist devices as a bridge to cardiac transplantation.

fested by changes in R_{in} among patients implanted with a univentricular Thoratec LVAD as a bridge to transplantation is displayed in Figure 2. Mean pulmonary arterial pressure fell 30%, from 37 ± 7 mm Hg before LVAD insertion to 26 ± 5 mm Hg during LVAD support, and R_{in} fell 53%, from 909 ± 279 to 428 ± 123 dyne sec/cm^5 during LVAD support. In patients with biventricular devices, mean pulmonary artery pressure was also reduced from 35 ± 11 mm Hg preoperatively to 27 ± 9 mm Hg during biVAD support.

Mechanical Anatomic Interactions

Because of the close mechanical coupling between the ventricles, forces that are generated in one chamber can be conveyed to the other. These forces can be transmitted in systole or diastole, and can be modulated by the pericardium and by intrathoracic pressures. An LVAD is capable of modifying these interactions substantially, either directly by unloading the left ventricle in relation to the right ventricle, or by changing the preload or afterload conditions of the right ventricle. Either of these can change the pressure-volume relationships of both ventricles.

During LVAD support, there can be significant unloading of the left ventricle that results in reductions in left ventricular volume and pressure. This is schematically illustrated in Figure 1, panel B, where there is a marked leftward shift of the interventricular septum due to changes in the transseptal pressure gradient during LVAD pumping. In theory, this mechanism can result in improved right ventricular diastolic compliance.[1,10] On the other hand, if peak left ventricular pressure is reduced, the interventricular septum may bulge into the left ventricle during right ventricular systole, resulting in reduced efficiency of right ventricular contraction.[1,12,20,21] Several experimental studies and theoretical models have supported this systolic ventricular interaction whereby the left ventricle normally contributes to right ventricular contraction[2,4,7,8,22]; unloading the left ventricle with an LVAD can, in theory, impair total effective right ventricular contractility.[10,20,21,23]

Experimental studies in *normal* hearts have failed to support the systolic ventricular interaction hypothesis.[12,20,24–28] For example, using a pulsatile LVAD to unload the normal porcine left ventricle, we showed that large reductions (90%) in left ventricular pressure result in changes in right ventricular geometry (leftward shift of the interventricular septum) but not in overall right ventricular function, as determined by global stroke work, regional preload recruitable stroke work, and end-systolic pressure-dimension relationships.[20] This is illustrated in Figure 3 where a parallel shift in the right ventricular preload-recruitable stroke work relationship was found during LVAD pumping, indicating a leftward septal shift but without change in overall right ventricular performance. Other investigators have reached the same conclusion with partial left ventricular unloading,[26] or have noted some reduction in measures of right ventricular contractility during left ventricular unloading,[27,28] but also with negligible alterations on overall right ventricular function. These findings are in accordance with computer models of ventricular interactions,[23] which predicted that, over the physiologic range of pressures and volumes studied, right ventricular stroke work was enhanced with the LVAD by isolated diastolic interaction (improved right ventricular compliance) and impaired by isolated systolic interaction (reduced right ventricular effective contractility). Due to the diametrically opposed nature of these forces, the final result was a negligible effect on right ventricular function (in the normal heart).

Hence, it appears that anatomic ventricular interactions are not responsible for the profound right heart failure that is seen in some patients receiving LVADs. Therefore, the third principle of right ventricular function with LVADs is that with reduced

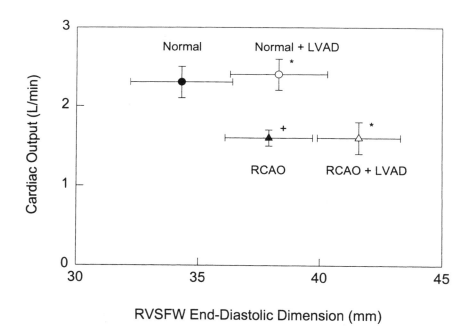

FIGURE 3. Cardiac output in pigs was significantly reduced during right ventricular (RV) ischemia produced by right coronary artery occlusion (RCAO), which also increased RV septal-to-free wall (RVSFW) end-diastolic dimension. Isolated use of a left ventricular assist device (LVAD), which also resulted in leftward septal shifting, was unable to improve hemodynamic conditions, thus mimicking the clinical situation of right heart failure during left heart assist. Systemic blood flow in this animal model was improved only upon use of RV or biventricular assistance. Modified from Reference 32.

left ventricular pressure and volume, there is a leftward septal shift and reduced contribution of the left ventricle to right ventricular contractility; however in normal hearts, the net result is a negligible effect on right ventricular function.

It should be noted that the same principles work in the opposite direction, and that a rightward shift of the interventricular septum during right ventricular unloading with isolated use of right ventricular assist device support has been documented.[29-31] It should also be noted that, due to concomitant reductions in pulmonary afterload during LVAD pumping, a leftward septal shift may not be as apparent, as both ventricles are reduced in size (Fig. 1, panel C).

Effects of Ischemia

Ischemia can result in significant right heart failure[31-34] and can affect the nature of ventricular interactions even in the presence of mechanical left ventricular unloading. Right ventricular free wall ischemia,[34] septal ischemia,[35] and global cardiac ischemia[33] have all been proposed as putative factors involved in the development of right ventricular failure that not uncommonly accompanies LVAD insertion. A porcine model of right ventricular ischemia produced by right coronary artery occlusion, with and without univentricular LVAD support, illustrates the problem of right ventricular failure during mechanical left ventricular support that occurs in some patients.[32] In this ischemic model, left ventricular pressure unloading with an LVAD produced a leftward septal shift under normal and ischemic conditions, increasing the right ventricular septal-to-free wall dimension (Fig. 3). But the effects due to ventricular interaction were negligible compared to the major detrimental effects of ischemia. LVAD support was unable to improve the impaired right ventricular cardiac output (produced by right ventricular ischemia) because of the inability of the right ventricle to pump sufficiently through the pulmonary vasculature (Fig. 3). With the addition of a right ventricular assist device or a biVAD, however, cardiac output in this model was significantly improved to control levels or slightly higher.[31]

Effects of Dilated Cardiomyopathy

In a pacing-induced model of biventricular heart failure, we found that dilated cardiomyopathy increases systolic but not diastolic ventricular interactions, and that the pericardium increases diastolic but not systolic interactions.[36] As shown in Figure 4, there was a marked reduction in diastolic interaction when the pericardium was opened in normal pigs and in pigs with pacing-induced heart failure. On the other hand, opening the pericardium had no significant effect on systolic ventricular interaction, whereas systolic interaction was significantly higher in heart failure pigs compared with normal pigs (Fig. 5). These results may explain why anatomic ventricular interactions had a more influential role in determining right ventricular function during left ventricular assist in dilated cardiomyopathy compared with the normal heart.[21] In this pacing-induced heart failure model, there was a significant impairment in right ventricular function observed as a direct result of left ventricular unloading with an LVAD (reduced cardiac output, global stroke work, and slopes of preload recruitable stroke work and end-systolic pressure-dimension relationships)

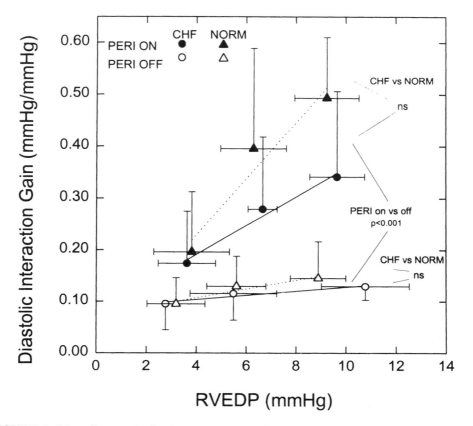

FIGURE 4. Diastolic ventricular interaction gains (a quantitative measure of the effects of pressure in one ventricle on the contralateral ventricle) as a function of right ventricular end-diastolic pressure (RVEDP) during volume loading. Diastolic interaction gains were significantly reduced when the pericardium (PERI) was opened, but there were no significant differences between pigs with congestive heart failure (CHF) and normal (NORM) pigs. Reproduced, with permission, from Reference 36.

(Fig. 6; CHF conditions). This impairment during left ventricular unloading is superimposed on the preexisting ventricular dysfunction produced by rapid ventricular pacing. In the normal heart,[20] the preservation of right ventricular function during left ventricular pressure unloading appears to be due to two competing effects of anatomic ventricular interactions: a detrimental effect of systolic interaction counterbalanced by a beneficial effect of diastolic interaction. In the congestive heart failure model, however, increased systolic interaction implies that the right ventricle is more dependent on the left ventricle for pressure generation, and under these circumstances, left ventricular unloading may lead to further decrease an already depressed right ventricle. Compensation would normally occur via diastolic interactions, but in the failing heart, which is already operating on the higher end of the Frank-Starling curve, there is decreased preload recruitable stroke work at higher end-diastolic pressures, decreased diastolic compliance, and consequently, overall decreased right ventricular performance. The mechanism for the enhancement of systolic interaction in failure situations is the relative elastance (or compliance) of the interventricular

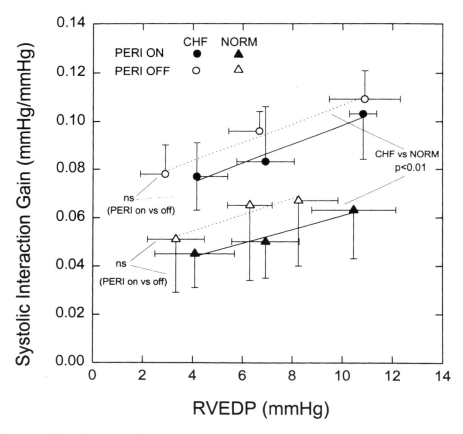

FIGURE 5. Systolic ventricular interaction gains as functions of right ventricular end-diastolic pressure (RVEDP) during volume loading. There was significantly higher systolic interaction in pigs with congestive heart failure (CHF) compared with normal (NORM) pigs, but there were no significant changes in systolic interaction gains when the pericardium (PERI) was opened. Reproduced, with permission, from Reference 36.

septum: systolic interaction is decreased during conditions in which the septal elastance is high (less compliant), such as hypertrophy, and is increased during conditions in which the septal elastance is low (more compliant), such as in dilated cardiomyopathy.[8,36]

Right Ventricular Function in LVAD Recipients

Although there are instances when biventricular support might be strongly indicated (eg, patients with biventricular infarction,[37] malignant arrhythmias,[38] low (<15%) right ventricular ejection fraction and large right ventricular volumes,[16] preexisting liver dysfunction,[39] or fixed elevated PVR), criteria for predicting which patients will require biventricular support are not well established. The need for biventricular support is dependent on the patient population, the devices available for use, and the philosophy of the investigators, with usage varying from less than

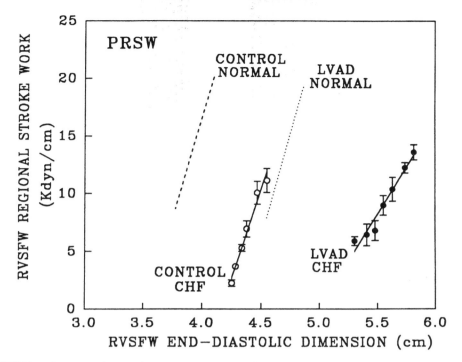

FIGURE 6. In normal pigs there is a parallel shift in the right ventricular (RV) preload recruitable stroke work (PRSW) relationship during left heart unloading with a left ventricular assist device (LVAD), indicating a leftward septal shift, but with no change in overall RV function. In contrast, an LVAD in pigs with pacing-induced congestive heart failure (CHF) also produced a leftward septal shift but resulted in impaired RV systolic pump function, indicated by a reduction in slope. Reprinted, with permission, from Reference 21.

10% to 85%.[37,39–42] In a direct comparison of LVAD and biVAD patients, the main finding was that patients receiving biventricular support were more severely ill preoperatively, and that the earlier the implant, the better the chances of succeeding with isolated LVAD support.[11] Experimental and clinical results to date also support the concept that anatomic ventricular interactions, altered by the LVAD either in diastole or systole, play a minor role and that preexisting right ventricular pathologic conditions such as ischemia, infarction, cardiomyopathy, or pulmonary hypertension, are the major factors that cause right ventricular failure. The extent of right ventricular dysfunction sometimes becomes apparent only after LVAD placement and the resultant increased venous return challenge an impaired right ventricle.

It has become clear that the main clinical effect of LVAD support on right ventricular function in most patients undergoing LVAD support as a bridge to transplantation is a beneficial one; namely, a significant reduction in right ventricular afterload. In an effort to obviate the need for additional RVAD support, LVAD patients receive treatments that attempt to offset any preexisting or developing pathologic conditions. Thus, patients with right coronary ischemia undergo concomitant bypass grafting. Hemostatic antifibrinolytic agents are administered during the implantation procedure to obviate the pulmonary hypertensive effects associated with massive blood product resuscitation. Patients with preexisting malignant arrhythmias are treated aggressively with antiarrhythmic and anti-ischemic agents to prevent further deterioration in ventricular function. Finally, patients with established pulmonary hypertension and elevated PVR receive intravenous and inhaled pulmonary vasodilators (ie, nitric oxide) to avoid the morbidity and mortality associated with the institution of mechanical right ventricular support.

Conclusions

There are two types of ventricular interactions relevant to ventricular assistance: hemodynamic interactions (eg, increased right ventricular venous return, reduced pulmonary pressures) and anatomic mechanical interactions (eg, leftward septal shift during left ventricular unloading). LVAD placement can be detrimental or beneficial to right ventricular function. In healthy animal models, these effects tend to balance, resulting in no overall change in right ventricular performance due to left heart unloading. In patients with end-stage heart disease who are undergoing LVAD placement as a bridge to cardiac transplantation, the beneficial trends dominate: a reduction in right ventricular afterload due to relief from passive pulmonary hypertension during LVAD support. Anatomic ventricular interactions appear to play a minor role in determining overall right ventricular function during LVAD support compared with the effects of preexisting pathologic conditions.

References

1. Farrar DJ, Compton PG, Hershon JJ, et al. Right heart interaction with the mechanically assisted left heart. *World J Surg* 1985;9:89–102.
2. Bove AA, Santamore WT. Ventricular interdependence. *Prog Cardiovasc Dis* 1981;23: 365–388.
3. Janicki JS, Weber KT. The pericardium and ventricular interaction, distensibility and function. *Am J Physiol* 1980;238:H494-H503.
4. Santamore WP, Burkhoff D. Hemodynamic consequences of ventricular interaction as assessed by model analysis. *Am J Physiol* 1991;260:H146-H157.
5. Slinker BK, Glantz SA. End-systolic and end-diastolic ventricular interaction. *Am J Physiol* 1986;251:H1062-H1075.
6. Slinker BK, Goto Y, LeWinter MM. Systolic direct ventricular interaction affects left ventricular contraction and relaxation in the intact dog circulation. *Circ Res* 1989;65:307–315.
7. Woodard JC, Chow E, Farrar DJ. Isolated ventricular systolic interaction during transient reductions in left ventricular pressure. *Circ Res* 1992;70:944–951.
8. Farrar DJ, Woodard JC, Chow E. Pacing-induced dilated cardiomyopathy increases left-to-right ventricular systolic interaction. *Circulation* 1993;88:720–725.
9. Farrar DJ. Ventricular interaction during mechanical circulatory support. *Semin Thorac Cardiovasc Surg* 1994;6:163–168.
10. Santamore WP, Gray LA Jr. Left ventricular contributions to right ventricular systolic function during LVAD support. *Ann Thorac Surg* 1996;61(1):350–356.
11. Farrar DJ, Hill JD, Pennington DG, et al. Preoperative and postoperative comparison of patients with uni- and bi-ventricular Thoratec VAD support as a bridge to heart transplantation. *J Thorac Cardiovasc Surg* 1997;113:202–209.
12. Farrar DJ, Compton PG, Dajee H, et al. Right heart function during left heart assist and the effects of volume loading in a canine preparation. *Circulation* 1984;70:708–716.
13. Hershon JJ, Farrar DJ, Compton PG, et al. Right ventricular dimensions with transesopha-

geal echocardiography during an operating room model of left heart assist. *Trans Am Soc Artif Intern Organs* 1984;30:129–132.

14. Farrar DJ, Compton PG, Hershon JJ, et al. Right ventricular function in an operating model of mechanical left ventricular assistance and its effects in patients with depressed left ventricular function. *Circulation* 1985;72:1279–1285.

15. Farrar DJ, Hill JD, Gray LA, et al. Heterotopic prosthetic ventricles as a bridge to cardiac transplantation. A multicenter study in 29 patients. *N Engl J Med* 1985;318:333–340.

16. Kormos RL, Gasior T, Antaki J, et al. Evaluation of right ventricular function during clinical left ventricular assistance. *Trans Am Soc Artif Intern Organs* 1989;35:547–550.

17. Gallagher RC, Kormos RL, Gasior T, et al. Univentricular support results in reduction in pulmonary resistance and improved right ventricular function. *ASAIO Trans* 1991;37: M287-M288.

18. Bennink GB, Noda H, Duncan JM, et al. Clinical evaluation of right ventricular function in patients with left ventricular assist device (LVAD). *Int J Artif Organs* 1992;15:109–113.

19. McCarthy PM. Hemodynamic and physiologic changes during support with an implantable left ventricular assist device. *J Thorac Cardiovasc Surg* 1995;109(3):409–418.

20. Chow E, Farrar DJ. Effects of left ventricular pressure reductions on right ventricular systolic performance. *Am J Physiol* 1989;257:H1878-H1885.

21. Chow E, Farrar DJ. Right heart function during prosthetic left ventricular assistance in a porcine model of congestive heart failure. *J Thorac Cardiovasc Surg* 1992;104:569–578.

22. Yamaguchi S, Harasawa H, Li KS, et al. Comparative significance in systolic interaction. *Cardiovasc Res* 1991;25:774–783.

23. Woodard JC, Farrar DJ, Chow E, et al. Computer model of ventricular interaction during left ventricular circulatory support. *Trans Am Soc Artif Intern Organs* 1989;35:439–441.

24. Farrar DJ, Compton PG, Verderber A, et al. Right ventricular end-systolic pressure-dimension relationship during left ventricular bypass in anesthetized pigs. *Trans Am Soc Artif Intern Organs* 1986;32:278–281.

25. Chow E, Brown CD, Farrar DJ. Effects of left ventricular pressure unloading during LVAD support on right ventricular contractility. *ASAIO J* 1992;38:M473-M476.

26. Elbeery JR, Owen CH, Savitt MA, et al. Effects of the left ventricular assist device on right ventricular function. *J Thorac Cardiovasc Surg* 1990;99:809–816.

27. Fukamachi K, Asou T, Nakamura Y, et al. Effects of left heart bypass on right ventricular performance. *J Thorac Cardiovasc Surg* 1990;99:725–734.

28. Moon MR, Castro LJ, DeAnda A, et al. Right ventricular dynamics during left ventricular assistance in closed-chest dogs. *Ann Thorac Surg* 1993;56:54–66.

29. Brunsting LA, Salter DR, Goldstein JP, et al. Ventricular interaction during right ventricular assist. *Trans Am Soc Artif Intern Organs* 1987;33:162–168.

30. Farrar DJ, Chow E, Wood JR, et al. Anatomic interaction between the right and left ventricles during univentricular and biventricular circulatory support. *Trans Am Soc Artif Intern Organs* 1988;34:235–240.

31. Farrar DJ, Chow E, Wood J, et al. Comparison of right ventricular and biventricular circulatory support in a porcine model of right heart failure. *ASAIO Trans* 1990;36:M522-M525.

32. Farrar DJ, Chow E, Compton PG, et al. Effects of acute right ventricular ischemia on ventricular interactions during prosthetic left ventricular support. *J Thorac Cardiovasc Surg* 1991;102:588–595.

33. Shuman TA, Palazzo RS, Jaquiss RBD, et al. A model of right ventricular failure after global myocardial ischemia and mechanical left ventricular support. *ASAIO Trans* 1991; 37:M212-M213.

34. Fischer EIC, Willshaw P, Armentano RL, et al. Experimental acute right ventricular failure and right ventricular assist in dogs. *J Thorac Cardiovas Surg* 1985;90:580–585.

35. Daly RC, Chandrasekaran K, Cavarocchi NC, et al. Ischemia of the interventricular septum: A mechanism of right ventricular failure during mechanical left ventricular assist. *J Thorac Cardiovasc Surg* 1992;102:1186–1191.

36. Farrar DJ, Chow E, Brown CD. Isolated systolic and diastolic ventricular interactions in pacing-induced dilated cardiomyopathy and effects of volume loading and pericardium. *Circulation* 1995;92:1284–1290.

37. Pennington DG, Merjavy JP, Swartz MT, et al. The importance of biventricular failure in patients with post-operative cardiogenic shock. *Ann Thorac Surg* 1985;39:16–26.

38. Farrar DJ, Hill JD, Gray LA Jr, et al. Successful biventricular circulatory support as a bridge to cardiac transplantation during prolonged ventricular fibrillation and asystole. *Circulation* 1989;80:III147-III151.
39. Reinhartz O, Farrar DJ, Hershon JH, et al. Importance of preoperative liver function as a predictor of survival in patients supported with Thoratec ventricular assist devices as a bridge to transplantation. *J Thorac Cardiovasc Surg* 1998;116(4):633–640.
40. Oz MC, Argenziano M, Catanese KA, et al. Bridge experience with long-term implantable left ventricular assist devices: Are they an alternative to transplantation? *Circulation* 1997; 95(7):1844–1852.
41. Portner PM, Oyer PE, Pennington DG, et al. Implantable electrical left ventricular assist system: Bridge to transplantation and the future. *Ann Thorac Surg* 1989;47:142–150.
42. Frazier OH, Rose EA, Macmanus Q, et al. Multicenter clinical evaluation of the HeartMate 1000 IP left ventricular assist device. *Ann Thorac Surg* 1992;53:1080–1090.

Chapter 3

Device Selection

Benjamin C. Sun, MD

Introduction

Selection of the appropriate mechanical support device for a given clinical situation depends on what is available in an institution and on the experience, comfort, and biases of the physicians. Although trends and anecdotes often guide this complex decision process, insufficient experience exists to unequivocally declare that a certain device, or combination of devices, is the perfect treatment for a given clinical scenario. Indeed, only two studies to date have attempted to compare outcomes between two long-term assist devices in a single institution.[1,2]

In addition to the intra-aortic balloon pump, five Food and Drug Administration (FDA)-approved cardiac assist systems can be used for different but overlapping indications. Each device has strengths and weaknesses in a given clinical scenario. Our institution has the benefit of extensively using four of the five FDA-approved assist devices. This chapter discusses the strengths and weaknesses of the available systems, to help the clinician decide which system would suit the needs of his or her institution and patients.

Issues that bear consideration during device selection include expected duration of support, type of support needed (right, left, or biventricular assist), overall cost, device-related morbidity, and patient-related issues. The recent change in United Network of Organ Sharing (UNOS) classification, which affects status I patients, may alter the support times in a region and affect device selection.

There are currently three major indications for mechanical assistance: 1) support to myocardial or hemodynamic recovery; 2) support to cardiac transplantation; and 3) permanent support for nontransplant candidates.

Each of the commercially available devices is designed to address these specific, though overlapping, indications. When a patient is in severe cardiogenic shock from a potentially reversible cardiac insult, an assist system may be used as a bridge to myocardial recovery. The assist system is implanted to decompress the injured myocardium, to allow cardiac recovery, and to provide physiologic support for the patient. Specific diagnoses include acute viral and postpartum cardiomyopathies,

From Goldstein DJ and Oz MC (eds). *Cardiac Assist Devices.* Armonk, NY: Futura Publishing Co., Inc.; ©2000.

postcardiotomy syndromes, and reperfusion injury in cardiac allografts. As the heart recovers and is able to sustain the circulation, the assist device may be weaned and subsequently explanted.

Cardiac transplant candidates who continue to deteriorate despite aggressive pharmacologic support can also become candidates for long-term assist support. The assist device is used as a bridge to cardiac transplantation and is explanted at the time of transplantation or, less commonly, after primary ventricular recovery.

The third indication for assist systems is as an alternative to cardiac transplantation, although this use is currently investigational. The current REMATCH (Randomized Evaluation of Mechanical Assist Treatment for Congestive Heart failure) trial is designed to compare outcomes for patients in New York Health Association Class IV heart failure supported with the Thermo Cardiosystems Inc. (Woburn, MA) vented electric (VE) left ventricular assist system (LVAS) with current maximal medical therapy.[3] Two additional trials will likely commence within the next 2 years with different assist systems from Arrow International (Reading, PA) and Baxter Healthcare Corporation (Oakland, CA).

Current Systems

Paracorporeal

There are two paracorporeal assist systems currently approved for use: the ABIOMED BVS 5000 (Abiomed, Danvers, MA) (described in detail in Chapter 18) and the Thoratec system (Thoratec Laboratories, Berkeley, CA) (described in detail in Chapter 19). Both systems are pulsatile and pneumatically actuated. The cannulae are internalized but the pumping chambers are extracorporeal. Both systems are versatile and can be configured for left ventricular, right ventricular, or biventricular support. Implantation involves cannulation of either an atrium or a ventricle for the inflow, and a graft anastomosis to either the aorta or pulmonary artery as the outflow. Although cardiopulmonary bypass (CPB) is generally used, these systems can be implanted without the aid of extracorporeal circulation. Both devices can be used in small patients with body surface areas (BSAs) as small as 0.8 m^2, although the low flow rates may require additional anticoagulation.

The ABIOMED BVS 5000 is a system that is logistically simple to initiate and maintain. Sandwiched between the cannulae is a dual-chambered drive unit separated by a polyurethane trileaflet valve. The "atrial" chamber fills passively and functions as a reservoir for the connected "ventricular" chamber. Attached to the ventricular chamber are another polyurethane trileaflet outflow valve and an air hose that is connected to the drive console. The console senses a 70 mL air displacement as the ventricular chamber fills; compressed air is then sent back through the same air hose to eject the blood out of the ventricular chamber into the patient. These pumping chambers are mounted on the side of the bed or onto intravenous (IV) poles. The configuration necessitates a fair amount of tubing that the blood must traverse as it flows through the system. Strict adherence to the manufacturer's anticoagulation regimen must be maintained to prevent thromboembolic complications.

The Thoratec system has been approved by the FDA for myocardial recovery and as a bridge to transplantation. The cannulae are internalized but traverse the abdominal wall to the externalized pumping chamber that rests on the upper abdomen of the patient. The blood chamber is a smooth seamless polyurethane sac housed within a transparent polysulfone shell. A fill switch is used to sense pump chamber filling, but is not integrated into the drive system of the console. In addition, appropriate emptying of the device is assured by manual inspection of the pumping chamber. The device is pneumatically actuated but is unique in employing suction for preload assistance. The suction should not be used as compensation for poor cannula placement, as hemolysis will become a major issue with high suction. An air hose connects the drive console with the pumping chamber as well as the electrical connector to the fill sensor. The system requires manual adjustments of ejection pressure, ejection duration, and vacuum levels to optimize output. This system requires some savvy to initiate support; however, once physiologic stability is achieved, few adjustments are required. Anticoagulation is also required to maintain an international normalized ratio (INR) 2.5 to 3.5 times normal and to assure a low thromboembolic rate. The Thoratec drive console is large and heavy and is not suited for extended patient mobility. Patients are relegated to the length and tether of their drive line for much of the day. A portable drive unit that addresses this limitation is currently under investigation.

Implantable Systems

There are currently three FDA-approved implantable assist systems: the Novacor LVAS (described in detail in Chapter 24) from Baxter Healthcare Corp, Oakland, CA, and two from Thermo Cardiosystems (Woburn, MA) (a pneumatically actuated [IP] HeartMate and a VE HeartMate) (see Chapter 23). The pumping chambers of these systems are internalized in the preperitoneal or peritoneal spaces of the patient. Not only is this approach aesthetically pleasing, but the decreased conduit length for the blood to traverse minimizes kinking of the inflow conduits during patient movement. This configuration also permits much better mobility and autonomous ambulation compared to the paracorporeal systems. All three systems are implanted in the same fashion and have percutaneous drive lines. The minimum patient BSA for receiving these implantable devices is 1.5 m². The Novacor and Thermo Cardiosystems VEs are electrically actuated and have wearable external controllers and rechargeable power sources. The electrical systems are currently the only devices approved for outpatient care.

The two Thermo Cardiosystems systems have identical pumping chambers and differ only in their size and method of device actuation. They incorporate a single pusher-plate system housed in a titanium shell. A Hall sensor detects the position of the pusher-plate at both end systole and end diastole. The pusher-plate drives a unique textured polyurethane diaphragm against a sintered titanium shell. The textured surface facilitates the attachment of a neointima along the blood-contacting surface of the diaphragm and effectively prevents thrombus formation. This is the only assist device that does not require anticoagulation. Despite no anticoagulation, the thromboembolic rate of this device is a very low (7% or less).[4,5]

The VE incorporates an electrical torque motor and is therefore larger and heavier. In the event of a catastrophic motor failure, the VE may be driven pneumatically. Device reliability during prolonged (>300 days) use is a concern for the VE. Bearing wear and motor failure has been seen in some patients requiring device change. There have been recent modifications to help address the evolving mechanical issues.

The Baxter Novacor LVAS is an electromagnetically powered driver attached to two symmetrically opposed pusher-plates. The blood chamber is a smooth seamless polyurethane sac straddled by two pericardial tissue valves enclosed in a fiberglass-reinforced shell. A percutaneous drive line houses the air vent and wiring, which is attached to an external controller and batteries.

The external controller and battery packs are worn similar to those of the HeartMate VE, allowing excellent patient mobility and relative independence. The Novacor LVAS requires systemic anticoagulation with coumadin to achieve an INR greater than 3.5. The elegant design of this LVAS has proven to be the most reliable of the implantable systems. Mechanical failure is rare and patients have been supported for over 3 years on their original pump. The Novacor LVAS has unfortunately been associated with high thromboembolic rate (up to 47%).[6] Modifications are being explored to help decrease the high incidence of thromboembolic events associated with this system.

Total Artificial Heart

The total artificial heart (TAH) (see Chapter 25 for a review of the currently available TAH) is implanted in the chest after removing the native heart. Early devices had marginal success rates, and enthusiasm for their use waned with the success of the evolving left ventricular assist devices (LVADs). Although the LVAD will likely remain the more widely used type of support system, there are certain patient groups that would most benefit from TAH support.

First, patients who have severe biventricular failure requiring long-term biventricular support or severe pulmonary hypertension may benefit from this type of support. Second, there are many patients who are poor candidates for LVAD support, for anatomic or physiologic reasons. Patients with large congenital or acquired intracardiac shunts are poor LVAD candidates. Patients with prosthetic aortic valves may be better served with a TAH. In these patients, placement of an LVAD will lead to little, if any, blood flow through the prosthetic valve, which then becomes a nidus for thrombus formation.

Certain patients would be better served with excision of their native heart, such as heart failure patients with endocarditis, a large ventricular thrombus, a large ventricular aneurysm, or those with malignant cardiac tumors.

A growing population of heart transplant recipients will develop graft vasculopathy (chronic allograft rejection) over time. This could potentially be the largest population for chronic TAH support, as there is presently no good treatment option for this patient population. Actuarial survival rates for retransplantation are 55% at 1 year as compared to 79% 1-year survival rates for first-time heart recipients. Many centers do not perform cardiac retransplantation for chronic allograft rejection because of the limited efficacy derived from this precious commodity. Placement of an LVAD for chronic or permanent support is suboptimal because immunosuppression would still need to be continued to maintain the graft, which could exacerbate infection concerns as well as other side effects associated with chronic immunosuppression. This rapidly growing patient population would certainly benefit from excision of their graft and chronic support with a TAH.

The CardioWest (Tucson, AZ) TAH is a pneumatic, implantable system that is currently the only such device in clinical use. The system is the current iteration of the widely publicized Jarvik-7–100 heart used in the patient Barney Clark, and has been used worldwide as a bridge to heart transplantation in 79 patients. A total of 55 patients (70%) have been transplanted, of which 50 survived (91% of patients transplanted) to discharge.[7] There are currently two programs supported by the National Heart, Lung, and Blood Institute (NHLBI) for developing a TAH: the Texas Heart Institute/ABIOMED TAH and the Penn State/3M Health Care TAH. Both systems are currently undergoing phase II in vivo testing.

Type of Support

Bridge to Recovery

The two paracorporeal systems are currently FDA-approved and are widely used to support patients when myocardial recovery is expected. Common indications include postcardiotomy syndromes, viral cardiomyopathies, anterior wall myocardial infarctions (with revascularization), and post-transplant reperfusion injury.

Both systems can be configured for either univentricular or biventricular support. Both systems are attached to the heart through proprietary cannulae that traverse the skin and attach to pumping chambers. Both require anticoagulation. The ABIOMED has the advantage of requiring minimal set-up and adjustment to initiate and maintain support, although it does limit patient mobility. The ABIOMED pump is significantly less expensive and costs one third as much as the Thoratec; however, Thoratec is initiating an aggressive pricing schedule, related to duration of support, to reduce the price differential. The Thoratec system requires a higher level of surgical sophistication to initiate and maintain support; however, resulting patient mobility is superior.

Centrifugal pumps (reviewed in detail in Chapter 17), with or without oxygenators, should not be overlooked as temporary support systems. There is no initial capital outlay and no training is required to initiate support. Peripheral cannulation and support can be rapidly initiated in the acute setting to resuscitate and stabilize dying patients. Once stabilized, the patient can be assessed for the potential of recovery or the need for further mechanical support. If additional mechanical support is not available, institutional transfer can be safely performed. Bleeding is the most frequent complication associated with centrifugal pump support, as the cannulae can be easily dislodged; therefore, the patient must remain immobile. A full-time perfusionist or technician is also required to continuously monitor the pump, adding to cost. These restrictions limit the usefulness of centrifugal pumps for long-term support. Nevertheless, they can be used to resuscitate and bridge a patient to another device.

If the patient's myocardium does not recover and the patient is a candidate for cardiac transplantation, the Thoratec system has an advantage over the ABIOMED due to its improved patient mobility and less stringent anticoagulation restrictions. Most transplant centers would explant the ABIOMED and implant one of the long-term assist systems for support to transplantation under these circumstances. Although a return to the operating room for a device change has added risk as well as cost, these may be offset by the ability to discharge the patient while awaiting transplantation.

Bridge to Transplantation

Four assist devices are currently FDA-approved for support to transplantation: the Thoratec system, the Baxter Novacor system, and Thermo Cardiosystems' IP and VE systems.

For univentricular assist, the implantable systems clearly have the advantage. Outpatient care and untethered mobility significantly enhance patient and family quality of life. Allowing patient discharge also offsets the higher cost of the electrical devices. Patients with potentially long support times (high panel reactive antibodies, large patient, blood group O) will likely benefit the most from both the quality of life and cost standpoints.

When outpatient management is not possible or if a short support time is anticipated, the HeartMate IP or Thoratec may be used. The HeartMate IP's drive console has the advantage of being much smaller than the Thoratec's and can be easily pushed by the patient. This facilitates better ambulation as well as some level of autonomy for the hospital-bound patient. There currently is a $10,000 cost premium for this advantage. For the smaller (<1.5 m^2 BSA) patient, the Thoratec is the best option.

When outpatient management is possible, either the HeartMate VE or the Novacor LVAS may be used. The cost premiums for these systems are currently $20,000 and $30,000, respectively, over the HeartMate IP. For the patient with a long anticipated wait time, 30 days or more of outpatient management could translate into a cost savings.

In the presence of right-sided circulatory failure, both the right ventricular stroke work (RVSW) and the pulmonary vascular resistance (PVR) should be assessed. If the RVSW is low and the PVR is also low, the patient can often do well with only left-sided support. Right-sided support may still be required in the immediate postoperative course, as the PVR rises from inflammatory-mediated events related to CPB. As the inflammatory response resolves, PVR returns to normal and right-sided support can be withdrawn. Inhaled nitric oxide is often the only therapy required to treat the PVR, thus avoiding the need for right ventricular assist device (RVAD) support.[8]

If, on the other hand, the RVSW is high and the PVR is also high, RVAD support is not commonly required. Although an LVAD removes the septal component of right ventricular contractility, and use of CPB will likely increase PVR in the short term, unloading the left ventricle with the device often more than compensates for these changes and the majority of patients will not require RVAD support.

Nonetheless, when right-sided support is required in the patient who is a transplant candidate, there are two configurations available: insertion of an implantable LVAD in combination with a paracorporeal RVAD (ABIOMED/Thoratec), or placement of a Thoratec in biventricular configuration.

Placing a paracorporeal RVAD in the patient with an implantable LVAD does require a return trip to the operating room to explant the RVAD in order to take advantage of the discharge potential of the implantable systems. For the patient who may have a long waiting time, and for whom discharge could be an option, the extra operative costs could be recovered when the patient is discharged. The improved mobility of the patient and improved quality of life with the current implantable systems could justify this approach. Implanting a Thoratec system on both right and left sides is a reasonable option for the patient who will not be discharged due to a short anticipated wait time and/or prohibitive distance to home.

The concept of "fixed PVR" has unclear meaning in this heart failure population. We and many others have observed "fixed" PVR of 7 or 8 Woods units decrease to 2 to 3 Woods units when the patient is on chronic LVAD support. If a patient is placed on chronic LVAD or biventricular assist device support and the PVR does not improve to acceptable levels, he or she should be assessed for options other than isolated orthotopic heart transplant.

Patient-Related Issues

Size

The current implantable systems are somewhat bulky and do require a certain body size (>1.5 m^2 BSA) as well as an appropriate body habitus for comfortable implantation of these devices. The size issue is not only related to the technical ability to implant the device, but also to the lowest rate the device will flow before increased thrombus risk develops. Patients as small as 0.8 m^2 BSA have been successfully supported by the Thoratec system and represent an ideal indication for this device. Large patients often have longer wait times and may benefit from early implantation of an electrically actuated pump.

Blood Type and Preformed Antibodies

The patient's blood type and the presence of preformed antibodies affect his or her waiting time to transplantation. The controversies surrounding preformed antibodies is addressed in Chapter 16. Nevertheless, if high preformed antibodies mandate cross-matching at your institution, an increased wait time will result. Placement of an implantable device would be advantageous, especially if discharge is an option.

Support

What type of support system does the patient have? Will he/she be able to learn how to manage the device at home? Will the patient be able to handle the psychosocial issues of outpatient management? Surgeons don't usually identify these issues personally when assessing the patient for device implant. Nonetheless, someone else likely has. If the support for outpatient management is not adequate and the patient is not likely to be discharged, cost savings can be realized by placing a pneumatic device and by providing the patient with a map of all of the power outlets in the hospital.

Discharge

The two electrically actuated systems are approved for outpatient support. Although the systems are costlier than the IP devices, outpatient management may offset their cost difference. Appropriate support networks must be established prior to discharge and will be addressed elsewhere. The recent change in the UNOS status I, will likely change the profile of transplant waiting times. Currently, patients who are placed on ventricular assist (excluding intra-aortic balloon pumps) are placed in status IA for 30 days after implant. Status IA receives the highest priority for donor offers and maximizes the possibility of receiving a heart. Unfortunately, patients transplanted within a month of device implantation have historically had poor outcomes. After 30 days, the patient is relegated to status IB, unless a device-related complication occurs. Centers with long anticipated wait times should consider investing in an electrical system that allows outpatient management.

Limitations

The current ventricular assist systems all require native outflow valves (aortic or pulmonary) in order to function appropriately. Even mild preoperative aortic insufficiency can be problematic, since patients in cardiogenic shock will have a low systemic pressure and a high left ventricular end-diastolic pressure and volume. The aortic transvalvular gradient will subsequently be trivial. With implementation of LVAD support, the left ventricular end-diastolic pressure will decrease and the mean aortic pressure will be higher; hence, the aortic transvalvular gradient will increase accordingly. Mild preoperative AI can become severe. The LVAD may sustain high flow rates and appear to be functioning well; however, the net forward "perfusion" flow will be low. The aortic valve must be addressed in this situation, but the approaches are controversial and there is insufficient experience to suggest a preferred method.

The presence of an aortic valve prosthesis has been considered a relative contraindication to LVAD support due to thromboembolic concerns, although authors have argued in favor of sealing these valves with sutures or patches.

Intracardiac thrombus and infection of the native heart are additional pathologies that are not well treated with current VAD options, and may warrant cardiac excision and TAH use.

What Device for My Institution?

Community Practice

For the community hospital that desires a device to support the infrequent cardiac disaster, the simplicity, versatility, and lower cost of the ABIOMED system should serve these needs. The ABIOMED system's "plug and play" ease of use and simple display allow the novice user to easily initiate and maintain good patient support. Although the Thoratec system has even greater versatility with the added capability to support a patient to transplantation, the novice user may find its drive console complex. Initiating support and troubleshooting device alarms can be difficult. The higher cost of the Thoratec system may also be an issue.

A relationship with a tertiary care center that may be the recipient of these patients should be established. Find out which short-term device(s) are used at your partner institution and consider purchasing them. Identify the surgeons who work with devices and establish lines of communication in advance. When a relationship has been established, the midnight phone call to try to transfer a patient is generally congenial.

Community Practice with a Heart Failure Program

At the minimum, these centers need a device for bridge to recovery. This allows the surgeons to have a "safety net" when performing high-risk procedures. As above, establish a relationship with the transplant center and find out what device(s) they are using and would like to receive in transfer.

As the incidence and prevalence of heart failure continues to grow, many large centers that do not offer transplantation would still like to offer implantable devices to their patients as a bridge to transplantation. "Link" programs are being established, where patients can be evaluated and listed for transplantation at the transplant center yet be managed by their local physician and local hospital. The local hospital may also implant the device and care for the patient until a heart becomes available, at which time the patient is transferred to the transplant center.

This type of arrangement not only allows the patient to be treated locally, but also allows the community hospital to become device savvy. This places them at considerable advantage when devices emerge that may be implanted as permanent support and not as bridge to transplantation.

Practice with Heart Transplant Program

Ideally, a practice should have a paracorporeal system as well as an implantable system. At the minimum, the capability to support patients for both bridge to recovery as well as bridge to transplantation is necessary. The least costly method of offering both is with the Thoratec system. Ideally, such centers should also be able to insert the implantable systems, which provide best quality of life. Cardiac transplant programs in this country that do not offer ventricular assist are not offering patients the current standard of care.

Many community practice hospitals will have the ABIOMED system as their short-term support system. Transplant centers should have this system as well to facilitate transfers.

Conclusions

Selecting the right device can be a complex matter requiring the consideration of patient-specific, institutional, and regional issues. There is often more than one correct device option for a patient; however, early institution of a system with which the surgical team is familiar is the hallmark of success. Every hospital should have access to at least one of the devices described above, and lines of communication with tertiary care centers specializing in the care of end-stage heart failure patients should be maintained.

References

1. Mehta S, Souza D, Boehmer J, et al. Comparison of Pierce-Donachy and TCI left ventricular assist systems as bridge to transplant–an institutional experience. *ASAIO J* 1999. In press.
2. El-Banayosy A, Arusoglu L, Kizner L, et al. *Novacor LVAS versus HeartMate as a Long Term Mechanical Circulatory Support Device in Bridging Patients: A Prospective Randomized Study.* American Association of Thoracic Surgery, 1999. Abstract.
3. Rose EA, Moskowitz AJ, Packer M, et al. The REMATCH trial: Rationale, design and endpoints. *Ann Thorac Surg* 1999;67:723–730.
4. Slater J, Rose EA, Levin HR, et al. Low thromboembolic risk without anticoagulation using advanced design left ventricular assist devices. *Ann Thorac Surg* 1996;62:1321–1327.
5. Rose EA, Levin HR, Oz MC, et al. Artificial circulatory support with textured interior surfaces: A counterintuitive approach to minimize thromboembolism. *Circulation* 1994;90: II87-II91.
6. Schmid C, Weyand M, Nabavi DG, et al. Cerebral and systemic embolization during left ventricular support with the N100 device. *Ann Thorac Surg* 1998;65:1703–1710.
7. Arabia FA, Copeland JG, Smith RG, et al. International experience with the CardioWest total artificial heart as a bridge to transplantation. *Eur J Cardiothorac Surg* 1997;11:S5-S10.
8. Yahagi N, Kumon K, Nakatani T, et al. Inhaled nitric oxide for the management of acute right ventricular failure in patients with a left ventricular assist system. *Artif Organs* 1995; 19(6):557–558.

Chapter 4

Options for Mechanical Support in Pediatric Patients

Tom R. Karl, MD and Stephen B. Horton, MD

Introduction

With an increasingly favorable experience in adults, ventricular assist device (VAD) support in various formats has become an accepted treatment for myocardial failure, either with an expectation of recovery or as a bridge to transplantation. Extracorporeal membrane oxygenation (ECMO) on the other hand, has been used less frequently in adults, due to a generally higher complication rate. This is perhaps related to the prevalence of multiorgan system failure in adults with respiratory distress syndrome and/or cardiac failure, and a stronger tendency toward thromboembolism.

The value of ECMO in children, however, is undisputed, with a large body of evidence supporting its use for various severe neonatal pulmonary problems, persistent fetal circulation, and, more recently, septic shock.[1,2] There has also been increasing interest in the use of ECMO for postoperative ventricular dysfunction in children of all ages. In fact, the majority of the world experience with extracorporeal life support for cardiac failure in children has been with ECMO, as detailed in the annual Extracorporeal Life Support Organization (ELSO) reports.[3]

In the last decade, a plethora of new VAD systems have been placed into clinical use, many being suitable for patients down to the 20 kg weight range. However, the experience with VAD support of smaller children (<20 kg) remains limited to date, partly due to technical considerations such as cannulation and limited space. Low flow rates in small patients may create a diathesis for thromboembolic complications when adult-sized systems are applied in this population.[4] There is also a longstanding perception that children with complex congenital heart disease will be unsuitable for univentricular support without an oxygenator. Many pediatric cardiac teams therefore feel that ECMO is the best alternative, especially since implantable VADs for small children are generally unavailable in many parts of the world.[5] Our own experience does not support this concept.[1,6–8] The purpose of this chapter is to review

From Goldstein DJ and Oz MC (eds). *Cardiac Assist Devices*. Armonk, NY: Futura Publishing Co., Inc.; ©2000.

our indications, technique, and outcome for short-term circulatory support in the pediatric population, with special emphasis on the use of centrifugal pump VAD and ECMO.[1,6–10]

Indications and Contraindications

Postoperative cardiac dysfunction has been the most common indication for circulatory support in our own unit. The majority of patients so treated underwent palliative or reparative open heart operations or cardiac transplantation and could not be weaned from cardiopulmonary bypass (CPB) despite optimization of intravascular volume, acid-base status, and inotropic support. A small subset of patients had refractory low cardiac output following initial satisfactory weaning from CPB. Rarely, low cardiac output not related to surgery was the primary indication. This latter group includes children with acute myocarditis, sepsis syndrome, cardiac trauma, and severe post-transplantation rejection.

A great deal of judgment on the part of the surgical and medical teams is required to decide on the optimal timing for institution of extracorporeal support, particularly since the devices themselves are not free of complications. In many published series, the strongest correlate of failure of extracorporeal support has been the presence of a residual cardiac defect, a finding corroborated in our own studies.[11] Ideally, technical failure of the operation should be ruled out prior to commencement of VAD or ECMO support, although in practice this may be quite difficult. Toward this end, there is a role for intraoperative transesophageal echocardiography, as well as direct cardiac chamber pressure measurements. One must ask whether there is a potential for recovery, and if not, whether transplantation is a realistic option. Family and social factors must be weighed, including whether conversion of an intraoperative death to an intensive care unit death several days later is a helpful or a punitive step for the particular family. Finally, one must consider which type of support is best for a given patient.

Numerous *relative* contraindications to the use of VAD and ECMO have been cited in the surgical literature. Examples are multiorgan system failure, severe coagulopathy, intracranial hemorrhage, neurologic impairment, uncontrolled sepsis, prolonged cardiac arrest, and the presence of a univentricular circulation. In practice, while all are relevant, most of these features are difficult or impossible to assess accurately in a child urgently needing placement of a support device, especially in the intraoperative setting. For example, addressing the sepsis issue, we have supported two patients with VAD and ECMO for essentially untreated endocarditis (with evidence of cerebral embolism) following emergency aortic valve replacement. Both had a prolonged but compete recovery. ECMO has also been employed in noncardiac patients specifically for the treatment of multiorgan system failure, with a 50% survival.[12] Every center using circulatory support in children could cite similar cases, and one might suggest that pediatric patients generally have a greater potential for recovery (without sequelae) than do adults. Therefore, in institutions that are capable of offering circulatory support, almost any child accepted for open heart surgery will also be a candidate for VAD or ECMO should the need arise. Other types of patients must be assessed on an individual basis.

Is mechanical support appropriate for resuscitation following cardiac arrest?

The main concern is neurologic outcome, and the prearrest status is obviously a critical factor for both the brain and the heart. Notably, recovery of cardiac function can occur well beyond the point of severe brain damage. We have initiated both VAD and ECMO support during prolonged (1 hour) cardiac arrest with good quality survival. In the Pittsburgh experience, 11 of 17 patients with cardiac arrest (6 of 11 who had >15 minutes of cardiac massage) survived to discharge following ECMO support.[13] Clearly, we have been obliged to rethink the issue of acceptable resuscitation times for children in the era of circulatory support.

The general aim of postoperative centrifugal pump VAD and ECMO support is recovery of the child within 5 days, although in selected cases there may be an option for a bridge to transplantation, with or without interim conversion to a pulsatile paracorporeal support system designed for longer term use.[13–17] For patients who weigh less than 20 kg, 2 weeks would be considered to be the maximal realistic projected duration of support in our own unit, although longer periods have been reported.

Pediatric experience with extracorporeal support for bridge to transplant has lagged well behind that in adults. Patients supported specifically for bridging (ie, those felt to have irreversible cardiac dysfunction) must prospectively meet institutional criteria for transplantation.[17] Factors such as size, blood group, and donor availability must be taken into consideration. This group typically includes patients with acute myocarditis, cardiomyopathy, and inoperable end-stage congenital heart disease.

Finally, there is a small subset of children with acute myocarditis who may recover (without transplantation) following prolonged VAD support.[17] If long-term mechanical support is deemed necessary, centrifugal pump VAD and ECMO are not the best options, although in most units a better system is not yet available.

The VAD Strategy

Our VAD circuit consists of a centrifugal pump head (Bio-Medicus, Eden Prairie, MN) mounted on a flexible drive cable (Fig. 1). Inlet and outlet pressure monitoring and an in-line arterial flow probe are routinely employed. The tubing length is minimized by mounting the pump head directly onto the patient's bed. In recent years we have favored the use of heparin-bonded circuits, although this is not considered essential.

The centrifugal pump is preferred over a roller pump, as it is simple in concept and it is designed to run at constant (but operator-determined) speed. There are no valves or diaphragms since the device output is nonpulsatile. The constrained vortex pump design results in subatmospheric pressure at the tip of the cone, establishing suction in the venous cannula (Fig. 2). Care must be taken to keep this pressure above −20 mm Hg, or excessive hemolysis can occur. In roller pumps, inlet obstruction results in a vacuum that is significant enough to cause collapse of the pump tubing. Roller pump ECMO circuits are therefore equipped with a collapsible bladder that servoregulates the circuit. This system could be used for VAD support, but pump support would stop if the bladder should collapse. With the centrifugal pump VAD system, a reduction in venous return will reduce pump output, with a reduction in inlet pressure. The operator must reduce the pump speed (rpm) at this point; this

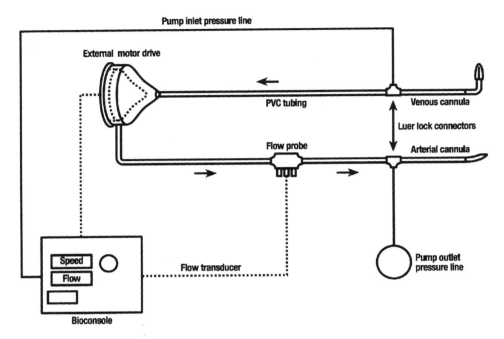

FIGURE 1. Schematic representation of the centrifugal pump ventricular assist device circuit used at the Royal Children's Hospital.

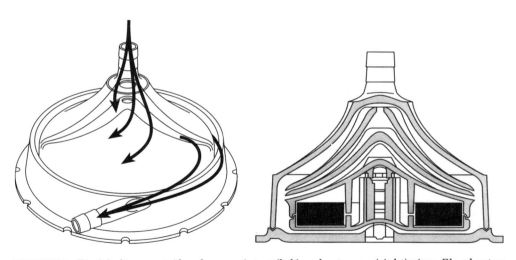

FIGURE 2. Bio-Medicus centrifugal pump, intact (left) and cut away (right) view. Blood enters at the apex of the cone and energy is implanted by the (constrained) vortex created by spinning cones along the vertical axis. Blood is ejected tangentially at the base of the cone. Mechanical energy is transferred to the cones by a spinning external magnet coupled to a second magnet inside the cone.

will not affect flow but will increase pump inlet pressure (ie, render it less "negative" or less subatmospheric). The alternative is to increase venous return to the pump by other means, primarily by increasing vascular volume. The centrifugal pump is most efficient (and least hemolytic) when revolutions are minimized for a given flow. Because roller pumps generate constant flow at a given speed, the above problems are averted. On the other hand, roller pumps have a higher incidence of hemolysis.

Benefits of the use of centrifugal pumps include reduced incidence of hemolysis and decreased risk of tubing rupture and embolism.[18] In addition, the battery back-up makes the pump convenient for transport of the patient and device during a period of assist. Most importantly, the centrifugal pump allows fine tuning of the peripheral circulation prior to and during weaning, as it is responsive (flow at a given pressure) to the patient's intravascular volume and resistance.

Centrifugal pumps can be configured for biventricular support. Cannulation of the right atrium and pulmonary artery can provide right-sided support, and simultaneous cannulation of the left atrium and aorta can result in biventricular support. Under these circumstances, the pump heads are adjusted for approximately 1:0.7 flow ratio. The biventricular support set-up, however, is technically cumbersome in a small child and, hence, we normally prefer ECMO in such a situation.

Is VAD support sufficient in patients with a univentricular circulation? While controversial, several investigators have successfully supported patients with VADs after the Norwood operation for hypoplastic left heart syndrome as well as after bidirectional cavopulmonary shunts performed as part of the treatment of other complex univentricular variants. In such cases, higher than normal flows (1.5 × calculated) may be required, as the assist device provides both pulmonary and systemic output. In our own practice, Blalock shunts have been left open during VAD (as well as ECMO) support in such cases.

The most common scenario for institution of VAD support in our unit has been intraoperative postcardiotomy failure. In this circumstance, cannulation is usually transmediastinal, using the left atrial appendage or left atrial body (at the right superior pulmonary vein junction) for drainage, and the ascending aorta for arterial return. For children with a univentricular circulation, the right atrial appendage and ascending aorta can be used. Standard or heparin-bonded cannulae designed to carry 150 mL/kg/min flow are employed. Cannulae are secured with purse-string sutures and tourniquets. The tourniquets are held fast with vascular clips, and left inside the mediastinum.

If VAD support is instituted for a postoperative cardiac arrest (ie, outside the operating room), then CPB may be required initially; in some cases, however, we have been able to place asystolic postoperative patients undergoing open cardiac massage directly onto left VAD (LVAD) support, with a successful outcome.

VAD support is commenced at minimum flows and quickly increased to 150 mL/kg/min. If the patient remains stable, flow is reduced to 70% of calculated output. We attempt to maintain a left atrial pressure of 3 to 4 mm Hg, allowing for some cardiac ejection if possible. In theory, this may reduce the risk of stasis and thrombus formation. Heparin can be reversed with protamine, and hemostasis can then be secured as for other CPB cases. However, administration of protamine to patients supported with a heparin-bonded (Carmeda, Medtronic Inc., Minneapolis, MN) circuit may neutralize some of the advantages of the Carmeda coating, and could result in a significantly greater heparin requirement or a higher risk for thrombus formation during VAD support.[15] When hemostasis has been secured (often a prolonged exercise), the skin is closed with cannulas exiting at either pole of the wound. Alternatively, a polytetrafluoroethylene (PTFE) membrane is sutured to the skin edges, leaving the sternum open in either case.

For some patients it is not clear whether univentricular support with a VAD will be sufficient. When biventricular failure is present, ECMO or biventricular assist device (biVAD) support are often required. The same could be said for patients with severe pulmonary hypertension or pulmonary dysfunction that complicates their clinical picture. It should be borne in mind, however, that the decrease in left atrial pressure afforded by LVAD support may dramatically improve pulmonary hypertension and right ventricular dysfunction in borderline cases, especially with the concurrent use of nitric oxide. As pointed out in Chapter 2, right ventricular function is sensitive to left ventricular function in a number of ways. By unloading the left ventricle with VAD support, right ventricular filling is improved and the decrease in chamber size and septal shift may improve tricuspid valve function as well.[19] Therefore, each case must be assessed on its own merits, and the simplest effective level of support should be first instituted (ie, VAD rather than ECMO).

An intraoperative algorithm has been developed to determine whether VAD support will be sufficient to sustain adequate perfusion. A venous cannula is placed in the left atrium and the right atrial or caval cannula used for CPB is clamped. This maneuver is used to assess the effect of partial left heart bypass. Right atrial and pulmonary artery pressure as well as right ventricular function are observed at 150 mL/kg/min pump flow. If all are satisfactory (right atrial pressure <12 mm Hg, pulmonary artery systolic pressure less than one-half systemic, no right ventricular dilation), then the patient is ventilated normally while gas exchange in the oxygenator is temporarily interrupted. If gas exchange, acid-base status, and hemodynamics remain acceptable, the patient is recannulated for VAD support. Otherwise, conversion to ECMO (or possibly biVAD) is undertaken.

During VAD support, patients are maintained fully sedated and ventilated. Inotropes are minimized to the level required to maintain optimal right heart function, as assessed by central venous pressure, oxygenation, and echocardiographic assessment. Hourly records of arterial pressure, VAD inlet/outlet pressure, right and left atrial pressure, total flow, and activated clotting time (ACT) are recorded. When postoperative bleeding subsides, systemic heparin anticoagulation is begun (approximately 20 international units [IU]/kg/h), keeping the ACT around 150 seconds.

Two different systems are commercially available for ACT measurement. One relies on the use of diatomaceous earth (Hemochron, International Technidyne Corporation, Edison, NJ) and the other on kaolin (Hemotec, Medtronic Inc.). We have found the latter more advantageous, as it requires only 0.2 mL of blood per sample to yield reproducible results. We have found the Hemochron ACT to be, on average, 1.1 times that obtained with the Hemotec equipment.

With Carmeda heparin bonding, the system theoretically can be operated without heparin or at reduced doses, particularly in situations of high flow in larger patients. However, clots may form in heparin-bonded circuits with or without anticoagulation, and this risk of thrombosis must constantly be weighed against the risk of bleeding.[20]

Inhaled nitric oxide is an effective and inexpensive treatment for pulmonary hypertension, and it is also useful for support of the right heart during low cardiac output states requiring support with a LVAD (Chapter 7). Even if pulmonary artery pressure is normal, some patients benefit from institution of nitric oxide therapy with improved left atrial filling and reduced ventilation/perfusion mismatch. Potential side effects such as methemoglobinemia and NO_2 toxicity are rare at the maximal clinically relevant dose of 20 ppm.

Normothermia is maintained during VAD support with a heating/cooling blanket and the heat generated by the centrifugal pump head itself. Peritoneal dialysis and/or venovenous hemofiltration are used as required for metabolic support and fluid removal. Vasodilators, parenteral nutrition, and antibiotics are also administered. In general, the measures used for metabolic support are much the same as those required for other critically ill cardiac patients who are not being supported with a VAD.

Plasma-free hemoglobin is monitored at least daily, and should remain below 60 mg/dL. Elevated plasma-free hemoglobin, especially in conjunction with noise or vibrations in the pump head, may be an indication of imminent mechanical failure. In this case, the pump head can be easily changed with only a very brief period off VAD support. In general, the pump head can be used for 7 days, after which it is routinely changed. Occasionally, a pump head is replaced earlier in the presence of signs of imminent failure. The median pump head life in our patients has been 71.5 hours (range 0.5 to 480 hours). A number of technical problems relating to centrifugal pump VAD support in children may be encountered (Table 1).

The ECMO Strategy

Our ECMO circuit for cardiac support mimics that used for neonatal pulmonary support (Fig. 3).[8,21] A closed venoarterial circuit powered by a Bio-Medicus (Medtronic-Bio-Medicus, Eden Prairie, MN) centrifugal pump is used. Both the Avecor membrane oxygenator and, more recently, the Medtronic Carmeda heparin bonded circuit (Minimax or Maxima oxygenator) have been used. Cannulation technique depends on circumstances surrounding the initiation of support. For patients who cannot be separated from CPB, the ascending aortic cannula used for CPB can be left in situ, and a second cannula placed in the right atrial appendage. Both cannulas should support 150 mL/kg flow with a pump inlet pressure of greater than -20 mm Hg and an outlet pressure of less than 200 mm Hg. When using ECMO in patients with minimal left ventricular ejection, left atrial or left ventricular decompression may be necessary to provide optimal cardiac support and to prevent hemorrhagic pulmonary edema.[13,22] A second venous cannula can be placed in the left atrial appendage or right superior pulmonary vein if further decompression is required to cope with the increased collateral return to the left side imposed by the ECMO circuit. Alternatively, balloon or blade septostomy has been used for this purpose in some nonsurgical patients.[22,23] Direct skin (or PTFE membrane to skin) closure is generally used, with cannulae exiting through the upper and lower poles of the wound. Patients without prior sternotomy generally undergo right cervical cannulation.[24] Permanent ligation of a carotid artery distal to the arterial cannula is unnecessary. With our current technique, reconstruction of the cervical vessels following decannulation has resulted in good long-term patency.[24]

Patients on ECMO support are cared for by a dedicated team. Sedation and

Table 1

Common Problems Encountered with Centrifugal Pump Support in Children, and Possible Solutions

Problem	Comments and Possible Solutions
High arterial outlet pressure	
• Acute	
-Cannula position has changed	Adjust cannula position
-Thrombus partly obstructing cannula	Recannulate, adjust ACT
-LV ejection above support provided by pump (equivalent of increased vascular resistance)	Consider weaning with flow reduction; vasodilator therapy
• Chronic	
-Flow too high for selected cannula	Recannulate with larger cannula
Low inlet pressure	
• Acute	
-Cannula position has changed	Adjust cannula position
-Thrombus partly obstructing cannula	Recannulate, adjust ACT
-Atrial wall collapsed around cannula	Reduce and increase flow slowly; infuse volume
• Chronic	
-Flow too high for selected cannula	Recannulate with larger cannula
-Failing RV, poor LA filling	Pulmonary vasodilators (NO), consider ECMO, RVAD
Inability to achieve nominal flow	
• Any combination of circumstances outlined above	As above
• Cardiac tempopade	Exploration, hemostasis, drainage
Excessive hemolysis	
• Low inlet pressure	As above
• Thrombus in pump head (especially if pump head is noisy)	Change pump head, adjust ACT
• Venous cannula is too small	Recannulate with larger cannula
Inconsistent ACT readings	
• Incorrect preparation of kaolin suspension	Mix suspension just prior to use
• Incorrect preparation of cuvettes	Store cuvettes at 2–25°C, warm to 37°C just before use
• Sensor contaminated with blood	Clean sensor with peroxide. Check for accurate clotting
• Concurrent platelet infusion	Increase heparin infusion by 10% during infusion
• Ongoing variation in heparin metabolism	Adjust heparin dose
Air in VAD circuit	
• Air entrapment around insertion site (very low inlet pressure)	Reduce support, infuse volume, revise cannulation site
• Open or faulty tap or connector in system	Change or close connectors or taps. De-air venous side
• Crack in pump housing	Change pump head
• Acute inlet obstruction with very low pressure	See above
Noisy pump head	
• Thrombus in pump head	Change pump head

LV = left ventricle; RV = right ventricle; LA = left atrium; ACT = activated clotting time; ECMO = extracorporeal membrane oxygenation; RVAD = right ventricular assist device.

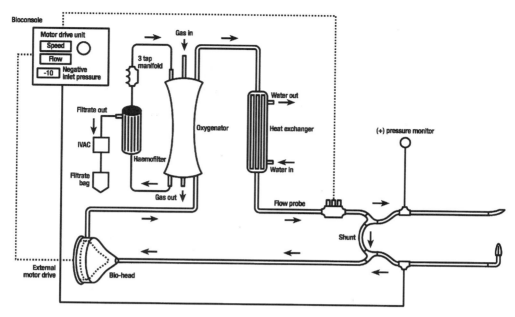

FIGURE 3. Schematic representation of centrifugal pump extracorporeal membrane oxygenation circuit used at the Royal Children's Hospital.

paralysis are generally required, along with antibiotics and total parenteral nutrition. Most of the principles outlined in the VAD strategy apply to ECMO patients as well. Flows on ECMO are initially set at 120 to 150 mL/min, but are sometimes higher in septic patients. Serum lactate is a useful guide to adequacy of flow. Heparin is infused to maintain the ACT between 160 and 180 seconds, or 140 to 150 seconds for heparin-bonded circuits. Inlet pressure is kept on the positive side of -20 mm Hg via appropriate cannula position, and normovolemia is ensured. Platelet counts are kept greater than $100,000/mm^3$ and epsilon-aminocaproic acid (Amicar, Immunex Corporation, Seattle, WA) is given by continuous infusion as required. We routinely employ hemofiltration via a shunt placed in parallel with the oxygenator, at 10 to 30 mL/min flow (Fig. 3). The volume of fluid removed can be controlled with a standard intravenous pump. Ventilator support is reduced to provide the lowest cardiac filling pressures, but must be increased as cardiac ejection improves to prevent coronary hypoxemia. Many of the problems and solutions noted for centrifugal VAD also apply to the centrifugal ECMO circuit; however some more complex issues may also arise due to the presence of the oxygenator. A guide for troubleshooting some of these problems is included in Table 2.

Weaning the Patient from Mechanical Support

The first sign of cardiac recovery is the appearance of a pulsatile systemic arterial pressure trace during full flow. Transeosophageal echo assessment is helpful at this

Table 2

Common Problems Encountered with Centrifugal Pump ECMO Support in Children, and Possible Solutions

Problem	Comments and Possible Solutions
1. **Air in venous side of circuit:** sources include IV infusions, cannulas, connectors, pressure monitoring lines	• Clamp arterial cannula and shunt, stop pump, ventilate • De-air with syringe via pump inlet pressure line tap • Reinstitute ECMO after securing point of air entry
2. **Air in oxygenator:** caused by membrane rupture, excess gas/blood flow ratio, air in venous line or pump head, entrainment from connectors or shunt line infusions	• Clamp ECMO lines between pump head and oxygenator, stop pump, ventilate patient and maintain cardiac output • De-air with syringe via tap in shunt manifold • Reinstitute ECMO after securing point of air entry or adjusting gas flow; may require circuit change for oxygenator failure
3. **Air in arterial side of circuit:** sources include membrane rupture, entrainment from connectors or hemofilter, major venous embolus	• Clamp arterial cannula and shunt, stop pump, ventilate • Trendelenburg position • Replace blood volume • De-air arterial cannula with syringe, then clamp line • De-air with syringe via arterial cannula tap • Secure air entry point, replace oxygenator if necessary • Reinstitute ECMO
4. **Decreased hemoglobin saturation** 　-Decreased flow 　-Anemia 　-Inadequate FiO_2 or ventilation 　-Excessive shunt flow 　-Pneumothorax 　-Oxygenator failure	 • Adjust flow • Transfuse • Increase FiO_2, optimize ventilation • Restrict shunt flow • Tube thoracostomy • Replace oxygenator
5. **Hypercarbia** 　Inadequate ventilation 　Pneumothorax 　Oxygenator failure	 • Optimize ventilation • Tube thoracostomy • Increase gas sweep. If ineffective, replace oxygenator
6. **Oxygenator failure** 　-Inadequate anticoagulation 　-Inadequate flow through oxygenator (high preoxygenator pressure indicates obstruction) 　-Membrane rupture 　-Plasma leak (hollow fiber oxygenator)	 • Adjust ACT • Clamp arterial cannula and shunt, stop pump, ventilate • New oxygenator and circuit can be connected via bridge in old circuit. De-air and recommence ECMO

IV = intravenous; FiO_2 = fraction of inspired oxygen; ECMO = extracorporeal membrane oxygenation.

point, to further evaluate the ventricular contractility and the response to volume loading. A Starling response suggests that weaning can proceed. Flow is reduced gradually down to a minimum total flow of 150 mL/min as the left ventricle begins to eject. Normal ventilation and low-dose inotropic support are maintained. Temporary augmentation of heparin may be required at low flows, and the cannulas may be heparin-flushed (5 IU/mL saline) to test the hemodynamics and pulmonary function with pump support discontinued. With an ECMO circuit, blood continues to circulate across the opened bridge. Decannulation is generally performed in the operating room, with concurrent sternal closure whenever possible.

Experience at the Royal Children's Hospital

Between 1989 and 1998, 53 infants and children (or approximately 1.2% of our CPB cases) were supported with a centrifugal pump VAD. The median age was 3.5 months (range 2 days to 19 years) and the median weight was 4 kg (1.9 to 70 kg). The diagnoses and operative procedures crossed the spectrum of congenital and acquired heart disease in children. Operations preceding VAD support included the Norwood procedure (n = 10), arterial switch (n = 8), aortic root procedures (n = 8), anomalous origin of the left coronary artery from the pulmonary artery (ALCAPA) repair (n = 5), repair of supravalvar aortic stenosis (n = 3), heart or heart lung transplant (n = 3), cavopulmonary connection (n = 3), mitral valve replacement (n = 2), and others. Of the 53 children supported, 38 were weaned from VAD (72%) and 24 (46%) were ultimately discharged from the hospital. Deaths following weaning generally reflected persistent cardiac dysfunction rather than morbidity specifically attributable to the VAD. Neither age, weight, timing of support (intra- versus postoperative), cyanosis, nor presence of a mechanical valve was associated with incremental risk ($P>0.05$ for all). The need for dialysis or ultrafiltration has been identified as a risk factor for death in other published series.[25] In our unit, both dialysis and ultrafiltration are used frequently during VAD and ECMO support, and have not emerged as independent risk factors. Actuarial survival at 1 year for all the VAD patients was 44% (CL = 0.31 to 0.58), suggesting a sharp decline in hazard function at the point of hospital discharge.

The median support time was 75 hours (range 19 to 428) for patients who could be weaned from VAD. For patients ultimately not weanable, it was 79.5 hours (range 2 to 114). For those discharged, the median support time was 71.5 hours (range 38 to 144), and for patients not discharged the median time was 88 hours (range 2 to 428). Thus, analyzed in various ways, VAD time was similar for survivors and nonsurvivors ($P=0.69$). The interpretation of support time data is possibly confounded by the fact that VAD was electively terminated in some children who showed no signs of ventricular recovery after 72 hours, in the absence of a realistic transplant option.

The VAD group of particular interest to us consists of children under 6 kg of weight, a technically challenging cohort whose options for support are more limited. It has been suggested that many of these patients are suitable only for ECMO.[1] We analyzed a subset of 34 of our patients, ages 2 days to 258 days (median 60 days) and weight 1.9 kg to 5.9 kg (median 3.7 kg). Twenty-four were unweanable from CPB, and 10 required support in the intensive care unit for postoperative refractory low cardiac output. Weaning and decannulation were performed in 22 of 34 (0.63; CL = 0.45 to 0.78), similar to the patients above 6 kg ($P=0.07$). One-year actuarial survival was 0.31 (CL = 0.17 to 0.47), with most deaths being due to irreversible cardiac disease. Within the group of children weighing less than 6 kg, neither age, weight, VAD duration, CPB duration, cross-clamp duration, nor the presence of univentricular anatomy proved useful in predicting hospital discharge ($P>0.05$).[10] The smallest patient in our series was a 19-day-old, 1.9-kg baby with Bing-Taussig anomaly and aortic arch obstruction who was placed on VAD postoperatively and survived with no neurologic sequelae despite a prolonged cardiac arrest.

Complications were frequent in VAD patients of all ages, as has been the case in most reported series. Bleeding that required exploration occurred in 15 patients. Three patients had sepsis with clinical signs and positive blood cultures, while positive blood cultures without clinical signs were found in another five. Transient neurologic defects were noted in three survivors, and two have had persistent mild neurologic complications. There have been no permanent renal sequelae. Mechanical complications were also frequent (20 patients) but usually manageable with appropriate surveillance and action. Included were pump head failure, cracked connectors, kinked cannulas, and air or clots in the circuit. Only four patients required an emergency circuit change as the primary intervention. The true incidence of all complications is underestimated, as assessment was incomplete in the nonsurvivors.

During the same time frame as our VAD experience, 40 children with cardiac or combined cardiopulmonary failure (not necessarily related to surgery) were supported with centrifugal pump ECMO.[9] Indications included failure to wean from CPB (n = 12), sepsis syndrome (n = 9), trauma/cardiomyopathy/myocarditis (n = 6), cardiopulmonary dysfunction not related to surgery (n = 6), and postoperative low cardiac output/arrest (n = 7). This analysis excludes children supported solely for pulmonary indications. Of the ECMO patients, 19 were weaned, 3 were bridged to transplant, and 19 were eventually discharged. Thus, although the weaning probability was better with VAD (0.71 versus 0.48; $P=0.014$), the discharge probability was similar with VAD and ECMO (0.46 versus 0.48; $P=1.0$). In interpreting these results, one must consider that most of the VAD patients could have been supported with ECMO, but the reverse would not generally apply. The ELSO results for ECMO are similar, and have been recently tabulated to July 1997. Of 16,098 patients supported to date by reporting centers, 2051 (42%) were in the "cardiac" category. Within this group, 1563 had cardiac surgery prior to support, 114 had a transplant-related indication, 57 had myocarditis, 95 had other cardiomyopathies, and 222 did not fall into any of these categories. Overall survival for the 2051 children supported was 0.42 (CL = 0.40 to 0.44). To date, ECMO support for noncardiac causes has met with better results than support for cardiac dysfunction (survival probability 0.75 versus 0.42; $P=0.0001$). The complications most frequently related to the ECMO circuit (primarily roller pump) were oxygenator failure, cannula problems, tubing rupture, and pump malfunction (1% to 6% of patients). The most frequently occurring patient-events were hemorrhage, arrhythmia, and renal insufficiency (16% to 28% of patients). Inotropes were required in 45% of patients during ECMO support.

Results of VAD and ECMO support have been remarkably similar across a number of published series,[14,15,20,26-29] suggesting that the patient population supported is more important than the method of support. At least for postoperative patients, a common feature in these series is that patients who are likely to recover tend to do so within the first few days. Beyond 2 weeks, complications of VAD such as sepsis and multiorgan system failure often supervene. A key question is whether paracorporeal pulsatile systems designed for longer term support can be used successfully as a bridge to recovery or transplantation should a heart donor become available.

Results with short-term VAD and ECMO in our own unit and in most others reflect a policy of expanding indications to include nearly all cardiac surgical patients who are not expected to survive without support. Whether this strategy is appropriate is a decision to be taken by each team in the context of local resources and philosophy. To most of us, a 30% to 40% long-term survival probability would immediately justify the effort and expense, especially if the child might have minimal or no disability. On the other hand, improvements in the technical aspects, safety, and efficacy of centrifugal pump VAD support may be somewhat obscured by the liberalization of indications for its use.

Centrifugal Pump VAD: Special Circumstances

Short-term circulatory support has been particularly effective for postoperative patients with ALCAPA, transposition of the great arteries (TGA) following arterial switch, and donor heart dysfunction following transplantation. Our patients with ALCAPA and TGA, as a group, had a 0.91 (CL = 0.59 to 1.0) overall survival probability ($P = 0.002$). The unifying thread in such cases is undoubtedly the presence of two anatomically normal ventricles, with one being temporarily (but critically) impaired. Conversely, patients whose cardiac abnormalities bear a poor prognosis without VAD (obstructive left heart syndromes, complex univentricular hearts) also fare poorly after VAD support. Some of these situations deserve further commentary.

Anomalous Origin of the Left Coronary Artery from the Pulmonary Artery

In this rare (approximately 10^{-5} of all infants) congenital anomaly, the entire left coronary system arises from the pulmonary artery. The basic pathophysiology is considered to be retrograde flow from the left coronary artery into the pulmonary artery that may increase as the pulmonary vascular resistance drops postnatally.[30,31] The result is a variable degree of myocardial ischemia, sometimes leading to extensive subendocardial or even transmural infarction. Despite its rarity, ALCAPA is the most common cause of myocardial infarction in children.[32] There is a tendency to develop papillary muscle dysfunction, which causes mitral insufficiency, exacerbated further by left ventricular dilation and loss of wall thickness (Fig. 4). The result may be severe low cardiac output syndrome, and the only effective treatment is surgery.

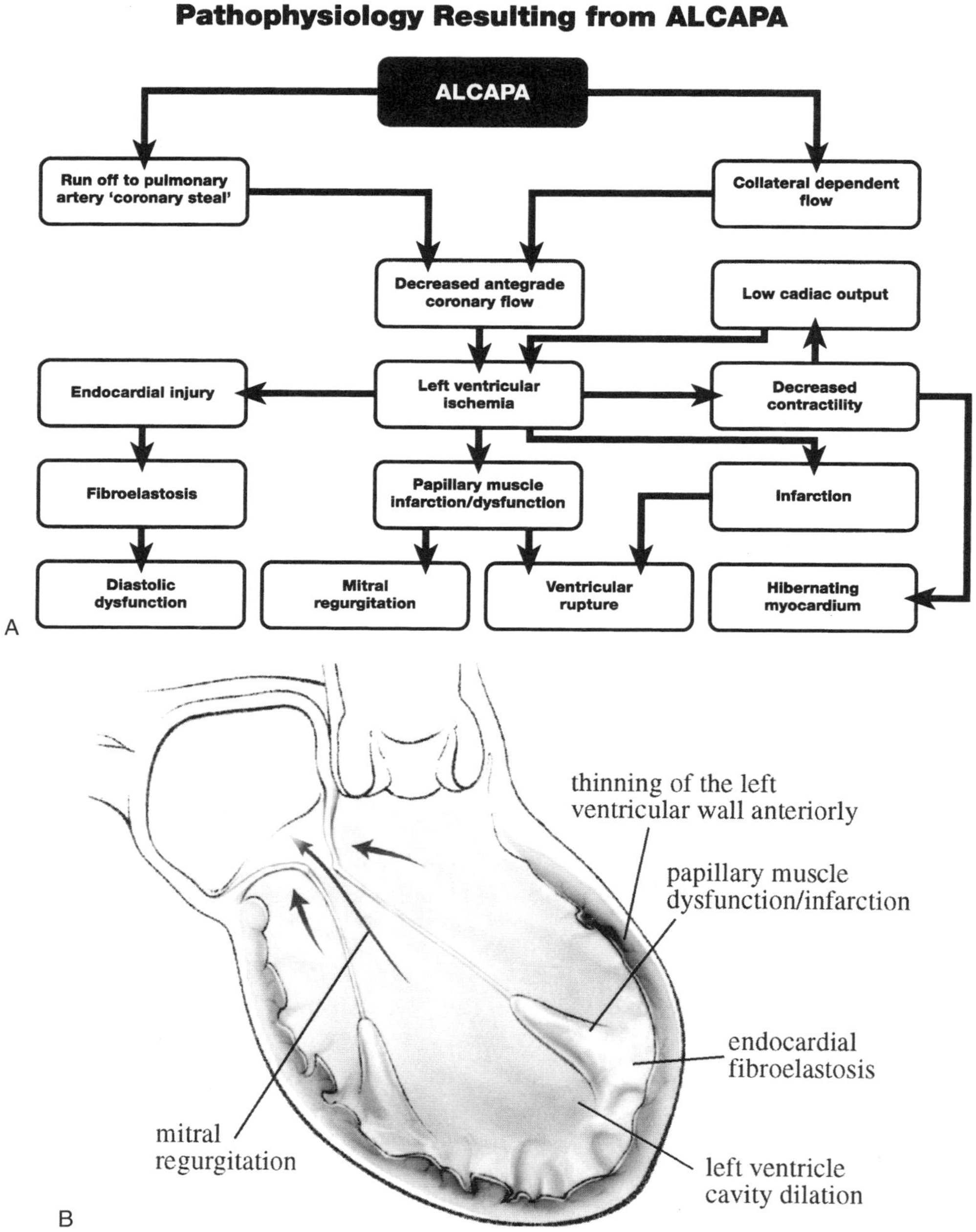

Pathophysiology Resulting from ALCAPA

A

B

FIGURE 4. Pathophysiology of anomalous origin of the left coronary artery from the pulmonary artery (ALCAPA). From Buxton B, Frazier OH, Westaby S. *Ischemic Heart Disease Surgical Management*. 1999: Mosby International Ltd. A. Sequence of events leading to severe low cardiac output. B. Anatomic changes which occur in the left ventricle as a result of the above.

The preferred surgical option is direct implantation of the anomalous left coronary into the aorta (Fig. 5).[32,33] An alternative approach consists of baffling the left coronary artery ostium within the pulmonary artery to the aorta (Fig. 5).[34] The anomalous left coronary artery may be connected to another systemic artery, or ligated to prevent run-off (least preferred option).

The ischemic time required for most of these repairs exacerbates the compromised preoperative condition and may render some infants unweanable from CPB or cause severe postoperative low cardiac output. Such patients are usually good candidates for centrifugal pump LVAD support, as recovery can be expected within a few days.

The mechanism of recovery appears to be reperfusion of areas of dysfunctional but viable myocardium, as in salvage of "hibernating" myocardium after revascularization of ischemic myocardium in adults. Typically, there will be an early return of myocyte contractile function and augmented β-adrenergic responsiveness during VAD support. Some extracardiac factors implicated in the progression of myocardial dysfunction, such as cytokine-mediated toxicity, unfavorable neurohormonal stimulation, and excessive hemodynamic loading conditions, are undoubtedly ameliorated as well. Because these mechanisms all have the potential to depress contractile function and promote myocyte loss through either ischemia or apoptosis, they also represent potential contributors to contractile improvement during and after VAD support. In ALCAPA patients, recovery of left ventricular function in the long term is very good, and the need for perioperative VAD does not predict a poor late functional status.[30]

We have operated on 21 patients with ALCAPA, ranging in age from 6 weeks to 10 years (median = 9 months). The operative strategy was reimplantation in 7 and the baffling procedure in 12. One patient had ligation of an isolated anomalous left circumflex, and another had an aortocoronary bypass. There were no perioperative deaths, but 5 patients required VAD support for 48 to 96 hours (median = 72). Long-term clinical outcome and left ventricular function have been good, despite severe dysfunction at presentation. At late follow-up (Fig. 6), the VAD patients are virtually indistinguishable from the remainder of the cohort, in terms of ventricular and mitral valve function as well as clinical status.[30]

Transposition of the Great Arteries

Timing is critical for the safe conduct of the arterial switch operation (ASO) for TGA. In babies with TGA and intact ventricular septum, an involution in muscle mass of the left ventricle takes place over the first month of postnatal life, as the pulmonary vascular resistance drops. The consequence is a deconditioned left ventricle that will not function adequately when placed acutely in the systemic circuit after the operation (Fig. 7). Since the early days of the arterial switch experience, it has been appreciated that the risk of operation increases after the second week of life unless left ventricular pressure is maintained at systemic levels by a large ventricular septal defect, a patent ductus, or left ventricular outflow tract obstruction. It has also been appreciated that in postnatal life, myocardial growth is characterized by an early hyperplastic phase of myocyte and capillaries, followed by myocyte hypertrophy. Pressure overload induces hyperplasia, hypertrophy, and angiogenesis in neonates,

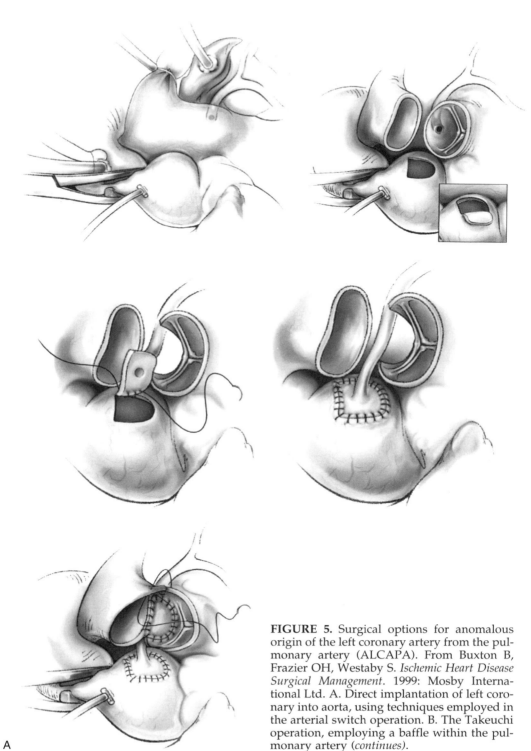

FIGURE 5. Surgical options for anomalous origin of the left coronary artery from the pulmonary artery (ALCAPA). From Buxton B, Frazier OH, Westaby S. *Ischemic Heart Disease Surgical Management.* 1999: Mosby International Ltd. A. Direct implantation of left coronary into aorta, using techniques employed in the arterial switch operation. B. The Takeuchi operation, employing a baffle within the pulmonary artery *(continues).*

A

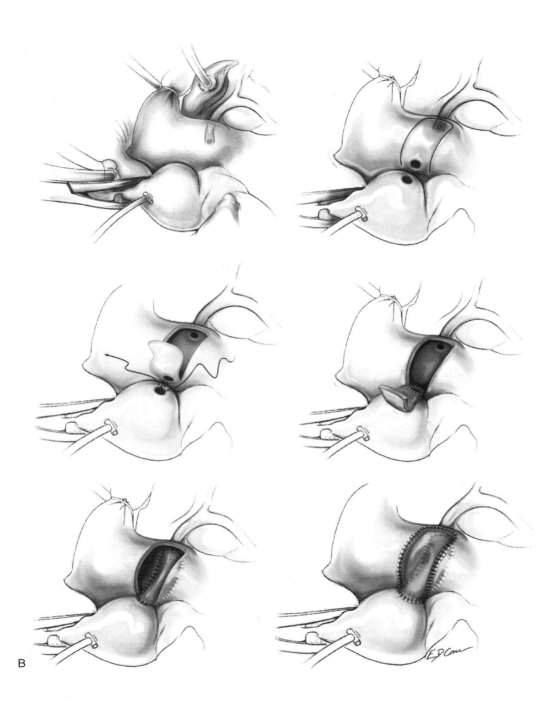

B

Late LV function: radionuclide studies
10 patients examined, 7 during exercise, 3 LVAD survivors

LVEF resting: 66 +/- 9 % (range 50 - 73 %)
       exercise: 76 +/- 8 % (range 66 - 87 %)

LVEF increased normally with exercise
       (mean increase 10%, p = .001)

Wall motion defect was seen in one patient

A   RVEF first pass: 65 +/- 6 % (range 57 - 76 %)

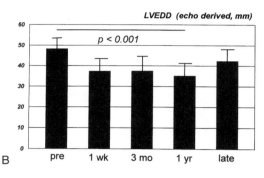

B

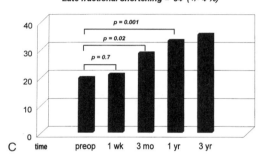

C

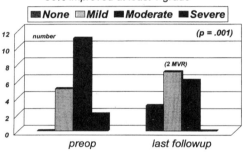

D

FIGURE 6. Outcome for anomalous origin of the left coronary artery from the pulmonary artery (ALCAPA) patients. Of 20 patients available for follow-up (total 147 patient years), 18 are in NYHA Class I and 2 are in Class II. Eight children had Bruce protocol exercise testing, and all scores were in the normal range (= 10th percentile for age). A. Summary of radionuclide studies. B and C. The time course for recovery of left ventricular function by echo measurements and fractional shortening. D. Outline of changes in the degree of mitral regurgitation. The need for VAD could not be predicted with preoperative variables, nor did it influence the late outcome.

but only myocyte hypertrophy later in life. The capacity for and rapidity of left ventricular hypertrophy may therefore decrease with increasing age.

Based on the above information, a two-stage approach has been used in many pediatric units for babies with TGA and intact ventricular septum presenting beyond 2 to 3 weeks of age.[35] A pulmonary artery band is placed and a modified Blalock-Taussig shunt is created to induce left ventricular hypertrophy while maintaining oxygenation. The ASO can usually be performed after a brief period of left ventricular conditioning, typically 2 weeks or less. During this time, left ventricular wall thickness and mass are seen to increase, based on echocardiographic studies. Our practice has been to perform a one-stage ASO for all babies presenting in the first 8 weeks of life, irrespective of left ventricular mass, pressure, or geometry.[36] LVAD support is used selectively as a means of rapid left ventricular conditioning postoperatively, since it is clear that there is potential for a very rapid increase in left ventricular mass in neonates up to this age. This approach is less suitable for older children,

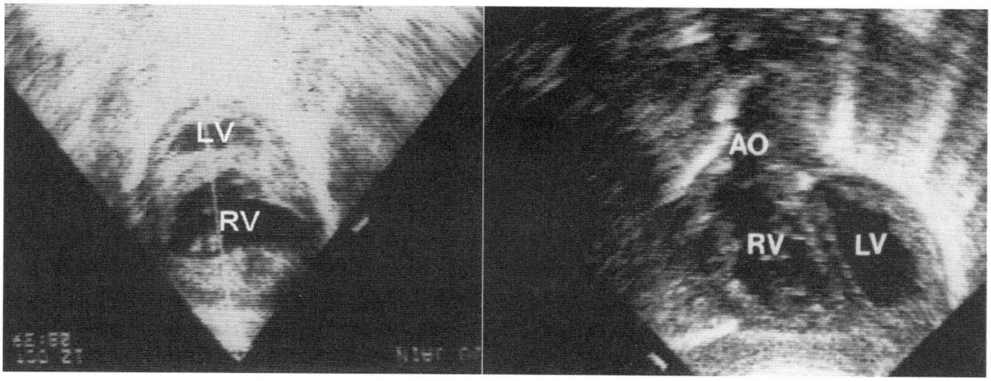

FIGURE 7. Echocardiographic assessment of the left ventricle in transposition of the great arteries with intact septum in a 4-week-old patient. Left: The postnatal drop in pulmonary vascular resistance results in low (pulmonary) pressure in the left ventricle: the interventricular septum bows into the left ventricle due to the high (systemic) pressure in the right ventricle. Right: A more normal geometry in a patient of similar age, but with a systemic left ventricular pressure maintained by the presence of a large ductus arteriosus.

who are likely to require a longer period of left ventricular conditioning than can be safely provided with a centrifugal pump VAD.

Twenty-five children in our unit had a one-stage ASO after 3 weeks of age. Four required postoperative VAD support for rapid left ventricular conditioning. Among the 25, there were two perioperative deaths, one related to a coronary artery technical problem, the other to extracardiac problems of prematurity. For this cohort, the results compare favorably with a two-stage approach, even if VAD should be required.

We have also used VAD support in older patients undergoing double switch (Senning and arterial switch) operations for discordant TGA in the presence of a deconditioned left ventricle, as well as in children with complex TGA whose main cause of left ventricular dysfunction was a poor preoperative condition or a long ischemic time. The favorable results with VAD in arterial switch patients have been obtained in other units as well.[37]

In any patient undergoing the ASO, a technical problem with a coronary anastomosis must be ruled out as the primary cause of left ventricular failure; otherwise, VAD support will not be helpful. Appearance of the heart and electrocardiogram are useful in this regard, but a great deal of judgment is required in deciding whether to use VAD or to revise the original repair, with the possibility of additional ischemic insult.

Donor Heart Dysfunction

In the last decade, the proliferation of cardiac transplant candidates and transplant teams has led to a generalized shortage of donor organs. Likewise, the use of pretransplant mechanical support has increased the urgency in many cases, especially since the outcome in such patients is potentially as good as in those with less advanced cardiac failure. In most centers, the magnitude of the problem increases inversely with the size of the patient. Consequently, the criteria for donor acceptability have been relaxed to the point that many units accept hearts with projected ischemic times greater than 6 hours, or hearts with compromised ventricular function in the donor. Although reversibility of donor dysfunction is predicted in such cases, it may appear in delayed fashion, preventing weaning from CPB. Short-term centrifugal LVAD support is ideal in such cases, especially if pulmonary vascular resistance is low. The problem is greatly compounded in patients with elevated pulmonary vascular resistance. Although post-transplant right ventricular heart dysfunction may improve with nitric oxide therapy and time, it can become critical in the immediate post-transplant period. Right ventricular centrifugal assist (isolated or as biVAD) has been used successfully for right ventricular failure following cardiac transplantation in such cases.

VAD versus ECMO for Children

Clearly, some patients are supportable only with ECMO, due to severe right heart failure, pulmonary problems, or complexity of the cardiac anatomy. However, in many children, even those with complex congenital heart disease, either type of system may be suitable. Previous institutional experience with neonatal ECMO for isolated pulmonary problems will have a strong influence on the choice of support systems, due to availability of equipment and trained personnel. One might consider the following points in decision making regarding centrifugal pump VAD versus ECMO:

- Simplicity: VAD is straightforward in concept and design and requires little technical attention following insertion. Only a few minutes are required to set up and prime the circuit, providing an advantage in the cardiac arrest situation. ECMO is more complex to set up, prime, and debubble. On the other hand, with ECMO, support can be established in some patients with peripheral closed chest cannulation, which is generally not possible with VAD in small children. The potential for complete left ventricular support with ECMO may be limited without the addition of a left ventricular vent, a maneuver which complicates the system considerably.
- Oxygenation: ECMO potentially provides pulmonary as well as cardiac support, although during periods of cardiac ejection the coronaries may be perfused with blood that has a hemoglobin saturation closer to the left atrial level than to that of the oxygenator outlet. Therefore, there is a potential for myocardial ischemia if pulmonary function is severely impaired. The oxygenator itself may contribute to this problem. Patients supported with VADs are totally dependent on the lungs for gas exchange, but pO_2 tends to remain uniform throughout the arterial circulation, barring residual intracardiac shunts at the ventricular level in patients with significant cardiac ejection. If an interatrial communication is present, significant right-to-left shunting (consequent to the low left atrial pressure) can cause uniform and significant arterial desaturation.
- Anticoagulation and blood elements: LVAD support requires little anticoagulation, especially at higher flows. Importantly, protamine may be administered to completely reverse anticoagulation before closure of the chest following intraoperative placement. By comparison, ECMO requires higher levels of anticoagulation, even with a heparin-bonded circuit. Also, the presence of the oxygenator results in more

platelet damage, platelet consumption, and hemolysis, even when the centrifugal pump is used. The data from the pre-Carmeda era in our own institution suggest that there was a lower blood and platelet transfusion requirement for VAD than for ECMO ($P<0.06$). The exact safe level of anticoagulation for either circuit may be difficult to establish, and an approach based on individual patient and circuit factors is required.

Is the Carmeda system likely to improve the results of extracorporeal circulatory support? The Carmeda process involves endpoint covalent bonding of fragmented heparin molecules to the circuit components, including oxygenator, tubing, pump head, cannulas, and all connectors.[38] The bioactive surface binds the polysaccharide containing the active sequence of heparin which is said to provide a uniform degree of thromboresistance. There is a need for continuous movement of blood over the surfaces of the circuit for the heparin-bonding process to be effective. Theoretically, there is a risk of increased thrombogenicity in patients with antithrombin-III deficiency. Carmeda-coated circuits may reduce the heparin requirement for both VAD and ECMO, but in small children the prospects for either type of support without heparin are still poor.[39,40] Accumulating experience in our own unit and elsewhere would suggest that postoperative bleeding is less with the heparin-bonded Carmeda system. Thus, the indications for ECMO and VAD may ultimately be extended to patients with hemorrhage, coagulopathy, respiratory distress syndrome from trauma, etc.[41] We have successfully supported two children with severe intrapulmonary hemorrhage using Carmeda components. This system is obviously attractive for intraoperative conversion of CPB to ECMO or VAD. However, even with a fully bonded circuit and moderate heparin doses, the problem of thrombus formation in the tubing and pump head has not been eliminated.[42]

The heparin-bonded circuit may have the added advantage of improved biocompatibility.[43–45] Recent studies in humans would suggest that serum concentrations of various inflammatory mediators during support are reduced with Carmeda circuits (using low-dose heparin) as compared to non-Carmeda circuits with higher dose heparin. In experimental models, CPB-induced pulmonary injury appears to be less severe with heparin-bonded circuits than with than nonbonded circuits.[45] Carmeda coating reduces complement[46,47] and thrombin activation[47,48] and granular release by neutrophils[48,49] during CPB. The clinical significance of these findings, however, has not been fully demonstrated.

The main disadvantage of commercially available Carmeda oxygenators is that because heparin cannot be bonded to the silicone polymers used in true membranes (eg, Avecor), a hollow fiber oxygenator is required. This latter type of oxygenator is subject to serum leakage with prolonged usage, and therefore is less suitable for long-term support. Whether the improved biocompatibility and decreased lung injury can offset this disadvantage is currently under study. In clinical practice, we have employed Carmeda circuits for up to 8 days, with a median time closer to 48 hours. This is in contrast to the Avecor non-heparin–bonded membrane, which has a median ECMO life of approximately 5 days. Our current ECMO protocol is to use Carmeda circuits for all patients requiring intraoperative or early postoperative support, or for patients who have significant bleeding/coagulopathy for other reasons, or for those who will require surgical procedures on ECMO. Other patients are supported with an Avecor membrane oxygenator. Detailed analysis awaits further clinical experience with these circuits.

Long-Term Support

Neither the centrifugal pump VAD nor the ECMO system is eminently suitable for long-term support in children. The limiting factor for both systems is the development of sepsis. Our longest successful VAD and ECMO supports have been 144 and 120 hours, respectively, although good metabolic support has been provided for up to 428 and 384 hours, respectively, in eventual nonsurvivors. A major limitation has been our inability to wean most patients from ventilator support during centrifugal pump VAD and ECMO, mobilize them, and make them independent of intensive care. The experience compares unfavorably to that in adults, in whom patient extubation and mobilization can often be accomplished with use of a number of devices. Long-term support (>30 days) is possible in the latter group, either by way of recovery or bridge to transplant, and some patients can even be discharged from the hospital prior to (or as an alternative to) transplantation.[17,50] In either case, the rehabilitation and improvement in end organ function can be dramatic. To date, this degree of mobilization has not been possible with small children, even with implantable devices designed for chronic support. We have experience with only three bridge-to-transplant cases to date, although other centers are reporting larger and more favorable experience,[13,51] even for postoperative patients whose initial plan was intracardiac repair. The question of when transplantation is a better option than continued extracorporeal support in a postoperative patient remains an intellectual challenge. At present, the majority of cardiac extracorporeal support in children is performed with a view to myocardial recovery. The usefulness of centrifugal pump VAD and ECMO as a bridge to transplant will depend heavily on the immediate availability of suitable donor hearts, a major problem in many parts of the world.

Cost

In our institution, LVAD support adds $234 per day to the patient's hospital costs, versus $1050 per day for ECMO. We currently employ two nurses per patient during ECMO support, but only one for management of both the VAD system and the patient. In either case, a perfusionist, a cardiac surgeon, and an intensivist are available for assistance in troubleshooting the system and for patient management problems.

Other Support Systems

The future of centrifugal pump VAD might be considered uncertain in light of recent advancements with paracorporeal or totally implantable pulsatile systems. The importance of pulsatile flow has been debated for many years, but the real issue is suitability for safe longer term support. Examples of systems that may be suitable for children, or in some cases infants, include the following: Berlin Heart[17] (see Chapter 21) the MEDOS/HIA assist,[15] the Toyoba and Zeon pumps,[52] the Thoratec VAD (see Chapter 19), the University of Pittsburgh mini centrifugal pump (not yet in clinical use),[53] the Pierce-Donachy pediatric system (not yet in clinical use),[54] the

Jarvik 2000 (see Chapter 26), and others. These devices may play an important role in the establishment of long-term support for recovery or for bridging to transplantation. Also, there are a number of devices available for children above 50 to 60 kg (flow >2.5 to 3l/min), who, from a technical point of view, are considered similar to adults (Table 3). For short-term support; however, the role of these devices remains controversial. The costs involved at the time of this writing for the clinically available systems are substantially greater than those for centrifugal pump VAD, both for the driving system and the disposable equipment required per ventricle per patient. We believe that for most cardiac surgical units, especially those not actively involved with transplantation, the simplicity, availability, cost effectiveness, and good outcome (in selected cases) will ensure the place of centrifugal pump VAD and ECMO in our surgical armamentarium for the foreseeable future.

Table 3

Extracorporeal Devices that Have Been Used Clinically for Pediatric Mechanical Support

Device	Technical Features	Type of Support	Pediatric Application	Availability
IABP[1]	Transfemoral or transaortic insertion	Left heart assist for patients with borderline output who do not have severe LV dysfunction	Limited, due to size constraints. Most effective with M mode echo timing. Short-term assist in older children	Worldwide
Hemopump[2]	Axila flow pump; transaortic valve positioning required; external console, percutaneous drive cable. 14F, 21F, and 24F sizes	Left heart assist; maximal flow 3.5 L/min short-term assist	Limited, due to complex insertion* technique	Europe, research stage in U.S
Centrifugal pump[3]	Constrained vortex pump, completely extracorporeal	Left, right or biVAD; short-term assist	Suitable for patients of all ages and weights	Worldwide
ECMO	Completely extracorporeal	Heart and lung support; may require left heart venting	Suitable for patients of all ages and weights	Worldwide
Berlin Heart and Medos/ HIA Heart assist system	Pneumatic paracorporeal VADs	Pulsatile for left, right, or biVAD.? Long-term assist	Suitable for patients of all ages and weights	Europe

[1] Intra-aortic balloon pump; Datascope, Paramus, NJ; [2] DLP; Medtronic, Grand Rapids, MI; [3] various devices in use.
ECMO = extracorporeal membrane oxygenation LV = left ventricular; biVAD = biventricular assist device.

Acknowledgment Many individuals at the RCH have contributed to the clinical work summarized herein, including Christian P.R. Brizard, Andrew D. Cochrane, Richard J. Mullaly, Clarke A. Thuys, Eve B. O'Connor, Alison Horton, and Roger B.B. Mee.

References

1. Karl TR. Extracorporeal circulatory support in infants and children. *Semin Thorac Cardiovasc Surg* 1994;6:154–160.
2. Butt WW, Karl TR, Horton AM, et al. Experience with extracorporeal membrane oxygenation in children more than one month old. *Anaesth Intensive Care* 1992;20:308–310.
3. Tracy TF Jr, DeLosh T, Bartlett RH. Extracorporeal Life Support Organization 1994. *ASAIO J* 1994;40:1017–1019.
4. Herwig V, Severin M, Waldenberger FR, Konertz W. MEDOS/HIA-assist system: First experiences with mechanical circulatory assist in infants and children. *Int J Artif Organs* 1997;20:692–694.
5. Frazier EA, Faulkner SC, Seib PM, et al. Prolonged extracorporeal life support for bridging to transplant: Technical and mechanical considerations. *Perfusion* 1997;12:93–98.
6. Karl TR, Horton SB, Mee RBB. Left heart assist for ischemic postoperative ventricular dysfunction in an infant with anomalous left coronary artery. *J Card Surg* 1989;4:352–354.
7. Karl TR, Horton SB, Sano S, Mee RBB. Centrifugal pump left heart assist in pediatric cardiac surgery: Indications, technique and results. *J Thorac Cardiovasc Surg* 1991;102:624–630.
8. Cochrane AD, Horton A, Butt W, et al. Neonatal and pediatric extracorporeal membrane oxygenation. *Austral As J Cardiac Thorac Surg* 1992;1:17–22.
9. Karl TR. Circulatory support in children. In Hetzer R, Hennig E, Loebe M (eds): *Mechanical Circulatory Support*. Berlin: Springer; 1997:7–20.
10. Thuys CA, Mullaly RJ, Horton SB, et al. Centrifugal ventricular assist in children under 6 kg. *Eur J Cardio Thorac Surg* 1998;13:130–134.
11. Warnecke H, Berdjis F, Hennig E, et al. Mechanical left ventricular support as a bridge to cardiac transplantation in childhood. *Eur J Cardio Thorac Surg* 1991;5:330–333.
12. Farmer DL, Cullen ML, Philippart AI, et al. Extracorporeal membrane oxygenation as salvage in pediatric surgical emergencies. *J Pediatr Surg* 1995;30:345–348.
13. Del Nido PJ, Armitage JM, Fricker FJ, et al. Extracorporeal membrane oxygenation as a bridge to pediatric heart transplantation. *Circulation* 1994;90: II66-II69.
14. Konertz W, Reul H. Mechanical circulatory support in children. *Int J Artif Organs* 1997; 20:657–658.
15. Ashton RC Jr, Oz MC, Michler RE, et al. Left ventricular assist device options in pediatric patients. *ASAIO J* 1995;41:M277-M280.
16. Konertz W, Hotz H, Schneider M, et al. Clinical expertise with the MEDOS HIA-VAD system in infants and children: A preliminary report. *Ann Thorac Surg* 1997;63:1138–1144.
17. Loebe M, Hennig E, Muller J, et al. Long-term mechanical circulatory support as a bridge to transplantation, for recovery from cardiomyopathy, and for permanent replacement. *Eur J Cardio Thorac Surg* 1997;11:S18-S24.
18. Horton AM, Butt W. Pump-induced hemolysis: Is the constrained vortex pump better or worse than the roller pump? *Perfusion* 1992;7:103–108.
19. Pavie A, Leger P. Physiology of univentricular versus biventricular support. *Ann Thorac Surg* 1996;61:347–349.
20. Costa RJ, Chard RB, Nunn GR, Cartmill TB. Ventricular assist devices in pediatric cardiac surgery. *Ann Thorac Surg* 1995;60:S536-S538.
21. Horton SB, Horton AM, Mullaly RJ, et al. Extracorporeal membrane oxygenation life support: A new approach. *Perfusion* 1993;8:239–247.
22. Hausdorf G, Loebe M. Treatment of low cardiac output syndrome in newborn infants and children. *Zeitschrift fur Kardiologie* 1994;83:91–100.
23. Alexi-Meskishvili V, Weng Y, Uhlemann F, et al. Prolonged open sternotomy after pediatric open heart operation: Experience with 1134 patients. *Ann Thorac Surg* 1995;59:379–383.
24. Karl TR, Iyer KS, Mee RBB. Infant ECMO cannulation technique allowing preservation of carotid and jugular vessels. *Ann Thorac Surg* 1990;50:105–109.

25. Pennington DG, Swartz MT. Circulatory support in infants and children. *Ann Thorac Surg* 1993;55:233–237.
26. Duncan BW, Hraska V, Jonas RA, et al. Mechanical circulatory support in children with cardiac disease. *J Thorac Cardiovasc Surg* 1999;117:529–542.
27. Kanter KR, Pennington DG, Weber TR, et al. Extracorporeal membrane oxygenation for postoperative cardiac support in children. *J Thorac Cardiovasc Surg* 1987;93:27–35.
28. Rogers AJ, Trento A, Siewers R, et al. Extracorporeal membrane oxygenation for postcardiotomy shock in children. *Ann Thorac Surg* 1989;47:903–906.
29. Ziomek S, Harrell JE, Fasules JW, et al. Extracorporeal membrane oxygenation for cardiac failure after congenital heart operation. *Ann Thorac Surg* 1992;54:861–868.
30. Cochrane AD, Coleman DM, Davis AD, et al. Excellent long term functional outcome after surgery for anomalous left coronary artery from the pulmonary artery. *J Thorac Cardiovasc Surg* 1999;117:332–342.
31. Karl TR, Cochrane AD, Brizard CP, et al. Coronary anomalies in children. In Buxton B, Frazier OH, Westaby S (eds): *Surgery for Ischemic Heart Disease: Surgical Management.* London: Mosby; 1997:261–287.
32. Neches WH, Mathews RA, Park SC, et al. Anomalous origin of the left coronary artery from the pulmonary artery. *Circulation* 1974;50:582–587.
33. Laborde F, Marchand M, Leca F, et al. Surgical treatment of anomalous origin of the left coronary artery in infancy and childhood. *J Thorac Cardiovasc Surg* 1981;82:423–428.
34. Takeuchi S, Imamura H, Katsumoto K, et al. New surgical method for repair of anomalous left coronary artery from pulmonary artery. *J Thorac Cardiovasc Surg* 1979;78:7–11.
35. Jonas RA, Giglia TM, Sanders SP, et al. Rapid two-stage arterial switch for transposition of the great arteries and intact ventricular septum beyond the neonatal period. *Circulation* 1989;80:1203–1208.
36. Davis A, Wilkinson JL, Karl TR, Mee RBB. Arterial switch for TGA.IVS after 21 days of life. *J Thorac Cardiovasc Surg* 1993;106:111–115.
37. Macha M, Litwak P, Yamazaki K, et al. In vivo evaluation of an extracorporeal pediatric centrifugal blood pump. *ASAIO J* 1997;43:284–288.
38. Bindslev L, Bohm C, Jolin A, et al. Extracorporeal carbon dioxide removal performed with surface-heparinized equipment in patients with ARDS. *Acta Anaesthesiol Scand* 1991;95: 125–130; discussion 130–131.
39. Muehrcke DD, McCarthy PM, Stewart RW, et al. Extracorporeal membrane oxygenation for postcardiotomy cardiogenic shock. *Ann Thorac Surg* 1996;61:684–691.
40. Schreurs HH, Wijers MJ, Gu YJ. Heparin-coated bypass circuits: Effects on inflammatory response in pediatric cardiac operations. *Ann Thorac Surg* 1998;66:166–171.
41. Rossaint R, Slama K, Lewandowski K, et al. Extracorporeal lung assist with heparin-coated systems. *Int J Artif Organs* 1992;15:29–34.
42. Bianchi JJ, Swartz MT, Raithel SC, et al. Initial clinical experience with centrifugal pumps coated with the Carmeda process. *ASAIO J* 1992;38:143–146.
43. Shigemitsu O, Hadama T, Takasaki H, et al. Biocompatibility of a heparin-bonded membrane oxygenator (Carmeda MAXIMA) during the first 90 minutes of cardiopulmonary bypass: Clinical comparison with the conventional system. *Artif Organs* 1994;18:936–941.
44. Fosse E, Moen O, Johnson E, et al. Reduced complement and granulocyte activation with heparin-coated cardiopulmonary bypass. *Ann Thorac Surg* 1994;58:472–477.
45. Redmond JM, Gillinov AM, Stuart RS, et al. Heparin-coated bypass circuits reduce pulmonary injury. *Ann Thorac Surg* 1993;56:474–478; discussion 479.
46. Mollnes TE, Videm V, Gotze O, et al. Formation of C5a during cardiopulmonary bypass: Inhibition by precoating with heparin. *Ann Thorac Surg* 1991;52(1):92–97.
47. Videm V, Mollnes TE, Garred P, Svennevig JL. Biocompatibility of extracorporeal circulation. In vitro comparison of heparin-coated and uncoated oxygenator circuits. *J Thorac Cardiovasc Surg* 1991;101:654–660.
48. Larsson R, Larm O, Olsson P. The search for thromboresistance using immobilized heparin. Blood in contact with natural and artificial surfaces. *Ann N Y Acad Sci* 1987;516:102–115.
49. Borowiec J, Thelin S, Bagge L, et al. Heparin-coated circuits reduce activation of granulocytes during cardiopulmonary bypass. A clinical study. *J Thorac Cardiovasc Surg* 1992;104: 642–647.
50. Fey O, El-Banayosy A, Arosuglu L, et al. Out-of-hospital experience in patients with im-

plantable mechanical circulatory support: Present and future trends. *Eur J Cardio Thorac Surg* 1997;11:S51-S53.

51. Dalton HJ, Siewers RD, Fuhrman BP, et al. Extracorporeal membrane oxygenation for cardiac rescue in children with severe myocardial dysfunction. *Crit Care Med* 1993;21: 1020–1028.

52. Takano H, Nakatani T. Ventricular assist systems: Experience in Japan with Toyobo pump and Zeon pump. *Ann Thorac Surg* 1996;61:317–322.

53. Litwak P, Butler KC, Thomas DC, et al. Development and initial testing of a pediatric centrifugal blood pump. *Ann Thorac Surg* 1996;61:448–451.

54. Daily BB, Pettitt TW, Sutera SP, Pierce WS. Pierce-Donachy pediatric VAD: Progress in development. *Ann Thorac Surg* 1996;61:437–443.

Chapter 5

Anesthetic Considerations During Left Ventricular Assist Device Implantation

Marc L. Dickstein, MD, Berend Mets, MB, ChB, FRCA, PhD, and Mark J.S. Heath, MD

Introduction

Several features distinguish left ventricular assist device (LVAD) placement from other procedures encountered by the cardiac anesthesiologist. These include the extreme degree of heart failure, the circulatory implications of LVAD therapy, device complications, and the high incidence of post-bypass right ventricular failure and bleeding. The purpose of this chapter is to describe these and other issues that arise during LVAD placement and to discuss a range of scenarios that can be encountered by the anesthesiologist in an active LVAD program.

Pathophysiology of Heart Failure

The cardinal feature of the patient presenting for LVAD implantation is the presence of decompensated heart failure that is refractory to medical management. Unlike the patient with heart failure presenting for other procedures, these patients typically display evidence of rapidly progressing end organ dysfunction and are likely to be hemodynamically fragile or frankly unstable. An understanding of the physiology of severe heart failure is therefore critical to the successful anesthetic management of these patients.

Heart failure is a chronic condition characterized by the physiologic consequences of impaired cardiac contractile function.[1,2] Depressed systolic function is evidenced by the Frank-Starling relationship that is shifted down and to the right, and by ejection fraction that is markedly reduced. The reduction in cardiac output and hence perfusion pressure initiates several compensatory mechanisms that pre-

From Goldstein DJ and Oz MC (eds). *Cardiac Assist Devices*. Armonk, NY: Futura Publishing Co., Inc.; ©2000.

dominantly serve to increase ventricular preload and blood pressure. Sympathetic activity results in increased circulating levels of catecholamines, renin, angiotensin, and vasopressin.[3,4] Ventricular preload is increased by venoconstriction, which redistributes blood volume to central compartments, and by renal fluid retention, which increases intravascular volume. Cardiac output is increased via the Frank-Starling mechanism as well as by increased resting heart rate.

Initially, increased preload stress is sufficient to maintain normal cardiac output; however, severe heart failure is characterized by preload insensitivity, as these hearts are operating on the flat portion of the Frank-Starling curve.[5] In contrast, the failing heart is particularly sensitive to changes in afterload.[6] Moreover, ventricular dilation is frequently associated with annular dilatation and mitral incompetence,[7] and mitral regurgitation amplifies the afterload sensitivity of ventricular function. In other words, as afterload is reduced, cardiac output is enhanced by greater fiber shortening, as well as a smaller regurgitant fraction.

These normal compensatory responses outlined above, however, lead to harmful changes over time.[8] Chronic elevations of circulating catecholamines lead to down-regulation of expression and function of β-adrenoceptors and $α_2$-receptors.[9] As a result, the responsiveness to β-adrenergic agonists is reduced and myocardial catecholamines are depleted.[10] Moreover, chronic elevations in left atrial pressure lead to changes in pulmonary vascular function and the development of increased pulmonary vascular resistance (PVR).[11] The resultant pulmonary hypertension poses a considerable afterload stress to the right ventricle, with the ultimate development of signs of right-sided failure. Hepatic congestion may lead to decreased synthetic function and coagulopathy. Symptoms of congestive heart failure (reduced exercise tolerance, dyspnea, orthopnea), however, are primarily attributable to pulmonary venous congestion.

How does this complex pathophysiology impact the intraoperative management of LVAD patients? The most important implications of congestive heart failure are elevated PVR, impaired right ventricular function, coagulopathy, renal insufficiency, and abnormal responsiveness to catecholamines. These considerations are discussed in the following section, which describes the stages of anesthetic management of LVAD placement.

Pharmacologic Considerations

The anesthesiologist should be aware of the potential for adverse interactions when heart failure patients who are taking angiotensin-converting enzyme (ACE) inhibitors[12] and/or amiodarone (Cordarone, Wyeth-Ayerst Laboratories, Philadelphia, PA)[13] are subjected to surgical stress and anesthesia. These agents are known to inhibit neurohormonal pathways that are crucial to maintaining blood pressure. The former are well known to increase vasoconstrictor requirements during cardiopulmonary bypass (CPB),[14] and Cordarone, a noncompetitive inhibitor of α- and β-receptors, has been associated with fatal vasodilatory shock.[15]

The cardiac failure patient with hepatic and renal impairment may exhibit altered pharmacokinetics of cardioactive drugs. The heart failure state is associated with a decreased volume of distribution and clearance for many drugs, resulting in elevated drug concentrations despite conventional dosing. The altered volume of distribution has been attributed to alterations in perfusion or protein binding, while the changes in drug clearance have been ascribed to impaired hepatic[16] and/or renal metabolism.

Impairment of hepatic drug clearance has been imputed to pathophysiologic mechanisms resulting from decreased perfusion. Reduced cardiac output results in parallel decreases in hepatic blood flow from shunting to more favored end organs, as well as from intrahepatic shunting induced by altered circulating catecholamine levels. Moreover, reduced hepatic perfusion and secondary intrahepatic hypoxia impair the metabolism of microsomal drugs.[17] Similarly, chronic renal hypoperfusions lead to altered drug elimination as a result of decreased glomerular filtration rate and redistribution of renal blood flow.

Preoperative Assessment

The decision to implant an LVAD is usually made because a patient on a heart transplant waiting list has begun the final stage of decompensation and has proven refractory to maximal medical therapy. For this reason, the first question that must be addressed in the perioperative evaluation is "why now?" The common precipitants of end-stage cardiac decompensation include infectious processes such as sepsis and pneumonia and cardiac events such as ischemia and arrhythmias. The degree of hemodynamic instability and respiratory compromise must be assessed with the focus on ensuring an "uneventful" transport to the operating room. Seemingly small details, such as the maintenance of adequate positive end-expiratory pressure during transport of the intubated patient, may mean the difference between routine cannulation versus emergent institution of CPB.

The remaining preoperative evaluation is similar to the evaluation performed for any patient with heart failure. Special attention is required to the airway, vascular access, the potential for ischemia on induction, and end organ involvement. Important points in the clinical history include etiology of heart failure, previous anesthetic experiences, previous cardiac surgery, presence of angina, the ability to lie flat, current medications, and allergies.

On physical examination, baseline cognitive function and presence of neuromuscular impairment are established; additionally, physical examination may reveal jugular venous distention, hepatojugular reflex (reflecting degree of right heart failure), an S3 gallop, and a laterally displaced point of maximal impulse (reflecting left ventricular failure and cardiomegaly). Important heart catheterization data include the transpulmonary gradient, PVR, the pulmonary vascular response to vasodilators (in patients with pulmonary hypertension), cardiac output, valvular function, and left ventricular filling pressure. Serum creatinine and liver function tests, including coagulation profiles, should be obtained to identify patients with impaired renal and liver function. Evaluation of hepatic synthetic capacity is important for gauging the need for perioperative transfusion of blood and coagulation factors. Serum electrolytes are often abnormal as a consequence of either alterations in the renin-angiotensin system or aggressive diuretic therapy. Moderate renal insufficiency is often present, and has an impact on pharmacologic management and the need for postoperative hemofiltration and hemodialysis.

Lining/Induction

The induction of anesthesia may be associated with hemodynamic instability as a result of negative inotropic and/or negative chronotropic actions, the vasodilatory effects of induction agents, the release of resting sympathetic tone, and the transition from spontaneous ventilation to positive pressure ventilation. Patients treated with ACE inhibitors have a higher risk of hypotension upon induction. Moreover, bolus administration of vasoactive agents used to counteract changes in vascular resistance will take considerably longer to have their desired effects, since circulation time is more than doubled in patients with congestive heart failure.[18] In general, induction agents are selected that are relatively devoid of negative inotropic or chronotropic effects. The bradycardia that often accompanies high-dose narcotic inductions may be poorly tolerated, as the increase in diastolic time period would not necessarily increase stroke volume in the failing heart. Even in the absence of inotropic or chronotropic changes, systemic blood pressure may drop as a result of vasodilation caused by release of resting sympathetic tone during the transition from the awake to the anesthetized state. While the concomitant reduction in venous return is usually well tolerated in the failing heart operating on the flat portion of the Starling curve, a reduction in left ventricular preload may be poorly tolerated in patients who have been subjected to aggressive diuretic therapy. Left ventricular preload may also be reduced as a result of the change from spontaneous ventilation to positive pressure ventilation; this increase in right ventricular afterload will decrease right ventricular output and decrease left ventricular filling. Furthermore, if there is a prolonged period of hypoventilation, hypercarbia may exacerbate pulmonary hypertension and further decrease left ventricular filling. For this reason, rapid sequence inductions are avoided despite the fact that many of these patients are considered to have full stomachs. Ventilation while maintaining cricoid pressure allows for a slower induction process than a true "rapid sequence,"[19] hypercarbia may be avoided, and induction agents may be more slowly titrated and their hemodynamic effects accommodated. Finally, unconsciousness must be ensured in these critically ill patients, while cardiac stability is maintained, as it is well recognized that cardiac surgical patients may experience recall after anesthesia.[20] Incorporating an end-tidal Isoflurane (Forane, Baxter Pharmaceuticals, Liberty Corner, NJ) concentration of 0.4% as part of the anesthetic technique may be useful in this regard.[20]

Typically, anesthesia is induced after placement of a large bore intravenous and a radial arterial line. Immediately after induction, a transesophageal echo probe is passed, and the right internal jugular vein is cannulated for placement of a Swan-Ganz catheter. Often, echocardiography is helpful in directing the Swan-Ganz catheter into the right ventricle, especially in patients with dilated right ventricle and significant tricuspid regurgitation. A 9F introducer is recommended, as smaller catheters are inadequate for volume resuscitation. While oximetric pulmonary artery catheters provide important data regarding the adequacy of oxygen delivery, the monitoring of continuous LVAD flows post implant may decrease the utility of continuous pulmonary oximetry. Continuous cardiac output catheters are unnecessary given the availability of continuous on-line LVAD flow. Right ejection fraction catheters (equipped with a rapid-response thermistor), in theory, provide useful physiologic information; however, the accuracy of this technique is questionable and it is therefore of little practical benefit.[21] Often, a second central line is placed and connected to a rapid infuser and used as a dedicated volume infusion line; this is especially important since these patients are at risk for massive hemorrhage.

Separation from CPB

After the completion of the inflow and outflow conduit anastomoses, preparations are made to separate from CPB. The pharmacologic management of these patients is directed toward providing inotropic support and afterload reduction for the right ventricle, and adequate systemic perfusion pressure. The combination of milrinone (Primacor, Sanofi Winthrop Pharmaceuticals, New York, NY) and dobutamine (Dobutrex, Eli Lilly & Company, Indianapolis, IN) provides effective inotropic support and also is effective in reducing PVR.[22] In situations requiring further reductions in PVR, inhaled nitric oxide is likely to be the most effective therapy.[23,24] In contrast to intravenous pulmonary vasodilators, inhaled nitric oxide has the important benefit of limiting pulmonary vasodilation to areas of ventilation, and thus improves V/Q matching and hence PaO_2.[25] Further, avid binding of nitric oxide by hemoglobin permits pulmonary vasodilation without negative inotropic effects or dilation of the systemic vasculature.[26] The expected hemodynamic responses in patients who benefit from this therapy include an increase in LVAD flow and a reduction in central venous pressure; pulmonary artery pressures may remain unchanged even in the presence of a positive response. However, dependency to nitric oxide may occur within hours due to suppression of nitric oxide synthase expression; it is thus important to discontinue therapy in patients who fail to respond. Finally, adequate systemic vascular tone may be achieved by the combination of norepinephrine (Levophed, Sanofi Winthrop Pharmaceuticals) and vasopressin (Pitressin, Parke-Davis, Morris Plains, NJ) infusions (for a full discussion of this agent, see Chapter 9). This combination, as compared to Levophed alone, increases renal perfusion and decreases PVR.[27]

Prior to separation from CPB, the presence of a patent foramen ovule (PFO), aortic insufficiency, and left ventricular decompression should be assessed (see Transesophageal Echocardiography [TEE] section below). Presence of a PFO should be identified prior to protamine administration in order to avert reheparinization. If present, the PFO can be repaired by inserting the right atrial venous cannula down the inferior vena cava and using the pump sucker to drain the superior vena cava. This approach preserves the vena cavae for bicaval cannulation during subsequent heart transplantation. Aortic insufficiency may be identified by color flow Doppler; if present, the magnitude of the recirculation may be appreciated by the discrepancy between LVAD flow and thermodilution cardiac output. The adequacy of left ventricular decompression must be frequently verified, as the lack of left ventricular decompression suggests a mechanical problem with either the LVAD inflow conduit (eg, malposition or graft kinking) or the device itself.

Right ventricular failure is a common and incompletely understood complication of LVAD implantation (see Chapter 7).[28] The cardinal features are low LVAD flows in the setting of elevated central venous pressure and a decompressed left ventricle. A sudden decompensation shortly after separation from CPB is likely to be the result of intracoronary air emboli. Corroborative signs include a sudden loss of rhythm, ST elevations, and the presence of air on TEE exam. The treatment strategy is to maintain a high coronary perfusion pressure while resting the heart on CPB. Another cause of right ventricular failure may be impaired contractile function. It is widely thought that the inflammatory responses to CPB, major surgery, and massive blood product infusion can produce negative inotropic effects on the right ventricle. Even in the absence of depressed myocyte function, right ventricular pump function may also be impaired by ventricular interactions. Since the two ventricles share a common wall, it is not altogether surprising that the emptying of the left ventricle by the LVAD has an impact on right ventricular performance; in fact, the direct ventricular interactions are more prominent in the dilated[29] and the failing heart (ventricular interactions are reviewed in detail in Chapter 2).[30]

Right ventricular failure may also be due to increased afterload. Two important determinants of right ventricular afterload are PVR and left atrial pressure. PVR may be elevated due to a variety of factors, most notably hypoxia, hypercarbia, elevated airway pressure, acidosis, inflammatory agents, and the effects of massive blood product transfusion.[31] PVR may be acutely elevated, thus negating the beneficial effects of the reduction in left atrial pressures achieved by the LVAD. Because of its thin wall, the normal right ventricle is highly sensitive to increases in its afterload; the failing right ventricle exhibits even more afterload sensitivity. For this reason, nitric oxide therapy may be highly efficacious in restoring adequate right ventricular output and avoiding the need for right ventricular mechanical assistance (RVAD).

In addition to right ventricular failure, a major concern of the anesthesiologist during LVAD placement is the potential for severe hemorrhage. Owing to the extent of the surgery and to the common presence of preoperative hepatic dysfunction and malnutrition, bleeding complications are prevalent. In the majority of patients, platelets and fresh frozen plasma transfusions are required to restore coagulation; it is important to aggressively infuse products soon after bypass to prevent dilutional coagulopathy. The magnitude of surgical dissection (both intrathoracic and abdominal), and the large amount of blood products and other fluids administered, place the patient at risk for hypothermia and its inherent complications. Adequate fluid warming equipment is required, and it is often helpful to have a dedicated central line for rapid administration of volume. LVAD recipients have a high rate of reexploration for bleeding, and are sometimes brought to the intensive care unit (ICU) with the chest open. We routinely employ the antifibrinolytic and platelet preserving agent aprotinin (Trasylol, Bayer Corporation, West Haven, CT) from the time immediately prior to CPB until bleeding has subsided in the ICU.[31]

Intraoperative arrhythmias are common following LVAD placement, and their hemodynamic effects are dependent on the effect on PVR (see Chapter 8). LVAD flow is entirely dependent on the output of the right heart, which is in turn a function of right ventricular function and right ventricular afterload. In the setting of normal PVR and decompressed left atrium, a moderate central venous pressure is sufficient to generate adequate blood flow through the lungs without any contribution from the right ventricle. As a result, some LVAD patients may tolerate severe arrhythmias, including ventricular fibrillation, without significant hemodynamic instability. However, LVAD recipients with high PVR are dependent on the right ventricle to drive blood through the pulmonary circulation, and even a slight rhythm abnormality may significantly impair right ventricular function and thus LVAD flow. Atrial fibrillation, junctional rhythm, and ventricular ectopy are common arrhythmias that may, in the pulmonary hypertensive patient, be very poorly tolerated.[32] Placement of atrioventricular sequential pacing wires can be highly valuable in these patients, and careful attention to pacemaker programming can lead to rewarding increases in right ventricular performance and LVAD flow.

Transesophageal Echocardiography

There are several aspects of the TEE exam that are particularly important before, during, and immediately after LVAD implantation.

Pre-Bypass

The competence of the aortic valve must be assessed in the pre-bypass period. Since regurgitant flow across the aortic valve causes recirculation through the LVAD (Fig. 1) (device to outflow cannula, retrograde into the left ventricle, back into the device via the inflow cannula), the incompetent aortic valve must be either replaced or oversewn. In view of the significant incidence of post-implantation right ventricular failure, it is important to evaluate the baseline right ventricular size, wall motion, and tricuspid valve function. Additionally, since dilated cardiomyopathy predisposes to left atrial and ventricular mural thrombi, their presence and mobility should also be assessed so they can, if necessary, be removed.

The presence of intracardiac shunts such as PFO should be investigated by a bubble study (agitated blood or saline injected into the right atrium) (Fig. 2). In these patients, left atrial pressure usually exceeds right atrial pressure throughout the entire cardiac cycle; hence, a PFO would not be evident under normal conditions. An important maneuver to reverse the atrial transseptal gradient is the sudden release of sustained airway pressure. This maneuver increases airway pressures and decreases blood flow across the lungs, thus reducing left atrial pressure; release of sustained

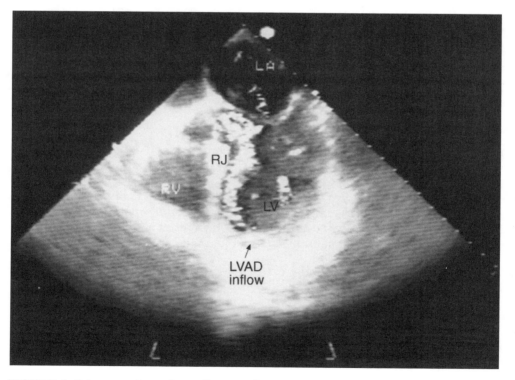

FIGURE 1. Intraoperative echocardiogram demonstrating significant aortic regurgitation with the left ventricular assist device (LVAD) in place. Thermodilution cardiac output was 2.3 L/min and the measured LVAD flow was 4.0 L/min after separation from cardiopulmonary bypass. Mild mitral regurgitation into the left atrium is also noted. LA = left atrium; LV = left ventricle; RJ = regurgitant jet; RV = right ventricle.

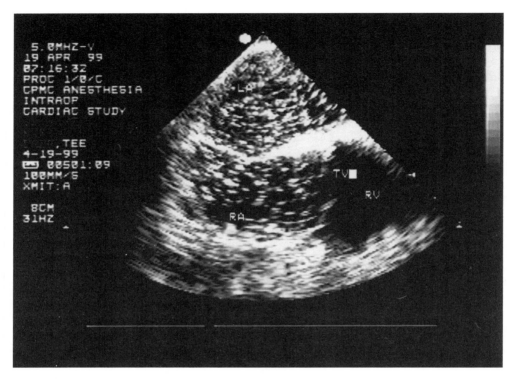

FIGURE 2. Intraoperative echocardiogram demonstrating the presence of a patent foramen ovale when a "bubble test" was performed. Echodense shadows from agitated saline injection into the right atrium are seen in the left atrium. LA = left atrium; RA = right atrium; RV = right ventricle; TV = tricuspid valve.

intrathoracic pressure also allows the sudden return of blood to the right atrium and further shifts the transseptal gradient. However, it is important to appreciate that the left atrial decompression associated with LVAD operation coupled with the often elevated right atrial pressures causes considerable bowing of the intra-atrial septum to the left; therefore, a PFO may not be demonstrable until separation from bypass. Failure to recognize and repair even a small PFO can result in drastic arterial desaturation owing to right-to-left shunting across the undiagnosed PFO.[33,34]

During Bypass

TEE can be used to assure that the apical inflow cannula of the LVAD is appropriately directed away from the intraventricular septum (to avoid inlet occlusion) and toward the mitral valve. It can also confirm that the selected cannula position allows complete left ventricular decompression.[35] Additionally, the TEE is extremely useful for determining the adequacy of chamber de-airing. This is of critical importance at the end of the bypass period, when filling and ejection of the LVAD often result in air entering the aortic root, coronary arteries, and systemic circulation. The right coronary circulation is particularly prone to air embolism because bubbles rise toward the right coronary ostium, leading to arrhythmias and right ventricular failure. Air tends to collect in the left ventricular apex, along the interventricular septum, and in the pulmonary veins; the device is also a major source of air bubbles. Because the anastomoses of the outflow conduit to the ascending aorta may be difficult to visualize with the TEE, it is useful to gauge the severity of intravascular air by interrogating the descending aorta.

Post Bypass

Upon weaning from CPB, the TEE becomes a key monitor of right ventricular function and tricuspid valve competence. Absence of significant aortic regurgitation (<2 L/min) and adequate left-sided chamber decompression must be reconfirmed. Left ventricular collapse and LVAD inlet occlusion can lead to subatmospheric pressure within the device, resulting in entry of air through otherwise airtight suture lines and graft interstices. Subsequent catastrophic air embolism may ensue.[36] Lastly, continuous wave Doppler and knowledge of outflow cannula dimensions can be used to derive an independent measure of LVAD flow.[36]

Management in the ICU

The ICU management of the LVAD recipient in many regards represents a continuation of the intraoperative care. Initially, the major problem is likely to be hemorrhage, and large amounts of blood products may be required. Coagulation studies, including activated clotting time, Hepcon, prothrombin time, partial thromboplastin time, fibrinogen, and ionized calcium, should be performed at frequent intervals to guide therapy. Trasylol infusion should be continued while bleeding persists, and normothermia should be maintained. In some instances the coagulopathy may be a result of a poorly understood response to the internal surface of the device, resulting in delayed bleeding.

As is the case in the operating room, LVAD flow is a key indicator of overall status, and the LVAD console/display should be situated where it can be easily monitored. Low LVAD flows can be corroborated by thermodilution cardiac output and mixed venous oxygenation measurement. Occasionally, a patient will display signs of hypoperfusion (such as low blood pressure, low urine output, low mixed venous pO_2) in spite of robust flows as reported by the LVAD monitor. In this setting it is important to perform an independent measurement of cardiac output (eg, by thermodilution) to rule out the possibility of recirculation through an incompetent aortic valve. Alternatively, color flow Doppler during TEE exam may be used to directly assess the competence of the aortic valve.

Hypovolemia (usually associated with hemorrhage) and right ventricular dysfunction remain the principal causes of low LVAD flow. As in the operating room, improvement of right ventricular performance may require volume, increased inotropic support, or reduction of PVR. Again, the combination of Primacor and Dobutrex for inotropy, and Pitressin and Levophed for support of systemic vascular resistance, is highly effective for supporting LVAD circulation. It is critical to maintain sufficient aortic pressure to adequately perfuse the right coronary artery. Nitric oxide is used if necessary, but should be weaned as soon as possible. In general, it is preferable to wean nitric oxide prior to inotropic support, thus accelerating extubation. When weaning nitric oxide, the parameters to monitor are LVAD flow and central venous pressure; transient shifts in other parameters are unlikely to cause problems.

Relative hypoxemia is frequently encountered postoperatively; adult respiratory distress syndrome and pulmonary edema, associated with the administration of large amounts of blood products, are common culprits. It may be prudent to repeat interrogation for a PFO, as increasing positive end-expiratory pressure will exacerbate shunt flow and paradoxically worsen hypoxemia. Otherwise, continuous venovenous hemofiltration may be useful for accelerating fluid removal and thus reducing the time to extubation.

If the major hurdles of right ventricular failure and hemorrhage can be avoided, it is often possible to extubate the LVAD recipient within 24 hours. Patients with more prolonged courses are likely to require intravenous sedation; this can be accomplished with infusions of agents such as propofol (Diprivan, Zeneca Pharmaceuticals, Wilmington, DE), midazolam (Versed, Roche Laboratories, Nutley, NJ), and fentanyl (Sublimaze, Elkins-Sinn Inc., Cherry Hill, NJ). Muscle relaxation with nondepolarizing agents should be avoided, as the prolonged ICU course and severity of illness places these patients at risk for critical illness polyneuropathy/myopathy.[37] This poorly understood entity, characterized by peripheral motor axon conduction deficits and muscle atrophy, has been associated with steroid administration, nondepolarizing muscle relaxants, prolonged immobility, sepsis, and multiple organ failure.[38] The diagnosis is usually suggested when a patient is hemodynamically robust but is unable to be weaned from respiratory support.

Summary

The complexities of end-stage heart failure and assisted circulation render LVAD implantation one of the most challenging procedures encountered by the adult cardiac anesthesiologist. At this point, much of what has been learned about these procedures is in the form of anecdotal experience and extrapolation from other types of cases. The completion of scientific studies and well designed outcome trials should provide further insight and guidance for the successful perioperative anesthetic care of LVAD implantation.

References

1. Braunwald E. Pathophysiology of heart failure. In Braunwald E (ed): *Heart Disease: A Textbook of Cardiovascular Medicine*. Philadelphia: W.B. Saunders Co.; 1992:393–418.
2. Kapoor AS, Laks H, Schroeder JS, Magdi Y. *Cardiomyopathies and Heart-Lung Transplantation*, ed 1. New York: McGraw-Hill, Inc.; 1991:511.
3. Francis GS, Goldsmith SR, Levine TB, et al. The neurohumoral axis in congestive heart failure. *Ann Intern Med* 1984;101:370–377.
4. Levine TB, Francis GS, Goldsmith SR, et al. Activity of the sympathetic nervous system and renin-angiotensin system assessed by plasma hormone levels and their relation to hemodynamic abnormalities in congestive heart failure. *Am J Cardiol* 1982;49:1659–1666.

5. Stevenson LW, Tillish JH. Maintenance of cardiac output with normal filling pressure in patients with dilated heart failure. *Circulation* 1986;74:1303–1308.
6. Levine TB. Role of vasodilators in the treatment of congestive heart failure. *Am J Cardiol* 1985;55:32A-35A.
7. Kono T, Sabbah HN, Stein PD, et al. Left ventricular shape as a determinant of functional mitral regurgitation in patients with severe heart failure secondary to either coronary artery disease or idiopathic dilated cardiomyopathy. *Am J Cardiol* 1991;68:355–359.
8. Packer M. Role of the sympathetic nervous system in chronic heart failure: A historical and philosophical perspective. *Circulation* 1990;82:11–16.
9. Spinale FG, Tempel GE, Mukherjee R, et al. Cellular and molecular alterations in beta-adrenergic system with cardiomyopathy induced by tachycardia. *Cardiovasc Res* 1994;28: 1243–1250.
10. Bristow M, Hershberger R, Port J, et al. Beta 1- and beta 2-adrenergic receptor-mediated adenylate cyclase stimulation in nonfailing and failing human ventricular myocardium. *Mol Pharmacol* 1989;35:295–303.
11. Kawaguchi A, Gandjbakhch I, Pavie A, et al. Cardiac transplant recipients with preoperative pulmonary hypertension: Evolution of pulmonary hemodynamics and surgical options. *Circulation* 1989;80:III90-III96.
12. Colson P, Saussine M, Seguin JR, et al. Hemodynamic effects of anesthesia in patients chronically treated with angiotensin-converting enzyme inhibitors. *Anesth Analg* 1992;74: 805–808.
13. Perkins M, Dasta J, Reilly T, Halpern P. Intraoperative complications of anesthesia in patients receiving amiodarone: Characteristics and risk factors. *DICP* 1989;23:757–763.
14. Tuman K, McCarthy R, O'Connor C. Angiotensin-converting enzyme inhibitors increase vasoconstrictor requirements after cardiopulmonary bypass. *Anesth Analg* 1995;80: 473–479.
15. Dyck MV, Baele P, Rennotte M, et al. Should amiodarone be discontinued before cardiac surgery? *Acta Anesthesiol Belg* 1988;39:3–10.
16. Wilkinson G. Pharmacokinetics of drug disposition: Hemodynamic considerations. *Ann Rev Pharmacol* 1975;15:11–27.
17. Mets B, Hickman R, Allin R, et al. Effect of hypoxia on the hepatic metabolism of lidocaine in the isolated perfused pig liver. *Hepatology* 1993;19:668–676.
18. Campione KM. Heart to head circulation time. *Illinois Med J* 1972;141:75–77.
19. Waterman PM. Rapid sequence induction technique in patients with severe ventricular dysfunction. *J Cardiothorac Anesth* 1988;2:602–606.
20. Ghoneim MM, Block RI. Learning and memory during general anesthesia: An update. *Anesthesiology* 1997;87:387–410.
21. Starling RC, Binkley PF, Haas GJ, et al. Thermodilution measures of right ventricular ejection fraction and volumes in heart transplant recipients: A comparison with radionuclide angiography. *J Heart Lung Transplant* 1992;11:1140–1146.
22. Chen EP, Bittner HB, Davis RDJ, Van Trigt PR. Milrinone improves pulmonary hemodynamics and right ventricular function in chronic pulmonary hypertension. *Ann Thorac Surg* 1997;63:814–821.
23. Fratacci MD, Frostell C, Chen TY, et al. Inhaled nitric oxide: A selective pulmonary vasodilator reversing hypoxic pulmonary vasoconstriction. *Circulation* 1991;83:2038–2047.
24. Argenziano M, Choudhri AF, Moazami N, et al. Randomized, double-blind trial of inhaled nitric oxide in LVAD recipients with pulmonary hypertension. *Ann Thorac Surg* 1998;65: 340–345.
25. Putensen C, Rasanen J, Lopez FA. Improvement in VA/Q distributions during inhalation of nitric oxide in pigs with methacholine-induced bronchoconstriction. *Am J Respir Crit Care Med* 1995;151:116–122.
26. Semigran MJ, Cockrill BA, Kacmarek R, et al. Hemodynamic effects of inhaled nitric oxide in heart failure. *J Am Coll Cardiol* 1994;24:982–988.
27. Shipley JB, Tolman D, Hastillo A, Hess ML. Milrinone: Basic and clinical pharmacology and acute and chronic management. *J Med Sci* 1996;311:286–291.
28. Frazier OH, Rose EA, Macmanus Q, et al. Multicenter clinical evaluation of the HeartMate 1000 IP left ventricular assist device. *Ann Thorac Surg* 1992;53:1080–1090.
29. Dickstein ML, Todaka K, Burkhoff D. Left-to-right systolic and diastolic ventricular interactions are dependent on right ventricular volume. *Am J Physiol* 1997;272:H2869-H2874.

30. Chow E, Farrar DJ. Right heart function during prosthetic left ventricular assistance in a porcine model of congestive heart failure. *J Thorac Cardiovasc Surg* 1992;104:569–578.
31. Goldstein DJ, Seldomridge JA, Chen JM, et al. Use of aprotinin in LVAD recipients reduces blood loss, blood use, and perioperative mortality. *Ann Thorac Surg* 1995;59:1063–1067.
32. Moroney DA, Swartz MT, Reedy JE, et al. Importance of ventricular arrhythmias in recovery patients with ventricular assist devices. *ASAIO Trans* 1991;37:M516-M517.
33. Shapiro GC, Leibowitz DW, Oz MC, et al. Diagnosis of patent foramen ovale with transesophageal echocardiography in a patient with a left ventricular assist device. *J Heart Lung Transplant* 1995;14:549–552.
34. Baldwin RT, Duncan JM, Frazier OH, Wilansky S. Patent foramen ovale: A cause of hypoxemia in patients on left ventricular support. *Ann Thorac Surg* 1991;52:865–867.
35. Hauptman PJ, Body S, Fox J, et al. Implantation of a pulsatile external left ventricular assist device: Role of intraoperative transesophageal echocardiography. *Am Heart J* 1992;124:793–794.
36. George S, Black J, Boscoe M. Intraoperative transesophageal echocardiography for implantation of a pulsatile left ventricular assist device. *Br J Anesth* 1995;75:794–797.
37. Thiele RI, Jakob H, Hund E, et al. Critical illness polyneuropathy: A new iatrogenically induced syndrome after cardiac surgery. *Eur J Cardiothorac Surg* 1997;12:826–835.
38. Nauwynck M, Huyghens L. Neurological complications in critically ill patients: Septic encephalopathy, critical illness polyneuropathy. *Acta Clin Belgica* 1998;53:92–97.

Chapter 6

Perioperative Management of Bleeding

Clifford H. Van Meter, Jr., MD

Introduction

The management of perioperative bleeding in ventricular assist device (VAD) recipients is one of the keys to operative survival and ultimate success of this technology. An understanding of the patient-related and device-related factors associated with this complication are essential to its management. While there are obvious initial consequences and complications caused by perioperative bleeding, the long-term repercussions are frequently underappreciated. In this chapter, a broad overview of this subject is presented and suggestions are offered for the management of perioperative hemorrhage, the most common source of early morbidity and mortality among VAD recipients.

Incidence and Predisposing Factors

Whether assist devices are used for postcardiotomy support[1] or as a bridge to transplant,[2,3] the incidence of perioperative bleeding following their insertion is significant and has historically ranged from greater than 50% in some of the earlier experiences to a current level of 15% to 35% in more recent reports.[4–8] Most combined registry data report a higher rate of bleeding in the postcardiotomy cohort than in those patients undergoing VAD insertion as a bridge to transplant.[4,5,9]

The factors that predispose to this complication are both related to the characteristics of the patient population and to the devices themselves (Table 1). It is well recognized that patients with prolonged heart failure have a variety of manifestations of this disease that directly contribute to the problem. Chronic passive congestion of the liver frequently leads to the loss of coagulation factor-dependent synthetic function. This defect is compounded by the frequent use of antibiotics and the presence of malnutrition in this patient population. Many patients have had prolonged

From Goldstein DJ and Oz MC (eds). *Cardiac Assist Devices.* Armonk, NY: Futura Publishing Co., Inc.; ©2000.

Table 1

Factors Predisposing to Postoperative Bleeding
Following LVAD Implantation

Prolonged heart failure
Passive hepatic congestion with loss of synthetic function
Prolonged or intermittent exposure to heparin
Platelet dysfunction or depletion (dilutional, drug-induced)
Chronic anemia
Previous surgery
Large nonendothelial blood-contacting surface
Extensive nature of LVAD implant surgery
Perioperative hypothermia

LVAD = left ventricular assist device.

and/or intermittent exposure to heparin, and platelet depletion and dysfunction are often present. Due to chronic illness and repeated laboratory testing, these patients are frequently anemic. Many patients have had previous surgery or, if receiving devices for postcardiotomy support, have already undergone extensive and prolonged procedures. Finally, the significant hematologic and immunologic derangements consequent to exposure to a large nonendothelial blood contacting surface continue to be evaluated and are yet to be fully understood. Studies have indicated that VAD systems strongly activate the coagulation, thrombolytic, and inflammatory systems.[10–12] Additionally, the decrease in physiologic coagulation inhibitors, especially protein C, implies that the device surfaces are activating and consuming these factors. Monocyte stimulation results in a release of inflammatory cytokines such as interleukin-8 (IL-8) and macrophage inflammatory protein-1α (MIP-1α), particularly when silicone is involved. Significant alterations in platelet morphology and function are induced due to the surface activation by these implanted devices.[11,13,14] Both silicone and polyurethane stimulate thrombocytes, resulting in the release of P-selectin and platelet-derived growth factors. Thus, the combination of predisposing factors and the impact of the extensive foreign blood contacting surface combine to create a milieu conducive to the development of a bleeding diathesis.

Consequences

Perioperative bleeding results in both short- and long-term sequelae. Perhaps the most overwhelming early consequence may be right heart failure. In almost every series reported, the incidence of perioperative bleeding is higher in patients supported with biventricular support than with univentricular support. While it has not been proven that extensive bleeding and transfusion requirements cause and/or contribute to the need for right heart support, the association between bleeding, blood use, and right heart failure is strong. Several mechanisms have been proposed to explain this observed clinical phenomenon. The most popular theory implicates an activated cytokine milieu. Indeed, the proinflammatory and immunoregulatory cytokine activity induced by hemorrhage and resuscitation clearly result in acute pulmonary injury.[15] The resultant exacerbation of frequently coexisting pulmonary hypertension and the hemodynamic and immunologic consequences of blood product transfusions can create an environment that is ripe for post-bypass right heart failure. The incidence of right heart failure following LVAD support has even been found to correlate with the type and amount of blood products required in the postoperative period.[16]

The consequences of right heart failure necessitating mechanical right heart support cannot be underemphasized. Many investigators believe that patients who require right ventricular support after left ventricular device implant have a poorer outcome than those who require initial biventricular support for biventricular failure diagnosed and anticipated preoperatively. In addition, patients who required subsequent right ventricular support for right heart failure were reported to have a markedly diminished survival to transplant compared to those requiring only left ventricular support without subsequent deterioration of right heart function.[7] Obviously, the need for reexploration for bleeding leads to additional technical complications of patient transportation and management as well as to an increased risk for infectious complications.

Additional long-term complications of perioperative bleeding include alterations in pulmonary function, including an adult respiratory distress-like syndrome. This may have an unfavorable impact on a patient's suitability for transplantation and on his or her post-transplant survival and functional capabilities. Repeated transfusions can lead to altered cytomegalovirus states and have led many investigators to use leukocyte depletion systems for autologous blood transfusions.

Finally, the amount and components of blood product transfusions have been correlated with an increased incidence of fungal infection and elevated panel reactive antibodies in device-supported patients. These factors can affect the duration and complication-free interval of device support and may affect the patient's chances for transplantation.

Management

Hemodynamics

The highest incidence of perioperative bleeding and need for right heart support has been correlated with compromised preoperative hemodynamic indices. Preoperative optimization of cardiac index and particularly right heart pressures is essential to avoid hemodilution and right heart volume overload, which can increase the probability of coagulopathy and lead to persistent venous bleeding in the early postoperative period. Optimization of fluid status preoperatively may necessitate the occasional use of continuous venovenous hemofiltration (CVVH) for removal of excess free water, minimization of hemodilution, and optimization of the patient's ability to tolerate needed perioperative component transfusion therapy.

Hematologic

The replenishment of diminished clotting factors in the immediate preoperative period can reduce the impact of the intraoperative coagulopathy and the requirement for massive product administration in the immediate postoperative period when other factors present are contributing to pulmonary and right heart dysfunction. Such adjuncts as intraoperative thromboelastography can be used to monitor factor depletion, platelet function, and platelet inactivation intraoperatively to anticipate immediate postoperative needs.

Humoral-Pharmacologic

Perhaps the most significant measure to reduce the perioperative complication of bleeding has been the introduction and use of aprotinin (Trasylol, Bayer Corporation, West Haven, CT). Trasylol is a serine protease inhibitor with antifibrinolytic and platelet-preserving properties. In addition, it has been found to reduce the inflammatory milieu associated with extracorporeal circulation by inhibiting neutrophil elastase. Use of Trasylol in patients undergoing conventional cardiac surgery has resulted in a dramatic reduction in blood loss and blood use.[17,18] Recent reports have indicated a decrease of as much as 60% in postoperative bleeding, as well as a 75% reduction in component transfusion requirements in patients in whom Trasylol is used as an adjunctive therapy during the insertion of ventricular assistance devices.[19,20] This has correlated with a decreased incidence of the requirement of right ventricular assistance in patients who were treated with Trasylol.[21] Concerns of anaphylaxis have been raised but they are extremely rare.[22,23] Repeated exposure, however, can increase this risk to 1% to 5%.[24] A recent experience with patients receiving repeat administration of Trasylol for staged cardiac transplantation (ie, LVAD implantation followed by cardiac transplantation) demonstrated a 4.8% incidence of anaphylaxis requiring emergent institution of cardiopulmonary bypass (CPB).[25] It appears that the potential for an anaphylactic response with subsequent exposure is increased by proximity to the initial treatment (6 to 9 months or less). Because of the ever present potential for these unpredictable anaphylactic reactions, some surgeons have abandoned the use of Trasylol during LVAD implantation, reserving its use for the reoperative cardiac transplant procedure. Others have modified their intraoperative administration by withholding the Trasylol loading dose during secondary exposure until the surgeons are ready to cannulate and institute CPB.[25] In theory, the use of other antifibrinolytic agents such as epsilon-aminocaproic acid (Amicar, Immunex Corporation, Seattle, WA) may augment the hemostatic actions associated with Trasylol use.

Avoidance of right heart dysfunction and especially elevated central venous pressures is helpful for avoiding the continuous venous bleeding that may be present postoperatively, especially in patients undergoing repeat surgical procedures. The use of nitric oxide to reduce pulmonary hypertension, the addition of vasopressin to maintain perfusion pressure while sparing conventional vasoconstrictor use, and the use of humoral therapies such as thyroid hormone to augment the function of depleted myocardium may aid in sustaining right heart function and avoiding the series of events leading to this complication.

Technical Aspects

Adjuncts to the CPB system may be helpful in reducing some of the previously discussed consequences of these procedures. Active hemofiltration to minimize hemodilution and remove excess free water from the chronically congested patient is often warranted. Additionally, leukocyte depletion systems in the CPB as well as cardioplegia administration systems have been shown to decrease the inflammatory response and consequent lung injury. Because of the well described effects of hypothermia on coagulation, efforts are made to administer warm intravenous fluids and to use surface warming devices.

Coagulation can be augmented by the use of substances such as topical Trasylol[26] and synthetic or autologous fibrin glues. Argon beam coagulation can be helpful for controlling the bleeding encountered in patients undergoing repeat operations. Buttressing of suture lines and purse-strings with felt, autologous pericardium, or porcine-derived pericardial substitutes can be helpful to secure suture lines and/or cannula purse-strings. Many surgeons have used low-porosity collagen-impregnated graft conduits as a substitute or to reinforce more porous grafts or conduits to minimize their potential for postoperative bleeding and extravasation. Most studies have indicated that sternal closure correlates with the reduced incidence of reexploration for bleeding. The use of heparin-coated extracorporeal circuits has resulted in a reduction of proinflammatory cytokine activation and, hence, represents an attractive option meriting further study.

Postoperative Management

Patients must be closely monitored for reperfusion acidosis. Many have been in an extended compensated state and, having undergone prolonged procedures, are often prone to reperfusion acidosis, which can lead to acute right heart dysfunction and predilection for bleeding. While the use of cell-savers is a helpful adjunct to component replacement, autotransfusion should be avoided due to the potential for induction or worsening of a proinflammatory and coagulopathic state. Many patients will experience reduced renal function in the immediate postoperative period. This has been variably attributed to preoperative low output state and concomitant use of nephrotoxic antibiotics, vasoconstrictors, and antifibrinolytic agents. The use of CVVH has revolutionized the management of these fluid-overloaded patients who often do not respond to conventional diuretic treatment. CVVH allows removal of excess fluid with little hemodynamic promise, thereby facilitating the required transfusion of components for correction of postoperative coagulopathies. Moreover, CVVH can be used for hemodialysis in anuric patients.

Most short-term devices and some long-term LVADs require the early institution of anticoagulant therapy to prevent disastrous thromboembolic events. An interval of time should be allowed for resolution of perioperative coagulopathy and decrease in postoperative mediastinal chest tube drainage before initiation of anticoagulation therapy. Many suggest the supplementation of low molecular weight dextran during an interval of at least 6 to 8 hours to allow diminution of mediastinal drainage prior to institution of heparin therapy.

Summary

Historically, the incidence of postoperative bleeding following the insertion of cardiac assist devices has been unacceptably high and has led to a spectrum of both short- and long-term consequences that have been frequently underappreciated. The predisposing factors for this are related to both the patient population and the nature of the devices and the procedure itself. Great strides have been made in understanding the factors leading to this problem and the steps that can be taken to address it. As knowledge and experience are acquired, devices become smaller, blood contacting surfaces become more biocompatible, and the circumstances of device implantation become more favorable, we anticipate a marked reduction in the incidence of postoperative bleeding. An appreciation of the multiple factors involved and the application of the adjuncts and suggestions derived from the cumulative experience of many surgical investigators are essential to the perioperative management of bleeding complications and to the success of mechanical cardiac assist therapy.

References

1. Pennington DG, Samuels LD, Williams G, et al. Experience with the Pierce-Donachy ventricular assist device in postcardiotomy patients with cardiogenic shock. *World J Surg* 1985; 9:37–46.
2. Farrar DJ, Hill D, Gray LA, et al. Heterotopic prosthetic ventricles as a bridge to cardiac transplantation–A multicenter study in 29 patients. *N Engl J Med* 1988;318:333–340.
3. Farrar DJ, Lawson JH, Litwak P, et al. Thoratec VAD system as a bridge to heart transplantation. *J Heart Transplant* 1990;9:415–423.
4. Oaks TE, Pae WE Jr, Miller CA, et al. Combined registry for the clinical use of mechanical ventricular assist pumps and the total artificial heart in conjunction with heart transplantation: Fifth official report–1990. *J Heart Lung Transplant* 1991;10:621–625.
5. Korfer R, El-Vanayosy A, Posival H, et al. Mechanical circulatory support: The bad Oeynhausen experience. *Ann Thorac Surg* 1995;59:S56-S63.
6. Farrar DJ, Hill JD, Pennington DG, et al. Preoperative and postoperative comparison of patients with univentricular and biventricular support with the Thoratec ventricular assist device as a bridge to cardiac transplantation. *J Thorac Cardiovasc Surg* 1997;113:202–209.
7. McCarthy PM, Smedira NO, Vargo RL, et al. One hundred patients with the HeartMate left ventricular assist device: Evolving concepts and technology. *J Thorac Cardiovasc Surg* 1998;115:904–912.
8. Koul B, Solem JO, Steen S, et al. HeartMate left ventricular assist device as bridge to heart transplantation. *Ann Thorac Surg* 1998;65:1625–1630.
9. Pennington DG, McBride LR, Swartz MT, et al. Use of the Pierce-Donachy ventricular assist device in patients with cardiogenic shock after cardiac operations. *Ann Thorac Surg* 1989;47:130–135.
10. Tanaka K, Wada K, Morimoto T, et al. Hemostatic alterations caused by ventricular assist devices for postcardiotomy heart failure. *Artif Organs* 1991;15:59–65.
11. Hasper D, Hummel M, Hetzer R, et al. Blood contact with artificial surfaces during BVAD support. *Int J Artif Organs* 1996;19:590–596.
12. Himmelreich G, Ullmann H, Riess H, et al. Pathophysiologic role of contact activation in bleeding followed by thromboembolic complications after implantation of a ventricular assist device. *ASAIO J* 1995;41:M790-M794.
13. Dewald O, Fischlein T, Vetter HO, et al. Platelet morphology in patients with mechanical circulatory support. *Eur J Cardiothorac Surg* 1997;12:634–641.
14. Livingston ER, Fisher CA, Bibidakis J, et al. Increased activation of the coagulation and fibrinolytic systems leads to hemorrhagic complications during left ventricular assist implantation. *Circulation* 1996;94(suppl II):II227-II234.
15. Shenkar R, Coulson WF, Abraham E. Hemorrhage and resuscitation induce alterations in cytokine expression and the development of acute lung injury. *Am J Respir Cell Mol Biol* 1994;10:290–297.
16. Kormos RL. *The Right Heart on LVAD support. The Heart Failure Summit, Cleveland OH,*

October 11–12, 1996. Cleveland OH: Cleveland Clinic Foundation, Dept. of Thoracic and Cardiovascular Surgery; 1996.

17. Massad MG, Cook DJ, Schmitt SK, et al. Factors influencing HLA sensitization in implantable LVAD recipients. *Ann Thorac Surg* 1997;64:1120–1125.
18. van Oeveren W, Jansen NJG, Bidstrup BP, et al. Effects of aprotinin on hemostatic mechanisms during cardiopulmonary bypass. *Ann Thorac Surg* 1987;44:640–645.
19. Blauhut B, Gross C, Necek S, et al. Effects of high-dose aprotinin on blood loss, platelet function, fibrinolysis, complement and renal function after cardiopulmonary bypass. *J Thorac Cardiovasc Surg* 1991;101:958–967.
20. Pae WE, Aufiero TX, Weldner PW, et al. Aprotinin therapy for insertion of ventricular assist devices for staged heart transplantation. *J Heart Lung Transplant* 1994;(suppl 56): 811–816.
21. Goldstein DJ, Seldomridge JA, Chen JM, et al. Use of aprotinin in LVAD recipients reduces blood loss, blood use, and perioperative mortality. *Ann Thorac Surg* 1995;59:1063–1068.
22. Freeman JG, Turner GA, Venables CW, et al. Serial use of aprotinin and incidence of allergic reactions. *Curr Med Res Opin* 1983;8:559–561.
23. Levy JH. Antibody formation after drug administration during cardiac surgery: Parameters for aprotinin use. *J Heart Lung Transplant* 1993;12:S26-S32.
24. Schulz K, Graeter T, Schaps D, et al. Severe anaphylactic shock due to repeated application of aprotinin in patients following intrathoracic aortic replacement. *Eur J Cardiothorac Surg* 1993;7:495–496.
25. Goldstein DJ, Choudhri AF, Argenziano M, et al. Repeat administration of aprotinin for staged cardiac transplantation. *J Circ Support* 1998;1:27–30.
26. Hariawala MD. Aprotinin: Topical or systemic delivery in left ventricular assist device implantation. *Circulation* 1997;96(8):2736–2737.

Management of Perioperative Right-Sided Circulatory Failure

Jonathan M. Chen, MD and Eric A. Rose, MD

Introduction

Despite advances in its perioperative management, right-sided circulatory failure (RSCF) that is unresponsive to standard pharmacologic interventions develops in 20% to 30% of left ventricular assist device (LVAD) recipients, and thereby represents a major source of postoperative morbidity and mortality in this population. The etiology of this phenomenon in patients with previously undiagnosed right ventricular dysfunction is multifactorial and is thought to be related to a number of anatomic, intraoperative, and perioperative factors. The purpose of this chapter is to discuss the phenomenon of RSCF in the setting of LVAD insertion, its diagnosis and perioperative management and future prospects for its earlier recognition, and potential prevention.

Right-Sided Circulatory Failure

Background

Since 1943, when Starr and coworkers[1] demonstrated little hemodynamic effect from extensive cauterization of the entire right ventricular free wall, many have supported the notion that normal right ventricular function may be unnecessary in the setting of normal lung physiology.[2] Indeed, additional evidence suggesting that the pulmonary circuit represents only 10% of the total peripheral resistance against which the heart performs (an additional load that is bearable by the left ventricle alone) further supported this contention.[3] This relative "dispensibility" has been perhaps no better demonstrated than in the numerous surgical procedures that have been developed that exclude the right ventricle from the pulmonary circulation,

From Goldstein DJ and Oz MC (eds). *Cardiac Assist Devices*. Armonk, NY: Futura Publishing Co., Inc.; ©2000.

such as that described by Fontan and Baudet.[4] However, the frequent finding of longstanding pulmonary disease in cardiac surgical patients has unequivocally demonstrated that the right ventricle is far more than a simple conduit for the passage of systemic venous blood to the lungs. In particular, in the setting of LVAD insertion, potential alterations in right ventricular blood flow, compliance, and anatomy can unmask otherwise occult mild right ventricular failure, accounting for the 20% to 30% incidence of RSCF consistently reported in a recent review of LVAD experiences nationwide.[5]

Pathophysiology

The precise mechanisms whereby left ventricular bypass and assistance result in right ventricular dysfunction have been the focus of extensive research and represent the subject of an additional chapter in this text (see Chapter 2). As Farrar et al[6] have suggested, the significant alteration of right ventricular loading conditions induced by a well functioning LVAD in parallel with a weak left ventricle may potentially have both beneficial and detrimental effects on the determinants of overall right ventricular function (Table 1).

First, changes in preload are primarily due to increased venous return from the increased cardiac output of the LVAD. A hypothetical advantage exists in the leftward shift produced by effective left ventricular unloading; however, this notion presumes a favorable transseptal force gradient generated by this shift.[6] Alternatively, as has been suggested by other investigators, this very loss of septal contribution to right ventricular systolic function (from left ventricular unloading) in patients without such favorable transseptal forces may account for a substantial component of perioperative RSCF.[7]

Second, because the major cause of right heart failure is left heart failure and passive overloading of the right ventricle, the beneficial contributions of LVAD support to right ventricular afterload are conceptually simple: relief of increased left atrial pressure decreases the afterload of the entire pulmonary bed, thereby decreasing overall right ventricular afterload.[8] Conversely, the concomitant presence of an elevated pulmonary vascular resistance due to intrinsic pulmonary disease could, in the setting of LVAD support, result in even greater right ventricular afterload and

Table 1

Potential Effects of Left Ventricular Assistance on Right Ventricular Function

	Beneficial Effects	Detrimental Effects
Preload	Increased RV diastolic compliance due to septal shift from LV unloading	Increased venous return
Afterload	Decreased PA pressures in response to decreased LA pressure	Increased PA pressure due to increased CO with high PVR
Contractility	Enhanced coronary perfusion pressure increases RV contractility	Decreased septal systolic contribution to RV ejection during LV unloading

RV = right ventricle; LV = left ventricle; PA = pulmonary artery; LA = left atrial; CO = cardiac output; PVR = pulmonary vascular resistance.
From Farrar et al, Reference 6.

volume, where LVAD-induced increased flow through the pulmonary bed will result only in further elevations in pulmonary arterial pressure and vascular resistance.

Finally, the beneficial effect of LVAD support in enhancing right coronary artery perfusion, and thereby contractility, is clear. Counterbalancing this increased perfusion, however, may be the presence of right coronary artery atherosclerosis, and a greater demand generated by the increased wall tension from right ventricular distension in the presence of a persistently increased right ventricular afterload.[9] Furthermore, the combination of LVAD support and septal ischemia has been shown to depress right ventricular function significantly in experimental models, a phenomenon that is reversible when the ischemia is reduced.[10]

Right ventricular contractility may also be altered anatomically by changes in the interventricular septum owing to left ventricular decompression. The loss of systolic left ventricular contribution to right ventricular systolic function has been demonstrated in a series of animal and isolated heart models. Yet, Moon and colleagues[11] have demonstrated no additional effect of left ventricular support on the impairment in right ventricular relaxation due to right ventricular ischemia. Farrar and others[10–12] have also shown minimal effects on overall right ventricular function from septal shifting due to left ventricular assistance when compared with the effects of right ventricular ischemia. However, the precise extent to which the pre-LVAD clinically diseased left ventricle (and therefore its septal components) contributes to overall right ventricular systolic function remains unclear.[13]

Preoperative and Perioperative Contributions

In addition to the previously mentioned direct hemodynamic effects, a number of potential factors can further contribute to the development of perioperative RSCF (Table 2).[6] Naturally, preoperative factors such as preexisting pulmonary hypertension or right coronary artery disease impact negatively on right ventricular contractility and increase the likelihood of RSCF. Furthermore, intraoperative factors including inadequate right ventricular and septal myocardial protection can have a great im-

---

Table 2

Potential Contributors to RSCF After LVAD Insertion

Preexisting Disease
 Pulmonary hypertension
 Right ventricular infarction
 Significant right coronary artery disease
Intraoperative Contributions
 Prolonged cardiopulmonary bypass
 Poor right ventricular myocardial protection
 Bleeding/blood product transfusion
 Use of intravenous vasopressors
 Shock

LVAD = left ventricular assist device; RSCF = right-sided circulatory failure.
From Farrar et al, Reference 6.

pact on right ventricular function. Other intraoperative forces that may contribute to pulmonary hypertension include the deleterious effects of prolonged cardiopulmonary bypass (CPB) (with its induction of thromboxane A_2 release), as well as bleeding and the need for extensive blood product transfusions.[14–17] Indeed, shock (an inclusion criteria for LVAD insertion) itself may lead to RSCF, owing to decreased right ventricular function and pulmonary compliance as well as increased pulmonary vascular resistance associated with this syndrome.[18] Finally, the treatment of shock with blood product transfusion and intravenous vasopressors also induces pulmonary hypertension and thereby increases right ventricular afterload.[18]

It is therefore through an imbalance of these beneficial and detrimental effects of LVAD support on overall right ventricular function, and against a background of additional pre- and perioperative contributing factors, that RSCF develops perioperatively in the LVAD recipient.[6,17]

Diagnosis

RSCF may be characterized by a constellation of hemodynamic and physical findings (Table 3). The former include right atrial pressure greater than 20 mm Hg, left atrial pressure less than 10 mm Hg, a cardiac index less than 1.8 L/min/m², and decreasing cardiac output (or LVAD pump flow) developing in the setting of high pulmonary artery and/or central venous pressures. Tricuspid regurgitation may contribute to right ventricular inefficiency and worsen RSCF. Intraoperatively, the right ventricle appears distended, a finding that often is correlated with echocardio-

---

Table 3

Clinical Findings in Right-Sided Circulatory Failure After LVAD Placement

Hemodynamic
Right atrial pressure ≥20 mm Hg
Left atrial pressure ≤10 mm Hg
Cardiac index ≤1.8 L/min/m²
Decrease in LVAD flow
Potential increase in pulmonary arterial pressure
Increase in pulmonary indices (PVR, TPG)

Echocardiographic
Tricuspid regurgitation
Septal "bowing"
Decrease in right ventricular ejection fraction

Physical examination
Gallop
Distended neck veins
Hepatomegaly

PVR = pulmonary vascular resistance; TPG = transpulmonary gradient; LVAD = left ventricular assist device.

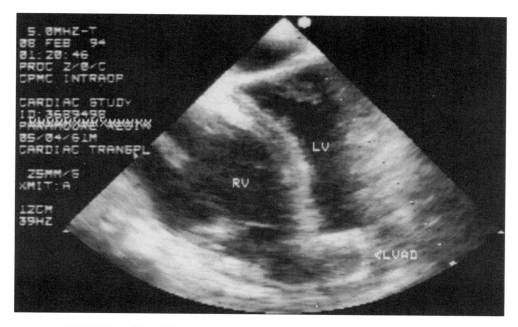

FIGURE 1. Septal "bowing" with left ventricular assist device in place.

graphic evidence of septal "bowing" into the left ventricle (Fig. 1). On physical examination, a gallop may be present on auscultation and the liver edge may be palpable (and tender) well below the costal margin, reflecting a significant degree of hepatic congestion.

Previous investigators have suggested hemodynamic parameters that may be predictive of postimplantation RSCF, including elevations in pulmonary vascular resistance and transpulmonary gradient. We have demonstrated that none of these parameters accurately distinguished survivors from nonsurvivors of right ventricular assist device (RVAD) support.[19] Similarly, other investigators have recently de-emphasized the correlation between preoperative hemodynamic criteria and the subsequent need for mechanical right ventricular assistance.[5,20] Interestingly, early data from the Cleveland Clinic (with the Thermo Cardiosystems HeartMate device, Woburn, MA), suggested that patients with elevated preoperative pulmonary indices (eg, transpulmonary gradient, right atrial pressure) were at lower risk for RVAD need and had a higher rate of survival to transplantation, a finding attributed to the likelihood that left-sided decompression would benefit right ventricular function.[21] Kormos et al[20] (working with the Novacor LVAD, Baxter Healthcare Corp., Oakland, CA) stratified the degree of post-LVAD RSCF, and demonstrated in a multivariable analysis that clinical surrogates of pre-implantation degree of illness (eg, fever) and perioperative factors that resulted in right ventricular ischemia or pulmonary hypertension were more predictive of the need for right ventricular support than either pre-implantation measures of ventricular function (eg, right ventricular ejection fraction) or hemodynamics. In a larger series, Nakatani[22] demonstrated right atrial pressure and transpulmonary gradient prior to LVAD insertion, and the acute decrease in pulmonary artery pressure after LVAD implantation to predict post-LVAD RSCF

Table 4

Sensitivity and Specificity for Predicting the Occurence of Right-Sided Ventricular Dysfunction after LVAD Implantation

	Sensitivity	Specificity
Preoperative RAP ≥20 mm Hg	64%	71%
Preoperative TPG ≥16 mm Hg	73%	65%
Change in PAP ≤10 mm Hg with LVAD	73%	65%
At least two of above	82%	88%

RAP = right atrial pressure; TPG = transpulmonary gradient; PAP = pulmonary artery pressure; LVAD = left ventricular assist device.
From Nakatani et al, Reference 22.

better than preoperative estimates of right ventricular ejection fraction. In this setting, while none of these factors was individually predictive of postoperative RSCF, a combination of two or three features was highly sensitive and specific (Table 4).[21,22]

It is important to note that pulmonary arterial pressures may occasionally be misleadingly low in the presence of LVAD-induced RSCF. This phenomenon reflects the low output state of the patient, rather than a true decrease in right-sided pressures. Lower than expected pulmonary arterial or central venous pressures therefore should not always constitute a contraindication to institution of right ventricular assistance (pharmacologic or mechanical) and, thus, the need for an RVAD may exist despite fictitiously low right-sided filling pressures. Indeed, in those patients who go on to require mechanical right ventricular support, such pressure may transiently increase as much as threefold during the initial periods of support, owing to the increased blood flow across the pulmonary beds.[19]

Treatment

Medical Therapy

Strategies for the treatment of post-LVAD perioperative RSCF parallel the potential etiologies contributing to its existence (Table 5).[6] Initial therapy for RSCF consists of volume loading in an attempt to raise right ventricular filling pressures and, therefore, right ventricular output. This pursuit is often limited by the risk of hepatic and splanchnic congestion. Although inotropic support may be used to enhance right ventricular contractility and reduce afterload via pulmonary vasodilatation, the typically used agents such as isoproterenol (Isuprel, Sanofi Winthrop Pharmaceuticals, New York, NY) and dobutamine (Dobutrex, Eli Lilly & Company, Indianapolis, IN) harbor a substantial risk for tachyarrhythmias. We have favored the use of phosphodiesterase inhibitors such as milrinone (Primacor, Sanofi Winthrop Pharmaceuticals); loading doses can be given during CPB in high-risk cases in order to reduce the likelihood of peripheral vasodilation that limits their administration. Efforts are made to obtain atrioventricular synchrony with the use of sequential pacing in cases in which LVAD flow may be compromised by the presence of bradycardias or junctional rhythms (Fig. 2).[6,23]

Table 5

Potential Strategies for the Treatment of Post-LVAD
RSCF

Medical Therapy
- Increase preload volume loading
- Increase contractility inotropes
- Decrease right ventricular afterload
   -nonselective: intravenous pulmonary vasodilators
   -selective: inhaled nitric oxide
- Optimize electrical activity
   -atrial pacing for sinus bradycardia
   -AV sequential pacing for junctional rhythms
- Treat pulmonary hypertension
   -use blood sparing agents (eg, antifibrinolytics)

Surgical Therapy
- Avoid long cardiopulmonary bypass time
- Pulmonary artery balloon counterpulsation
- Extracorporeal membrane oxygenation
- Creation of right-to-left shunt
- Right ventricular assist device

AV = atrioventricular; LVAD = left ventricular assist device; RSCF = right-sided circulatory failure.
From Farrar et al, Reference 6.

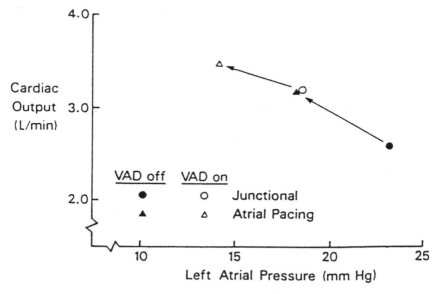

FIGURE 2. Atrial pacing postoperatively produced a marked improvement in right and left ventricular function in a 72-year-old left ventricular assist device (LVAD) recipient. With atrial pacing on and the LVAD off, cardiac output was increased and left atrial pressure was decreased to the same level as with the LVAD alone. Further improvements were seen with the LVAD plus pacing. Reprinted with permission from the Society of Thoracic Surgeons (*The Annals of Thoracic Surgery* 1991;51:658–660).

Reducing Pulmonary Hypertension

The treatment of potential contributing causes of pulmonary hypertension is of paramount importance. The induction of a coagulopathy during LVAD support has been well established, and bleeding with subsequent extensive blood product transfusion has also been associated with pulmonary hypertension.[5,24,25] We have favored the use of the Thermo Cardiosystems HeartMate device because its shorter, wider inflow cannula substantially reduces the residual left ventricular pressure, ultimately leading to fewer bleeding complications. Moreover, we rely on the use of the plasmin inhibitor aprotinin (Trasylol, Bayer Corporation, West Haven, CT), as it has been shown to reduce blood loss, blood use, and the need for right ventricular assistance after LVAD insertion.[26] Lastly, the use of thromboxane A_2 inhibitors holds promise for the reduction of CPB-induced pulmonary hypertension.[14,15]

Inhaled nitric oxide has received much attention for the treatment of postcardiotomy pulmonary hypertension, including that seen in the postoperative LVAD recipient.[27-29] Pulmonary hypertension is associated with diminished expression of endothelial nitric oxide synthase, a phenomenon thought to contribute to pulmonary vasoconstriction and, further, to account for the pulmonary vasoreactivity to inhaled nitric oxide.[20] Nitric oxide is a selective pulmonary artery vasodilator that crosses the alveolus easily and is absorbed into the bloodstream, where it is rapidly bound to hemoglobin and converted into nitrate and nitrite moieties by the enzyme methemoglobin reductase. Nitric oxide has no appreciable systemic vasodilatory effects at concentrations that generate pulmonary vasodilation, and it is metabolized in one pass through the lungs.

In a recent experience,[29] 11 LVAD recipients were randomized to receive either inhaled nitric oxide (at a dose of 20 ppm) or nitrogen alone. Hemodynamics were evaluated before and after commencement of support, and if no hemodynamic effect was noted within 15 minutes, a cross-over was performed. Effect on hemodynamics is depicted in Figures 3 through 5. The cumulative data of the 11 patients who received nitric oxide appear in Table 6. As shown, nitric oxide significantly reduced mean pulmonary artery pressure and increased both mean arterial pressure and LVAD flow in LVAD recipients with elevated pulmonary vascular resistance. While

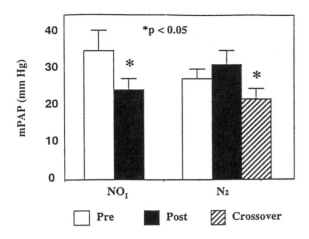

FIGURE 3. Effects of nitric oxide (NO$_I$) and nitrogen (N$_2$) on mean pulmonary arterial pressure (mPAP).

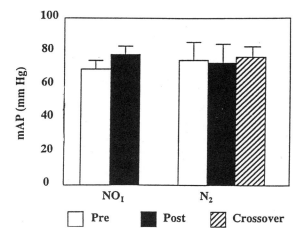

FIGURE 4. Effects of nitric oxide (NO_I) and nitrogen (N_2) on mean arterial pressure (mAP).

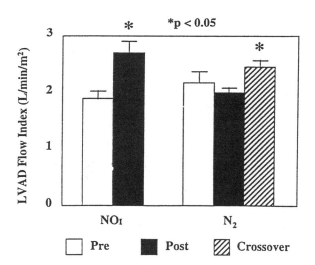

FIGURE 5. Effects of nitric oxide (NO_I) and nitrogen (N_2) on mean left ventricular assist device (LVAD) flow.

Table 6		
Hemodynamics of 11 Recipients of LVADs Before and After Treatment with Inhaled Nitric Oxide (iNO)		
Variable	Before iNO	After iNO
Mean pulmonary artery pressure (mm Hg)	33 ± 4	23 ± 3*
LVAD flow index (L/min/m^2)	1.9 ± 0.1	2.6 ± 0.2§
Mean arterial pressure (mm Hg)	71 ± 6	77 ± 5

* $P = 0.03$; § $P = 0.005$. LVAD = left ventricular assist device.

these findings have been confirmed by other investigators, there exists a subgroup of patients who do not respond so dramatically (or at all) to inhaled nitric oxide therapy. The further characterization of this subgroup of LVAD recipients as well as those who are exquisitely sensitive to its administration form the basis of ongoing research efforts.

Persistent pulmonary hypertension that is refractory to intravenous vasodilators and inhaled nitric oxide therapy generally represents a fatal condition. First, severe fixed pulmonary hypertension (presumably due to longstanding pulmonary architectural changes) can often markedly limit the ability of the right ventricle—mechanically supported or not—from generating sufficient left ventricular preload to support LVAD flow. Second, the cascade of events surrounding severe pulmonary hypertension (eg, the need for increased vasodilators in the setting of hypotension, or ongoing bleeding and the need for transfusion) generally leads to continued clinical deterioration. Thus, the aggressive management of pulmonary hypertension is of supreme importance in the perioperative period.

Surgical Therapy

Surgical options for the treatment of perioperative RSCF include 1) augmentation of right ventricular function with pulmonary artery balloon counterpulsation (PABC) or RVAD insertion; 2) bypass of the right ventricular and pulmonary bed functions with extracorporeal membrane oxygenation (ECMO); and 3) decompression of elevated right-sided filling pressures with right-to-left shunts (Table 5).

Pulmonary Artery Balloon Counterpulsation   While PABC represents a compelling technique that could potentially be modified into a percutaneous method, it has largely been surpassed by the RVAD. Early case reports of PABC involved the use of a device that placed a standard intra-aortic balloon pump into a graft sewn to the pulmonary artery as a reservoir for blood and the balloon (Fig. 6).[30–33] Although investigations with the device progressed from animal models into the clinical arena, most concur that PABC should be reserved for the treatment of mild RSCF, since it is not efficient enough to ameliorate severe RSCF.[33,34]

Extracorporeal Membrane Oxygenation   The use of ECMO has mainly been reserved for the pediatric population, for whom other modes of mechanical support are very limited (see Chapter 4). Recently, however, ECMO has received increasing recognition as an important adjunct in extracorporeal life support for adult patients in cardiogenic shock, for whom it may provide excellent hemodynamic and pulmonary support.[35] This modality is described in detail in Chapter 20.

A large series report from the Cleveland Clinic revealed comparable mortality in those patients treated with ECMO and those supported with centrifugal pump assistance for right ventricular failure, a finding in keeping with others that demonstrate a 25% to 35% survival rate in patients who are unable to be weaned from bypass.[35–37] These investigators further reported the use of ECMO for the treatment of perioperative RSCF following LVAD implantation.[38] Interestingly, in this group,

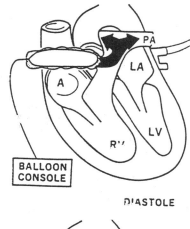

FIGURE 6. The action of pulmonary artery balloon counterpulsation. In diastole, balloon inflation ejects blood from the graft into the pulmonary circulation. In systole, the right ventricle fills the graft after balloon deflation; there is almost no flow through the pulmonary circulation. Reprinted with permission from the Society of Thoracic Surgeons (*The Annals of Thoracic Surgery* 1985;39:329–335).

while the overall survival rate to transplantation was noted to be 45%, 8 of their 12 patients supported with ECMO required subsequent RVAD placement.

In summary, ECMO represents mainstay therapy for the support of the pediatric patient who requires mechanical assistance. The use of ECMO for the treatment of RSCF has met only with mixed success and most often it is employed as a bridge to RVAD support.

Right-to-Left Venoarterial Shunting The benefits of right-to-left shunting were first realized by Austen et al[39] more than 30 years ago, and were later clinically applied by Connolly et al[40] and Wakabayashi et al.[41] Their work was initially prompted by the recognition of the protective effect of an intracardiac defect in patients with Eisenmenger's syndrome subjected to acute stress when compared with individuals with primary pulmonary hypertension. In this setting, the intracardiac defect allowed for decompression of the right heart and subsequent maintenance of left ventricular output during stress. Indeed, these clinical considerations led to the use of atrial septostomy in patients with terminal cor pulmonale caused by pulmonary vascular disease, and of prophylactic fenestrated atrial septal defects during Fontan operations in patients considered to be at high risk for RSCF.[42,43]

Investigators at our institution have pursued right-to-left venoarterial shunting as a novel approach to treat the RSCF that develops in the setting of LVAD implantation and after orthotopic cardiac transplantation. In a series of animal models of RSCF, or in the setting of LVAD implantation, we have demonstrated that a controlled right atrial to right femoral artery, or right femoral vein to right femoral artery shunt improves hemodynamics and cardiac output with minimal effects on systemic oxygenation.[44–48] The shunt decreases right-sided pressures, thereby decreasing right ventricular size and improving diastolic perfusion.

In this system, systemic blood pressure is maintained at the expense of arterial saturation; oxygen saturation and the cardiac index should increase if the additional blood pressure generated contributes to coronary perfusion and thus allows reduction of vasopressor medications. Ideally, as the reactive pulmonary vascular bed (and resultant RSCF) resolves, the shunt becomes less necessary and can be weaned. Others have demonstrated in model analysis that when the total cardiac output increases after the creation of such a shunt, the latter will have little effect on systemic venous oxygen saturation. Hence, a decrease in the systemic venous oxygen saturation implies an inadequate increase in cardiac (LVAD) output or a decrease in pulmonary flow owing to the creation of the shunt.[47]

We have used this system in two patients, one after cardiac transplantation (right atrium to right femoral artery), and one after LVAD implantation (femoral vein to LVAD outflow).[48] This system can be easily inserted (and removed) at the bedside, it selectively infuses desaturated venous blood to the lower extremities while maintaining cerebral and cardiac perfusion with oxygen-rich blood, it reduces the risk of paradoxical emboli, and it allows for a known and adjustable degree of shunting (a major advantage when compared with an atrial septal defect).

Despite this, our clinical experience with right-to-left shunting has been disappointing. Indeed, the recent introduction and success of inhaled nitric oxide therapy in conjunction with RVAD support has led us to abandon this mode of surgical therapy.

Right Ventricular Assist Devices Institution of RVAD support remains the standard treatment for severe right ventricular impairment that is unresponsive to medical therapies. The incidence of severe biventricular failure in those patients who require an LVAD is substantial, as illustrated in a review by Pennington et al,[49] in which there were no survivors in the cohort of 16 LVAD recipients whose RSCF was treated medically, compared to a 30% survival rate for those treated with biventricular assist device support. These findings demonstrate the devastating impact of biventricular failure on survival in LVAD recipients; even in the setting of right-sided mechanical support, a 70% mortality persists.

A number of short-term devices are available to support the failing right ventricle in the setting of LVAD implantation, with inflow established via the right atrium or ventricle and outflow to the pulmonary artery. However, no system currently available completely decompresses the right heart, and indeed, if severe pulmonary vascular hypertension exists, substantial right ventricular distension can result from RVAD flow against a high afterload.

In a review of our institutional experience with RVAD support for RSCF after transplantation or LVAD implantation, we demonstrated substantial improvements

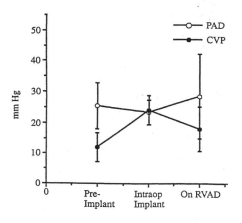 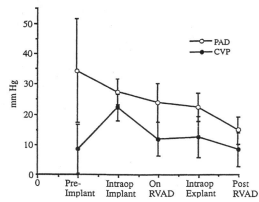

FIGURE 7. Changes in the pulmonary artery diastolic pressure (PAD) and central venous pressure (CVP) in survivors (right) and nonsurvivors (left) of RVAD support. Differences between pre-implant, on RVAD support, and after RVAD support were statistically significant. Reprinted with permission from the Society of Thoracic Surgeons (*The Annals of Thoracic Surgery* 1996;61:305–310).

in right-sided filling pressures in survivors only (Fig. 7).[19] The RVAD also clearly improved end organ function in survivors, as indicated by increases in urine output, and a resolution of elevated serum transaminase levels (Fig. 8).[19] These improvements have similarly been demonstrated by others with regard to LVAD-induced impairment in renal function that improves with the institution of RVAD support.[50]

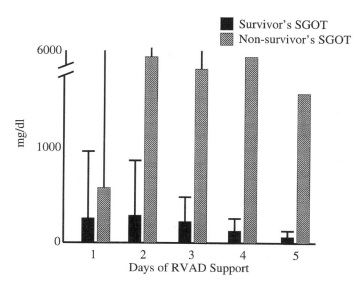

FIGURE 8. Daily serum transaminase levels for survivors and nonsurvivors over the first 5 days of right ventricular assist device (RVAD) support. Serum glutamic-oxaloacetic transaminase (SGOT) levels tended to decrease in survivors throughout the period of support. A similar trend was present in nonsurvivors; however, the absolute values of SGOT were nearly 10-fold higher. Reprinted with permission from the Society of Thoracic Surgeons (*The Annals of Thoracic Surgery* 1996;61:305–310).

With regard to renal failure, we have also reported the use of continuous veno-venous hemofiltration (CVVH) and hemodialysis for volume removal and correction of electrolyte imbalances while on RVAD assistance.[51] In these patients, the period of RVAD support represents a temporary therapeutic window during which certain factors (eg, intravascular volume, electrolytes, acid-base balance) may be optimized prior to RVAD explantation. Of particular importance is the maintenance of a net diuresis with CVVH, despite a normal urine output and serum creatinine. We have found that aggressive management of fluid status during the period of RVAD support is mandatory to wean the device; even with excellent renal function and a net urine output of 1 liter per day, the LVAD patient in RSCF would take 1 month to diurese the 20 to 30 liters of excess perioperative fluid necessary to maximize pulmonary function and weaning of the RVAD. Indeed, the ease with which a venovenous apparatus can be incorporated into the RVAD circuit renders its application simple and virtually standard at our institution (Fig. 9). We additionally splice a blood saturation monitor in line to provide continuous mixed venous saturation data.

Interestingly, although one might expect a patient who is undergoing biventricular support to have a higher incidence of thrombotic, infectious, cannulation-related, and mechanical complications than a patient who is undergoing univentricular support only, this has not been demonstrated in recent reviews.[19,52] In our series, the predominant causes of death were intractable coagulopathy, multisystem organ failure, and sepsis. A particular note must be made of those patients in whom a fixed pulmonary vascular resistance may herald the development of acute pulmonary edema with the institution of mechanical right ventricular assistance.

In recent years, we have preferred the use of a pulsatile device (ABIOMED BVS 5000, ABIOMED, Danvers, MA) over the centrifugal pumps for mechanical right ventricular assistance for two reasons. First, their cannulae are easier to manage after implantation and are made for longer term support. Second, the ABIOMED closed-loop control system avoids the cost associated with continuous need for trained bedside personnel that is required with centrifugal pumps. Novel approaches to the implantation of the outflow cannula for right ventricular assistance via the right outflow tract have resulted in less perioperative complications (Fig. 10).[53,54]

Several investigators have suggested hemodynamic criteria on which to base the withdrawal of right mechanical support in LVAD recipients; these include LVAD filling rates, which are themselves coupled closely to right ventricular ejection.[55] The ABIOMED device, when used in combination with hemodynamic and echocardiographic monitoring, allows bedside weaning attempts that provide a reasonable estimate of "recovered" right ventricular function prior to RVAD removal. In general, we do not close the sternum in our RVAD recipients. While this decision limits perioperative mobility of the patients, it allows easy access for reexploration should bleeding or tamponade ensue.

Several lessons have been learned during our experience with RVAD support for the treatment of RSCF. First, RVADs work most effectively if implanted early enough so as to avoid significant and potentially irreversible end organ injury. Second, we liberally employ venovenous hemofiltration (and/or dialysis) in line with the RVAD circuit to optimize intravascular volume status, acid-base balance, and electrolyte profile. Third, we minimize the use of heparin in the immediate postoperative period to avoid the attendant risks of bleeding and the need of transfusions; the risk of potential embolism to the pulmonary bed in this setting remains unclear. Once perioperative bleeding subsides, efforts are made to maintain an activated

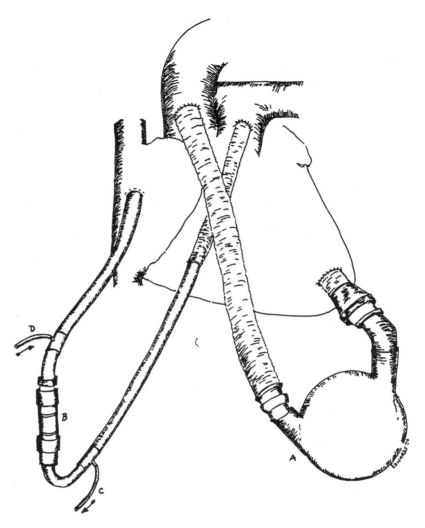

FIGURE 9. Illustration demonstrating the use of continuous venovenous hemofiltration and dialysis (CVVH-D) in the right ventricular assist device circuit. A. Thermo Cardiosystems LVAD; B. ABIOMED BVS 5000; C. inflow to CVVH-D; D. outflow from CVVH-D. Reprinted with permission from the Society of Thoracic Surgeons (*The Annals of Thoracic Surgery* 1996; 61:305–310).

clotting time of 180 to 200 seconds. It cannot be overemphasized that reduction in bleeding and transfusion requirements is mandatory for RVAD removal; the cascade of events attendant to ongoing bleeding and transfusion (eg, pulmonary hypertension and the systemic inflammatory response) are prohibitive to clinical success in this regard. Fourth, we keep patients sedated so as to decrease oxygen consumption. Finally, we continue RVAD support until the patient displays signs of hemodynamic and end organ recovery as heralded by 1) a decrease in central venous and/or pulmonary artery diastolic pressure; 2) an increase in urine output; and 3) a decrease in transaminase levels. In our experience, the length of RVAD support averages 5 days.

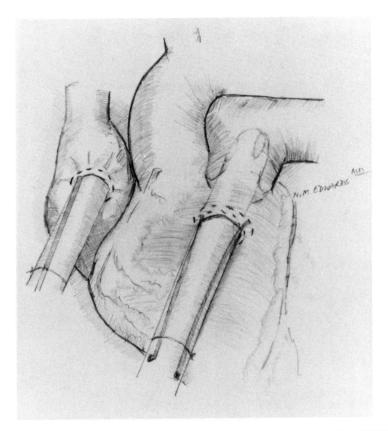

FIGURE 10. Illustration demonstrating our approach to placement of the ABIOMED BVS 5000 right ventricular assist device outflow cannula. Placement into the pulmonary artery via the right ventricular outflow tract allows easy insertion and removal under direct vision, easier reinforcement for bleeding, and simpler removal for transplant if required. Reprinted with permission from the Society of Thoracic Surgeons (*The Annals of Thoracic Surgery* 1998; 66:1829–1830).

In summary, the RSCF that develops following LVAD implantation is multifactorial in etiology. The resultant morbidity and mortality are substantial and continue to represent a major complication of LVAD insertion.[56] At present, the management of RSCF in centers specialized in the care of end-stage heart disease patients revolves around the use of volume loading, inotropic support, and, most importantly, inhaled nitric oxide. Should these measures fail, RVAD support is instituted. With improving therapy, the incidence of clinically significant RSCF has fallen to less than 20% with a resultant increase in overall operative survival.

References

1. Starr I, Jeffers WA, Meade RH. The absence of conspicuous increments of venous pressure after severe damage to the right ventricle of the dog, with discussion of the relation between clinical congestive heart failure and heart disease. *Am Heart J* 1943;26:291–301.

2. Sade RM, Castaneda AR. The dispensable right ventricle. *Surgery* 1975;77(5):624–631.
3. Furey SA, Zieske HA, Levy MN. The essential function of the right ventricle. *Am Heart J* 1984;107:404–410.
4. Fontan F, Baudet E. Surgical repair of tricuspid atresia. *Thorax* 1971;26:240–248.
5. Mc Carthy PM, Savage RM, Fraser CD, et al. Hemodynamic and physiologic changes during support with an implantable left ventricular assist device. *J Thorac Cardiovasc Surg* 1995;109:409–418.
6. Farrar DJ, Compton PG, Hershon JJ, et al. Right heart interaction with the mechanically assisted left heart. *World J Surg* 1985;9:89–102.
7. Waldenberger F, Kim Y, Laycock S, et al. Effects of failure of the right side of the heart and increased pulmonary resistance on mechanical circulatory support with use of the miniaturized HIA-VAD displacement pump system. *J Thorac Cardiovasc Surg* 1996;112: 484–493.
8. Weber KT, Janicki JS, Shroff SG, et al. The right ventricle: Physiologic and pathophysiologic considerations. *Crit Care Med* 1983;1:323–328.
9. Hendry PJ, Nathan H, Rajagopalan K. Right ventricular blood flow during left ventricular support in an experimental porcine model. *Ann Thorac Surg* 1996;61:1199–1204.
10. Daly RC, Chandrasekaran K, Cavarocchi NC, et al. Ischemia of the interventricular septum. A mechanism of right ventricular failure during mechanical left ventricular assist. *J Thorac Cardiovasc Surg* 1992;103:1186–1191.
11. Moon MR, DeAnda A, Castro LJ, et al. Effects of mechanical left ventricular support on right ventricular diastolic function. *J Heart Lung Transplant* 1997;16:398–407.
12. Farrar DJ, Chow E, Compton PG, et al. Effects of acute right ventricular ischemia on ventricular interactions during prosthetic left ventricular support. *J Thorac Cardiovasc Surg* 1991;102:588–595.
13. Santamore WP, Gray LA Jr. Left ventricular contributions to right ventricular systolic function during LVAD support. *Ann Thorac Surg* 1996;61:350–356.
14. Smith WJ, Murphy MP, Appleyard RF, et al. Prevention of complement-induced pulmonary hypertension and improvement of right ventricular function by selective thromboxane receptor antagonism. *J Thorac Cardiovasc Surg* 1994;107:800–806.
15. Friedman M, Wang SY, Sellke FW, et al. Pulmonary injury after total or partial cardiopulmonary bypass with thromboxane synthesis inhibition. *Ann Thorac Surg* 1995;59:598–603.
16. Cave AC, Manch A, Derias NW, Hearse DJ. Thromboxane A$_2$ mediates pulmonary hypertension after cardiopulmonary bypass in the rabbit. *J Thorac Cardiovasc Surg* 1993;106: 959–967.
17. Wong C, Huval W, Hechtman LT, Demling RH. Effect of hemorrhagic shock on endotoxininduced pulmonary hypertension and increased vascular permeability in unanesthetized sheep. *Circ Shock* 1984;12:61–71.
18. Cryer HG, Mavroudis C, Yu J, et al. Shock, transfusion, and pneumonectomy. Death is due to right heart failure and increased pulmonary vascular resistance. *Ann Surg* 1990; 212(2):197–201.
19. Chen JM, Levin HR, Rose EA, et al. Experience with right ventricular assist devices for perioperative right-sided circulatory failure. *Ann Thorac Surg* 1996;61:305–310.
20. Kormos RL, Gasior TA, Kawai A, et al. Transplant candidate's clinical status rather than right ventricular function defines need for univentricular versus biventricular support. *J Thorac Cardiovasc Surg* 1996;111:773–783.
21. Smedira NG, Massad MG, Navia J, et al. Pulmonary hypertension is not a risk factor for RVAD use and death after left ventricular assist system support. *ASAIO J* 1996;42:M733-M735.
22. Nakatani S, Thomas JD, Savage RM, et al. Prediction of right ventricular dysfunction after left ventricular assist device implantation. *Circulation* 1996;94(suppl II):II216-II221.
23. Haffajee CI, Love J, Gore JM, Alpert JS. Reversibility of shock by atrial or atrioventricular sequential pacing in right ventricular infarction. *Am Heart J* 1984;108:5–13.
24. Livingston ER, Fischer CA, Bibidakis EJ, et al. Increased activation of the coagulation and fibrinolytic systems lead to hemorrhagic complications during left ventricular assist implantation. *Circulation* 1996;94(suppl II):II227-II234.
25. Shenkar R, Coulson WF, Abraham E. Hemorrhage and resuscitation induce alterations in cytokine expression and the development of acute lung injury. *Am J Respir Cell Mol Biol* 1994;10:290–297.

26. Goldstein DJ, Seldomridge JA, Chen JM, et al. Use of aprotinin in LVAD recipients reduces blood loss, blood use, and perioperative mortality. *Ann Thorac Surg* 1995;59:1063–1068.
27. Chang J, Sawa Y, Ohtake S, et al. Hemodynamic effect of inhaled nitric oxide in dilated cardiomyopathy patients on LVAD support. *ASAIO J* 1997;43:M418-M421.
28. Yahagi N, Kumon K, Nakatani T, et al. Inhaled nitric oxide for the management of acute right ventricular failure in patients with a left ventricular assist system. *Artif Organs* 1995; 19(6):557–558.
29. Argenziano M, Choudhri AF, Moazami N, et al. Randomized, double-blind trial of inhaled nitric oxide in LVAD recipients with pulmonary hypertension. *Ann Thorac Surg* 1998;65: 340–345.
30. Skillington PD, Couper GS, Peigh PS, et al. Pulmonary artery balloon counterpulsation for intraoperative right ventricular failure. *Ann Thorac Surg* 1991;51:658–660.
31. Letsou GV, Franco KL, Detmer W, et al. Pulmonary artery balloon counterpulsation: Safe after peripheral placement. *Ann Thorac Surg* 1993;55:741–746.
32. Moran J, Oprovil M, Gorma A. Pulmonary artery balloon counterpulsation for right ventricular failure II. Clinical experience. *Ann Thorac Surg* 1984;38:254–259.
33. Spence PA, Weisel R, Easdown J, et al. The hemodynamic effects and mechanism of action of pulmonary artery balloon counterpulsation in the treatment of right ventricular failure during left heart bypass. *Ann Thorac Surg* 1985;39:329–335.
34. Spence PA, Peniston CM, Mihic N, et al. A rational approach to the selection of an assist device for the failing right ventricle. *Ann Thorac Surg* 1986;41:606–608.
35. Muehrcke DD, McCarthy PM, Stewart RW, et al. Extracorporeal membrane oxygenation for postcardiotomy cardiogenic shock. *Ann Thorac Surg* 1996;61:684–691.
36. Kawahito K, Ino T, Adachi H, et al. Heparin coated percutaneous cardiopulmonary support for the treatment of circulatory collapse after cardiac surgery. *ASAIO Trans* 1994;40: 972–976.
37. Tracy TF Jr, DeLosh T, Bartlett RH. Extracorporeal life support organization 1994. *ASAIO Trans* 1994;40:1017–1019.
38. Wudel JH, Hloe CC, Smedira NG, McCarthy PM. Extracorporeal life support as a post left ventricular assist device implant supplement. *ASAIO J* 1997;43(5):M441-M443.
39. Austen WG, Morrow AG, Berry WB. Experimental studies of the surgical treatment of primary pulmonary hypertension. *J Thorac Cardiovasc Surg* 1964;48:448–455.
40. Connolly JE, Bacaner MB, Bruns DL, et al. Mechanical support of the circulation in acute heart failure. *Surgery* 1958;44:255–262.
41. Wakabayashi A, Nakamura Y, Murphy KJ, et al. Controlled venoarterial bypass without oxygenation in the treatment of cardiogenic shock. *ASAIO* 1973;19:511–515.
42. Nihill MR, O'Laughlin MP, Mullins CE. Effects of atrial septostomy in patients with cor pulmonale due to primary pulmonary vascular disease. *Cathet Cardiovasc Diagn* 1991;24: 166–172.
43. Mavroudis C, Zales VR, Backer CL, et al. Fenestrated Fontan with delayed catheter closure. *Circulation* 1992;86(suppl II):II85-II92.
44. Slater JP, Goldstein DJ, Ashton RC, et al. Right-to-left veno-arterial shunting for right-sided circulatory failure. *Ann Thorac Surg* 1995;60:978–985.
45. Slater JP, Yamada A, Yano OJ, et al. Creation of a controlled venoarterial shunt. A surgical intervention for right-sided circulatory failure. *Circulation* 1995;92(suppl II):II467-II471.
46. Goldstein DJ, Ashton RC Jr, Slater JP, et al. Venoarterial shunting for the treatment of right sided circulatory failure after left ventricular assist device placement. *ASAIO J* 1997; 43:171–176.
47. Santamore WP, Austin EH, Gray L Jr. Overcoming right ventricular failure with left ventricular assist devices. *J Heart Lung Transplant* 1997;16:1122–1128.
48. Oz MC, Slater JP, Edwards NM, et al. Desaturated venous-to-arterial shunting reduces right-sided heart failure after cardiopulmonary bypass. *J Heart Lung Transplant* 1995;14: 172–176.
49. Pennington DG, Merjavy JP, Swart MT, et al. The importance of biventricular failure in patients with postoperative cardiogenic shock. *Ann Thorac Surg* 1985;39(1):16–26.
50. Akamatsu H, Arai H, Sakamoto T, Suzuki A. Effects of right ventricular failure on renal function during pneumatic left ventricular assist. *Artif Organs* 1996;20(3):240–246.
51. Chen JM, Levin HR, Catanese KA, et al. Use of a pulsatile right ventricular assist device

and continuous arteriovenous hemodialysis in a 57 year old man with a pulsatile left ventricular assist device. *J Heart Lung Transplant* 1994;14(1 Pt. 1):186–191.

52. Pennington DG, Reedy JE, Swartz MT, et al. Univentricular versus biventricular assist device support. *J Heart Lung Transplant* 1991;10:258–263.
53. Dewey TM, Chen JM, Spanier TB, Oz MC. Alternative technique of right sided outflow cannula insertion for right ventricular support. *Ann Thorac Surg* 1998;66:1829–1830.
54. Krause TJ. Abiomed BVS 5000 system: Repair of venous cannulation site for excessive bleeding. *Ann Thorac Surg* 1998;66:1817.
55. Mandarino WA, Winowich S, Gasior TA, et al. Assessment of timing right ventricular assist device withdrawal using left ventricular assist device filling characteristics. *ASAIO J* 1997;43:M801-M805.
56. Goldstein DJ, Oz MC, Rose EA. Implantable left ventricular assist devices. *N Engl J Med* 1998;339:1522–1533.

Chapter 8

Perioperative Management of Arrhythmias in Recipients of Left Ventricular Assist Devices

Mathew Williams, MD and James Coromilas, MD

Introduction

Arrhythmias represent an interesting and relatively common problem among recipients of cardiac assist devices. Depending on the series, 19% to 43% of patients will experience at least one episode of a malignant arrhythmia (ventricular tachycardia, ventricular fibrillation, or asystole) during support.[1–5] The occurrence of arrhythmias in this population is generally well tolerated compared to that in their nonsupported counterparts. Nonetheless, arrhythmias still require prompt recognition and treatment to prevent potentially deleterious consequences. A high index of suspicion must be maintained for arrhythmias, as they frequently do not present themselves clinically in the unmonitored patient. Indeed, even an asymptomatic patient may be found to have ventricular fibrillation. This chapter addresses the perioperative management of arrhythmias in patients with assist devices. The theoretical sequelae of device placement are examined and the sparse data on recurrent malignant arrhythmias as an indication for device placement are reviewed.

Preoperative

According to the data from the Thermo Cardiosystems (TCI) Woburn, MA) trials, as many as 50% of patients requiring left ventricular assist device (LVAD) placement experienced some type of arrhythmia prior to implantation. Unfortunately, the type or duration of arrhythmia was not specified (personal communication. Thermo Cardiosystems Inc., Woburn, MA. 1999). In smaller trials, 16% to 64% of patients experienced a malignant ventricular arrhythmia preoperatively. These numbers should not be surprising, as it is well known that patients with both ischemic (acute and chronic) and idiopathic cardiomyopathy are prone to develop potentially

From Goldstein DJ and Oz MC (eds). *Cardiac Assist Devices*. Armonk, NY: Futura Publishing Co., Inc.; ©2000.

fatal arrhythmias. In fact, arrhythmias represent the most common cause of death in this population.[6] Fifty percent of patients with New York Heart Association Class III or IV heart failure will have unsustained ventricular tachycardia on a 24-hour continuous electrocardiogram. The mortality for all of these patients is approximately 40%; half of these deaths are sudden and thus likely related to arrhythmias.[7] It is therefore reasonable to anticipate that a large proportion of LVAD patients either have experienced or will experience some type of ventricular arrhythmia. For this reason, patients who present for LVAD placement will frequently be taking a number of different antiarrhythmic medications. Often, several antiarrhythmic agents will have already been tried; it is important to be aware of this history, as it may prove to be useful in the postoperative management.

Preoperatively, patients should continue on their antiarrhythmic regimen through device placement. For patients with documented atrial fibrillation in the preoperative period, great care should be exercised at the time of implant to avoid any embolization of intracardiac thrombus into the device. Transesophageal echocardiography can prove to be particularly useful in this regard.

The presence of arrhythmias in their own right can represent an indication for assist device placement. Several studies have demonstrated the use of intra-aortic balloon counter pulsation for therapy of uncontrollable ventricular arrhythmias.[8] It is expected that this benefit is due to increased coronary perfusion and, thus, reversal of ischemia. There have also been two case reports of patients who received assist devices due to intractable arrhythmias with otherwise stable hemodynamics.[9,10] In both instances, ischemic disease was present. One patient was a transplant candidate with recurrent arrhythmias that were unresponsive to conventional therapies, and the other was a patient who developed refractory malignant ventricular arrhythmias following coronary artery bypass grafting. Both patients had no further episodes of arrhythmias after device placement. One patient was weaned from support and the other went on to successful transplantation. The resolution of these patients' arrhythmias was possibly due to improved coronary perfusion. Assist devices should be considered for select patients with intractable ventricular arrhythmias that are unresponsive to cardioversion, pharmacologic therapy, overdrive pacing, and optimization of coronary perfusion. While no significant literature exists to support this contention, recurrent arrhythmias will result in inadequate circulation and further myocardial damage from persistent arrhythmias and from repeated attempts at cardioversion. There certainly are theoretical reasons why these patients will experience improvement of their arrhythmias after device placement, but the inability to maintain adequate circulation is reason enough to justify artificial circulatory support. Additionally, it appears that patients who are placed on devices due to recurrent arrhythmias will have a reduction in the incidence of arrhythmias, particularly if improvement of myocardial ischemia occurs.

Postoperative Management

The post-implantation period is the most challenging time in arrhythmia management. As previously stated, up to 43% of LVAD recipients will experience a malignant ventricular arrhythmia. In the largest published series, the incidence of malignant arrhythmias was similar before (16%) and after (19%) device implantation.[4] A patient's ability to tolerate the arrhythmia is related to various factors, but in general there is a remarkably low incidence of mortality attributed to malignant ventricular arrhythmias during assist device support, and there are only a few reported deaths.

The reason for the propensity for patients with prior arrhythmias to maintain or develop arrhythmias after artificial support has been achieved is unclear, and conflicting data exist in the literature.[1-4] There is also no agreement as to whether ischemic or nonischemic cardiomyopathies will lead to a greater probability of arrhythmia development, although as one might expect, there appears to be a higher incidence in patients with ischemic myopathy. One study[1] reports an 8% incidence of malignant arrhythmia in nonischemic cardiomyopathy patients compared with a 44% incidence in ischemic cardiomyopathy patients post device. This is in agreement with the cardiology literature demonstrating a greater likelihood of developing malignant ventricular arrhythmia in ischemic syndromes.[16] Additionally, one might expect that patients with old myocardial infarctions and persistent arrhythmias may continue to have arrhythmias, as the focus of arrhythmogenicity is not likely affected by device implantation. This is in contrast to acute coronary syndromes with viable myocardium that might have improvement in arrhythmogenicity due to reversal of ischemia. Preoperative inotropic agents, antiarrhythmic agents, intra-aortic balloon pump support, and mechanical ventilation appear to be factors that identify patients who are more likely to develop post-implant arrhythmias, although no statistical significance has been demonstrated nor have odds ratios been established.[2]

Numerous reports exist describing survival of patients with assist devices during malignant ventricular arrhythmias.[1-5,12] The earlier studies demonstrated success using biventricular assist, as it was felt that, in the presence of malignant arrhythmias, right-sided assist was necessary in order to fill the left-sided device. More recently, several reports have demonstrated that ventricular arrhythmias are well tolerated with only left-sided assistance. Thus, these patients exhibit essentially the equivalent of a Fontan circulation with central venous pressure being the driving force for pulmonary flow. In one series of 58 patients, 11 developed malignant ventricular arrhythmias and all patients were maintained only with left ventricular assist with no mortality related to arrhythmias or associated sequalae.[4] Patients have survived ventricular arrhythmia of 12 days' duration on left-sided support and 22 days with biventricular support.

The symptomatology of these patients is also intriguing. Most reported a sense of lethargy, but there were no episodes of syncope; 67% of the patients were fully ambulatory. In fact, one arrhythmia was not diagnosed until the patient presented as an outpatient to undergo transplantation. The presenting symptoms in patients with biventricular devices have not been described. The difference between these populations lies in the device flows during the arrhythmia. Patients with only left-sided assist demonstrated a statistically significant decrease in device flows with concomitant decreases in mean arterial pressure and central venous pressure during the arrhythmia,[3] whereas patients with biventricular support demonstrated no appreciable change in device flows.[2] It may be inferred that the right-sided circulation is affected by the arrhythmia but not to the point of circulatory collapse.

Although arrhythmias are remarkably well tolerated, there is a group of patients that, as a result of an arrhythmia, either does not survive or encounters dangerous decreases in device flows. This group is characterized by arrhythmias early after device implantation in the setting of elevated pulmonary pressures. There are two reported cases of mortality with left-sided assist only, both occurring in the operating room in patients with ventricular fibrillation and profound right heart failure.[3] In another series, two patients were noted to have dangerous decreases in flows at the time of arrhythmia; both of these occurred within 48 hours of device implantation, and right-sided failure was also present.[3] From a mechanical standpoint, it is obvious why the presence of an arrhythmia and right heart failure could be deleterious. The physiologic explanation for the early postoperative time course can be extrapolated from the cardiac transplant population. It has been demonstrated that heart failure patients often exhibit elevated pulmonary vascular resistance (PVR), largely due to a reactive component to left-sided failure. Within 1 week of transplantation, and with normalization of left-sided pressures, the reactive component of the PVR resolves[14] and only the fixed component remains. It is for this reason that PVR is a good predictor of right heart failure in cardiac transplant candidates. Similarly, LVAD recipients should manifest normalization of elevated PVR as a result of left heart unloading. However, it has been demonstrated that in LVAD patients PVR is not a predictor of right-sided failure. This is due to the fact that these patients are using the same right ventricle that has become accustomed to elevated pulmonary pressures; indeed it is right-sided function that is a predictor of right heart failure in these patients.[13] In other words, a heart transplant patient does not tolerate an elevated PVR, as the new heart is not accustomed to a high right ventricular afterload, whereas an LVAD patient maintains a right ventricle that is accustomed to elevated PVR. In LVAD recipients, and in the early postoperative period in particular, the coexistence of arrhythmias and elevated PVR renders the otherwise compensated right ventricle dysfunctional. Thus, much like Fontan patients, they are unable to maintain adequate circulation in the presence of elevated pulmonary artery pressures or vascular resistance. As the patient progresses beyond the first 48 hours to 7 days, it is expected that he or she will better tolerate malignant ventricular arrhythmias, due to the normalization of right-sided afterload secondary to unloading of the left heart. It is for this reason that special attention must be paid to early right heart function in these patients, particularly if they are experiencing arrhythmias. LVAD patients will not infrequently require some type of intervention for the failing right heart. These include β-agonists (which can be arrhythmogenic), phosphodiesterase inhibitors , inhaled nitric oxide, and even right-sided assist devices. It is important that patients with recurrent arrhythmias and right heart failure requiring an intervention not be weaned from that intervention until the arrhythmia is controlled. In patients with persistent arrhythmias in the setting of right heart failure, serious consideration should be given to the use of a right-sided assist device.

Despite the general tolerance of malignant ventricular arrhythmias, it is still important to make an early diagnosis and to undertake effective treatment. With correction of the arrhythmia, the patient realizes several benefits. First, in a normal sinus rhythm, device flow is clearly optimized. Second, arrhythmias increase the likelihood of developing an intracardiac thrombus with the potential for subsequent embolic consequences. Finally, the presence of an arrhythmia such as ventricular fibrillation may cause prolonged deterioration of right-sided function. At the time of arrhythmia recognition, prompt intervention is warranted. If the patient is using a device such as the TCI HeartMate that does not require anticoagulation, then low-dose intravenous heparin should be initiated to prevent embolic complications. To date, there has been no reported case of an embolic complication precipitated by an arrhythmia in an assist device patient.

VT Algorithm

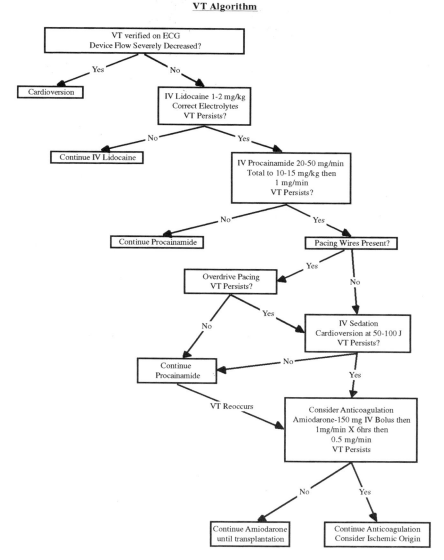

FIGURE 1. Algorithm for the management of ventricular tachycardia (VT) in left ventricular assist device recipients at our institution.

Sustained ventricular tachycardia (Fig. 1) is the most common malignant arrhythmia in LVAD patients. Since sustained ventricular tachycardia is virtually always well tolerated, there is time to obtain a 12-lead electrocardiogram and to verify that the wide-complex tachycardia indeed represents ventricular tachycardia (rather than supraventricular tachycardia with aberrancy). Although intravenous procainamide (Procan, Elkins-Sinn Inc., Cherry Hill, NJ) is far superior to Lidocaine (Elkins-Sinn Inc.) for terminating sustained monomorphic ventricular tachycardia, we routinely administer Lidocaine (1 to 2 mg/kg intravenously) first because of its ease of administration and the lack of arrhythmogenic effect. If Lidocaine does not terminate the ventricular tachycardia, Procan is administered at a rate of 20 to 50 mg/min to a total of 10 to 15 mg/kg. Administration of Procan requires a minimum of approximately 20 minutes. If ventricular pacing wires are present, one can attempt to overdrive pace and terminate ventricular tachycardia. If all of the above measures are unsuccessful, electrical cardioversion with 50 to 100 joules is attempted. If sustained ventricular tachycardia becomes recurrent despite pharmacologic therapy and after correction of electrolyte imbalances (ie, potassium, magnesium), we administer intravenous amiodarone (Cordarone, Wyeth-Ayerst Laboratories, Philadelphia, PA) with an initial bolus of 150 over 10 minutes, followed by a 1-mg/min infusion for 6 hours and a 0.5-mg/min infusion thereafter.

If ventricular tachycardia becomes incessant despite the above measures, the diagnosis of ischemia must be considered. In this situation, intravenous esmolol (Brevibloc, Ohmeda Pharmaceuticals, Liberty Corner, NJ) can sometimes be very effective in controlling incessant ventricular tachycardia. The ischemia may be the result of recent infarction with resultant damaged but not necrotic myocardium.

The syndrome of torsades de pointes ventricular tachycardia, consisting of a characteristic "twisting of the points" polymorphic ventricular tachycardia in the presence of a long QT interval, should be recognized and treated with intravenous magnesium, pacing, and identification and removal of the precipitating factors. At times, a typical torsades de pointes ventricular tachycardia occurs in the absence of any identifying precipitating factors such as a potassium channel blocking drug and sometimes even in the absence of a long QT interval. In these cases, recent infarction is often the cause and β-blocker therapy is often effective.

Regardless of hemodynamic status, ventricular fibrillation always requires electrical cardioversion. Since LVAD patients are usually awake, intravenous sedation is required before electrical defibrillation. In the absence of correctable factors, Lidocaine is usually started for prophylaxis of further episodes of ventricular fibrillation. If ventricular fibrillation reoccurs, amiodarone therapy is instituted.

Patients who are responsive to pharmacologic therapy for arrhythmias should be switched to the appropriate oral dose when they are able to take medications by mouth. Antiarrhythmic therapy should be continued until the time of transplant, provided no intolerable side effects develop. Should the latter occur, the agents should be withdrawn and close monitoring for evidence of arrhythmia recurrence should be instituted.

A significant number of LVAD candidates have undergone prior automatic implantable defibrillators. These devices can be activated in the postoperative period and can be useful for terminating ventricular arrhythmias with antitachycardia pacing algorithms or low-energy cardioversion. The role of automatic implantable defibrillator implantation in LVAD patients, as more of these patients go home with electronically implanted LVADs, remains to be determined.

Atrial fibrillation is an arrhythmia that has received little attention in the LVAD literature. The incidence of this arrhythmia has not been characterized in this population. As in other cardiac surgery procedures, new-onset atrial fibrillation should be met with standard pharmacologic techniques to convert to sinus rhythm. Patients with chronic atrial fibrillation have a theoretical possibility of converting to sinus rhythm due to reduction in left atrial distention; however, this is unlikely, due to the chronic electrophysiologic changes that occur in the atrium that favor perpetuation of the arrhythmia. In these patients, anticoagulation should be initiated if not already required by the type of assist device being used, and ventricular rate should be controlled with digoxin, β-blockers, or calcium channel blockers as appropriate for the individual patient.

Electrophysiologic Effects of Device Placement

Circulatory assist likely plays two significant roles in altering the electrophysiologic performance of the heart. First, as discussed above, it increases coronary perfusion and thereby decreases the incidence of ischemic-induced arrhythmias. A more exciting possibility is that of modulation of electrical properties via contraction-excitation feedback. Contraction-excitation feedback is the process by which changes in mechanical loading conditions can directly alter myocardial refractoriness and excitability. This has been studied in several animal models and in some clinical scenarios.[16–20] Volume loading of the ventricle shortens action potential duration, and does so more in scarred areas of the heart, causing an increase in dispersion of refractoriness. The increased load may also cause a reduction in membrane potential and an increase in afterpotential. The decrease in volume and tension that occurs with LVAD placement may therefore reverse these abnormalities. The changes at the cellular level are not as well understood but probably are related to intracellular calcium processing. One case report in which an assist device was placed for arrhythmia management postulated that this was the mechanism by which the patient's arrhythmias resolved.[10] Current experience does not support a lower incidence of arrhythmia after device placement except perhaps in patients with nonischemic cardiomyopathy; however, other factors may be at play. It may be, for example, that the outflow cannulation/sewing ring serves as an arrhythmogenic focus either through local ischemia early after implant or from scar formation thereafter. Also, particularly during the initial days of device support, patients with assist devices often have concomitant metabolic abnormalities or inotropic dependence that may precipitate arrhythmias. Patients with ischemic cardiomyopathy may have had recent infarcts, which predispose the patients to recurrent arrhythmia.

Conclusion

Arrhythmias represent an important component in the management of patients with assist devices. Arrhythmias are remarkably well tolerated by these patients provided the patients are able to maintain transpulmonary flow, be it from a right-sided device or from a favorable pulmonary vasculature. Early postoperative right heart function should be closely monitored, particularly in the setting of arrhythmias and high PVR, and early consideration should be given to mechanical support of the right heart.

The clinician must maintain a high index of suspicion and the presence of an arrhythmia must be ruled out in any situation of unexplained decrease in device flow. Arrhythmias should be diagnosed and treated promptly to maximize device filling, reduce the risk of thromboembolism, and prevent further deterioration of cardiac function.

References

1. Arai H, Swartz MT, Pennington G, et al. Importance of ventricular arrhythmias in bridge patients with ventricular assist devices. *ASAIO Trans* 1991;37:M427-M428.
2. Farrar J, Hill D, Laman A, et al. Successful biventricular circulatory support as a bridge to cardiac transplantation during prolonged ventricular fibrillation and asystole. *Circulation* 1989;80(suppl III):III147–III151.
3. Oz M, Rose E, Slater J, et al. Malignant ventricular arrhythmias are well tolerated in patients receiving long-term left ventricular assist devices. *J Am Coll Cardiol* 1994;24:1688–1691.
4. Oz M, Argenziano M, Catanese K, et al. Bridge experience with long-term implantable left ventricular assist devices: Are they an alternative to transplantation? *Circulation* 1997; 7:1844–1852.
5. Moroney D, Swartz MT, Reedy J, et al. Importance of ventricular arrhythmias in the recovery of patients with ventricular assist devices. ASAIO Transactions 1991;37:M516–17.
6. Weiss J, Nademanee K, Stevenson W, Singh B. Ventricular arrhythmias in ischemic heart disease. *Ann Intern Med* 1991;114:784–797.
7. Bigger JT. Why patients with congestive heart failure die: Arrhythmias and sudden cardiac death. *Circulation* 1987;75:IV-28–35.
8. Hanson E, Levine F, Kay H, et al. Control of postinfarction ventricular irritability with intraaortic balloon pump. *Circulation* 1980;62(suppl I):I130-I137.
9. Geannopoulos C, Wilber D, Olshansky B. Control of refractory ventricular tachycardia with biventricular assist devices. *PACE* 1991;14:1432–1434.
10. Kulik D, Bolman M, Salerno C, et al. Management of recurrent ventricular tachycardia with ventricular assist device placement. *Ann Thorac Surg* 1998;66:571–573.
11. Parmley W. Factors causing arrhythmias in chronic congestive heart failure. *Am Heart J* 1987;114:1267–1272.
12. Holman W, Roye D, Bourge R, et al. Circulatory support for myocardial infarction with ventricular arrhythmias. *Ann Thorac Surg* 1995;59:1230–1231.
13. Bourge R, Kirklin J, Naftel D, et al. Analysis and predictors of pulmonary vascular resistance after cardiac transplantation. *J Thorac Cardiovasc Surg* 1991;101:432–445.
14. Levin H, Burkhoff D, Oz M, et al. Preoperative right ventricular stroke work is a major determinant of right heart failure in patients after left ventricular assist device implantation. *J Heart Lung Transplant* 1994;13:S73.
15. Lab M. Contraction-excitation feedback in myocardium: Physiological basis and clinical relevance. *Circ Res* 1982;50:757–767.
16. Taggart P, Sutton P, Treasure T, et al. Monophasic action potentials at discontinuation of cardiopulmonary bypass: Evidence for contraction-excitation feedback in man. *Circulation* 1988;77:1266–1275.
17. Gornick C, Tobler G, Pritzker M, et al. Electrophysiologic effects of papillary muscle traction in the intact heart. *Circulation* 1986;73:1013–1021.
18. Calkins H, Maughan L, Weisman H, et al. Effect of acute volume load on refractoriness and arrhythmia development in isolated, chronically infarcted canine hearts. *Circulation* 1989;79:687–697.
19. Levine J, Guarnieri T, Kadish A, et al. Changes in myocardial repolarization in patients undergoing balloon valvuloplasty for congenital pulmonary stenosis: Evidence for contraction-excitation feedback in humans. *Circulation* 1988;77:70–77.

Chapter 9

Management of Vasodilatory Hypotension After Left Ventricular Assist Device Placement

Michael Argenziano, MD
and Donald W. Landry, MD, PhD

Background

Distributive shock is defined as systemic hypotension and organ hypoperfusion caused by loss of vascular tone, or "vasomotor collapse," and is characterized by low systemic vascular resistance and normal or elevated cardiac output. Clinical conditions classically associated with distributive or vasodilatory shock include sepsis and anaphylaxis, but cardiopulmonary bypass (CPB) with pump oxygenation also induces a systemic inflammatory response and, in many patients, a vasodilatory shock state.[1,2] CPB-induced vasodilatory shock is usually mild, and requires moderate amounts of pressor support as CPB is weaned and through the next 24 to 36 hours. Some patients, however, develop profound vasodilatory shock and require high-dose catecholamine and fluid therapy. Severe forms of vasodilatory shock are more common after extensive cardiac surgical procedures, with prolonged CPB time, and in patients with preoperative congestive heart failure.[3]

All three of these risk factors are frequently present in patients undergoing left ventricular assist device (LVAD) insertion for end-stage cardiac failure, and the incidence of vasodilatory shock in this population can approach 40%. In these patients, perioperative catecholamine pressor therapy is standard, but long-term management options are sometimes limited by the well described adverse effects of these agents, which include renal, coronary, and gastrointestinal hypoperfusion, peripheral vascular ischemia, and increased cardiac work and oxygen consumption. These effects promote lactic acidosis, leading to myocardial depression and catecholamine receptor insensitivity. The factors responsible for the loss of vascular tone in these cases are unknown but there is evidence to suggest that a deficiency in the vasoconstrictor hormone vasopressin may play a role.

Arginine vasopressin (AVP) is an intriguing hormone in that it has little vasoconstrictor effect in normal subjects, but is an important component of the homeostatic

From Goldstein DJ and Oz MC (eds). *Cardiac Assist Devices.* Armonk, NY: Futura Publishing Co., Inc.; ©2000.

pressor response when arterial pressure is threatened. Studies performed in canine models of hypotension have suggested that the hypothalamic-hypophyseal AVP system might function as a rapidly acting mechanism for maintenance of blood pressure in low flow states,[4,5] in some cases potentiating the effects of endogenous catecholamines. The importance of endogenous vasopressin in the maintenance of vascular tone is further supported by studies demonstrating that animals with diabetes insipidus are more susceptible than normals to hypotension after mild hemorrhage,[6] and that physiologic concentrations of vasopressin reverse hypotension in dogs after hypophysectomy.[7] Furthermore, while the administration of supraphysiologic doses of AVP does not alter blood pressure in normal subjects,[8] the pressor sensitivity to exogenous AVP is greatly enhanced under certain conditions, such as after baroreceptor denervation,[9] ganglionic blockade,[10] and in primary autonomic failure.[11] In the case of autonomic failure, the increased sensitivity to exogenous AVP is associated with a deficiency of endogenous hormone, and the severity of orthostatic hypotension has been correlated to the degree of AVP deficiency.[12]

Prompted by a clinical observation of AVP sensitivity in a patient with sepsis syndrome (unpublished observation, DWL), our laboratory has investigated the role of AVP deficiency and hypersensitivity in vasodilatory septic shock. In a study of 19 patients with vasodilatory septic shock requiring catecholamines,[13] plasma AVP concentrations were markedly depressed in comparison to a group of 12 patients with cardiogenic shock matched for degree of hypotension, dose of catecholamines, and plasma osmolality. In another study,[14] vasopressin was administered to a subgroup of 10 patients with catecholamine-resistant septic shock. Administration of this hormone in minute quantities (0.04 U/min) resulted in a significant rise in blood pressure within minutes, allowing rapid discontinuation of catecholamine support.

We have subsequently observed AVP pressor hypersensitivity in a series of patients with vasodilatory shock after CPB uncomplicated by infection.[15–18] This experience suggests that vasopressin deficiency might play a role in the vasodilatory state often seen after high-risk cardiac surgical procedures, particularly in patients with congestive heart failure and those undergoing LVAD placement or heart transplantation. The purpose of this chapter is to review our clinical experience with AVP in LVAD recipients and heart failure patients.

AVP for Vasodilatory Shock in LVAD Patients

In a clinical trial performed at our institution,[15] patients with vasodilatory hypotension after placement of an LVAD were randomized to low-dose vasopressin infusion or saline control. All patients undergoing LVAD insertion for end-stage heart failure over a 1-year period were enrolled, with the exception of those with active peripheral or mesenteric vascular disease or prior exposure to exogenous AVP. Upon weaning from CPB, subjects were selected for a mean arterial pressure ≤ 70 mm Hg, norepinephrine administration in excess of 8 µg/min, and LVAD-assisted cardiac index greater than 2.5 L/min/m². Consecutive eligible subjects were blindly randomized 5 minutes after bypass to receive intravenous vasopressin (Pitressin, Parke-Davis, Morris Plains, NJ) at 0.1 U/min or normal saline placebo. A plasma sample for vasopressin measurement was collected at the time of randomization. A clinical response was defined as an increase in mean arterial pressure (>20 mm Hg) without an increase in norepinephrine administration and/or a decrease in norepinephrine requirement (>5 µg/min) without a decline in mean pressure, in the absence of other pharmacologic or surgical interventions. In the absence of a clinical response after 15 minutes of infusion, subjects were eligible for blinded administration of the alternate solution. If a clinical response was observed, the assigned infusion was continued postoperatively. Upon arrival in the intensive care unit, vasopressin infusions were decreased to maintain mean arterial pressure above 70 mm Hg.

Hemodynamic Effects of AVP in LVAD Patients

Over the 12-month study period, 10 of 23 LVAD recipients met inclusion criteria for vasodilatory shock, with decreased mean arterial pressure (60 ± 2 mm Hg), increased cardiac index (2.9 ± 0.1 L/min/m^2), and a requirement for exogenous norepinephrine (19.7 ± 5.4 µg/min) to maintain blood pressure. Despite administration of catecholamine pressors, systemic vascular resistance was decreased (828 ± 70 dyne-sec/cm^5). The study group consisted of eight men and two women, with a mean age of 52 years, mean ejection fraction of $15 \pm 2\%$, and mean CPB time of 120 ± 13 minutes. Etiology of heart failure was ischemic cardiomyopathy in seven cases and idiopathic dilated cardiomyopathy in three cases. These patients did not differ significantly from the 13 patients who did not meet criteria for vasodilatory shock, with respect to etiology of heart failure, ejection fraction, preoperative medication regimens, CPB time, or other basic demographic data. Five subjects were randomized to receive intravenous vasopressin, and five to saline placebo; hemodynamic responses are summarized in Table 1. Vasopressin rapidly (<15 minutes) and significantly increased mean arterial pressure (57 ± 4 to 84 ± 2 mm Hg; $P<0.001$) and systemic vascular resistance (813 ± 113 to 1188 ± 87 dyne-sec/cm^5; $P<0.05$). Cardiac index was not significantly changed and, thus, the pressor effect of the hormone was due solely to vasoconstriction. These increases in mean arterial pressure coincided with decreased norepinephrine administration (26.7 ± 9.0 to 10.7 ± 10.7 µg/min). Norepinephrine was discontinued in 4 of 5 subjects during the initial 15-minute

---

Table 1

Hemodynamic Responses and Catecholamine Requirements of Randomized Patients

Parameter	Randomized to AVP (n = 5)		Randomized to NS (n = 5)		Cross-over (NS to AVP) (n = 3)	
	pre-AVP	post-AVP	pre-NS	post-NS	pre-AVP	post-AVP
MAP (mm Hg)	57 ± 4	$84 \pm 2^*$	63 ± 3	65 ± 5	69 ± 8	93 ± 4
SVR (dynes-sec/cm^5)	813 ± 113	$1188 \pm 87^{**}$	843 ± 95	857 ± 63	898 ± 95	1443 ± 72
LVAD flow (L/min)	4.2 ± 0.2	4.4 ± 0.3	4.2 ± 0.4	4.3 ± 0.4	4.7 ± 0.6	4.7 ± 0.6
NE dose (µg/min)	26.7 ± 9.0	10.7 ± 10.7	12.8 ± 5.2	12.2 ± 5.1	16.8 ± 7.7	1.8 ± 1.8

* $P <0.001$ versus pre-AVP; ** $P <0.05$ versus pre-AVP.

AVP = ariginine vasopressin; NS = nornal saline; MAP = mean arterial pressure; SVR = systemic vascular resistance; LVAD = left ventricular assist device; NE = norepinephrine.

period of vasopressin administration; the fifth was tapered off norepinephrine over several hours.

Subjects who received saline placebo showed no significant change in arterial pressure, systemic vascular resistance, or catecholamine dose after 15 minutes (Table 1). In three subjects who were blindly crossed over to AVP infusions, vasopressin increased mean arterial pressure (69 ± 8 to 93 ± 4 mm Hg) and systemic vascular resistance (898 ± 88 to 1443 ± 72 dyne-sec/cm^5) while decreasing norepinephrine requirements (16.8 ± 7.7 to 1.8 ± 1.8 mg/min). Two of the three subjects were tapered off catecholamines within 15 minutes; the third was tapered off catecholamines over several hours despite a mean arterial pressure of 100 mm Hg.

In the eight subjects who received vasopressin (5 at initial randomization and 3 after cross-over), the hormone increased mean arterial pressure (61.3 ± 12.1 to 87.4 ± 7.0; $P < 0.05$) and systemic vascular resistance (845 ± 212 to 1284 ± 208 dyne-sec/cm^5; $P < 0.05$), with all patients weaned from catecholamines (and 6 of the 8 within the first 15 minutes of administration). Despite these significant increases in systemic arterial pressure, vasopressin administration did not significantly alter mean pulmonary artery pressures (25.9 ± 2.9 mm Hg to 23.7 ± 3.7; $P = NS$). For subjects who maintained a mean arterial pressure greater than 70 mm Hg without catecholamine support, vasopressin was tapered to 0.01 U/min and then discontinued. The median duration of vasopressin infusion was 36 hours (range 1 hour to 7 days), and no subjects required reinstitution of norepinephrine. No complications were associated with vasopressin administration. There was one perioperative death, occurring on postoperative day 3, due to intractable hemorrhage in a patient with multisystem organ failure and severe coagulopathy.

Vasodilatory Shock in LVAD Patients is Associated with Vasopressin Deficiency

The plasma vasopressin concentrations of the 10 randomized subjects varied widely (Fig. 1) and were inappropriately low for the immediate postbypass period,

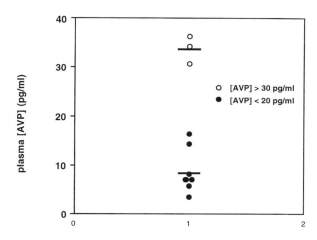

FIGURE 1. Plasma vasopressin (AVP) levels in vasodilatory shock after cardiopulmonary bypass in 10 left ventricular assist device patients.

during which levels of 100 to 200 pg/mL are reported.[19-24] Based simply on the degree of hypotension, levels greater than 20 pg/mL would be expected for these subjects[13,25]; however, the majority (n = 7) fell below this level, with a mean of 8.8 ± 4.7 pg/mL (Fig. 1, closed circles). A second group (n = 3) clustered above 30 pg/mL, with a mean of 33.7 ± 1.6 pg/mL (Fig. 1, open circles). Preoperative medication regimens, hemodynamics, plasma sodium concentrations, and serum osmolality did not differ significantly between the groups. None of the subjects manifested diabetes insipidus, and the low AVP levels were consistent with a defect in baroreflex-mediated secretion of the hormone.

Five of the eight subjects who ultimately received vasopressin had levels below 20 pg/mL (mean 8.4 ± 2.1 pg/mL) prior to randomization. These five subjects had a mean arterial pressure of 57 ± 4 mm Hg that rose 28 ± 6 mm Hg upon administration of vasopressin ($P<0.01$) (Fig. 2). Finally, in the three subjects with elevated plasma vasopressin levels prior to randomization, mean arterial pressure was higher (68 ± 8 mm Hg) on less norepinephrine, and increased by a smaller increment (18 ± 6 mm Hg) after administration of vasopressin.

In summary, we demonstrated in a blinded, placebo-controlled, randomized trial that vasopressin is a generally effective pressor for LVAD recipients who have vasodilatory shock after CPB; it significantly increases mean arterial pressure while rapidly reducing catecholamine requirements. The marked pressor sensitivity of these patients to vasopressin contrasted with their diminished sensitivity to catecholamines, and a similar pattern may contribute to the recently described effectiveness of vasopressin in patients suffering from cardiopulmonary arrest.[26] All subjects in this study, regardless of pretreatment vasopressin level, responded to vasopressin administration, but the severity of shock and the magnitude of the hemodynamic response to exogenous hormone appeared to be related to the degree of vasopressin deficiency.

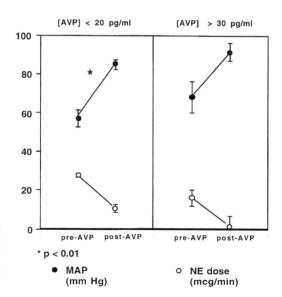

FIGURE 2. Relationship of pretreatment vasopressin (AVP) level to hemodynamic effect of vasopressin administration in vasodilatory shock after cardiopulmonary bypass in 8 left ventricular assist device patients.

AVP in Other Cardiac Surgical Populations

Incidence and Predictors of Vasodilatory Hypotension in Cardiac Surgical Patients

As described above, vasodilatory hypotension can be a significant problem after LVAD insertion, and AVP is an effective pressor in this setting. However, LVAD insertion comprises a small fraction of the total number of cardiac operations performed each year, and the general incidence of post-bypass vasodilatory shock is not known. For this reason, we investigated the incidence and clinical predictors of vasodilatory shock in a general population of cardiac surgical patients. In this study,[17] 145 patients undergoing CPB were followed prospectively. As in other studies, vasodilatory hypotension was defined as mean arterial pressure less than 70 mm Hg, cardiac index greater than 2.5 L/min/m^2, and norepinephrine dependence. Preoperative ejection fraction, medications, and perioperative hemodynamics were recorded, post-bypass serum AVP levels were measured, and predictors of this vasodilatory hypotension were investigated by logistic regression analysis.

Eleven of 145 general cardiac surgery patients (8%) met criteria for post-bypass vasodilatory hypotension. In these patients, mean arterial pressure was 64.6 ± 6.6 mm Hg and cardiac index was 2.7 ± 0.3 L/min/m^2. By multivariate analysis, ejection fraction less than 0.35 and angiotensin-converting enzyme (ACE) inhibitor use were independent predictors of this complication (relative risk of 9.1 and 11.9, respectively). In addition, vasodilatory hypotension was associated with inappropriately low serum AVP concentrations (12.0 ± 6.6 pg/mL). By comparison, nine patients with cardiogenic shock (mean arterial pressure of 68.0 ± 1.2 mm Hg and cardiac index 1.0 ± 0.6 L/min/m^2) had a mean serum AVP level of 29.3 ± 15.0 pg/mL (Fig. 3). We concluded that vasodilatory hypotension occurred in a significant proportion of

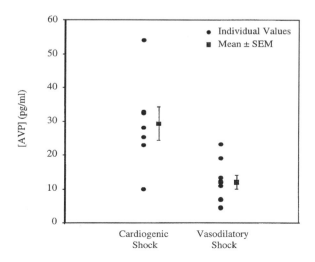

FIGURE 3. Distribution of vasopressin (AVP) levels in 20 patients with cardiogenic and vasodilatory shock after cardiopulmonary bypass.

patients undergoing cardiac surgery, was more likely in the setting of heart failure or ACE inhibitor use, and was associated with a relative vasopressin deficiency.

AVP in Patients Undergoing Heart Transplantation

After demonstrating the efficacy of vasopressin therapy in LVAD patients, we sought to characterize AVP responsiveness in other cardiac surgical populations. Since heart failure is an important pathophysiologic determinant of post-bypass vasodilation, we chose to study patients who were undergoing heart transplantation. Also, because the risk of AVP-induced coronary vasoconstriction was undefined, we sought to avoid patients with significant coronary artery disease. As reported in a recent article,[27] vasopressin was administered to 20 patients undergoing orthotopic heart transplantation at our institution who met criteria for post-bypass vasodilatory hypotension. These patients were characterized by a mean arterial pressure of 60 ± 15 mm Hg, systemic vascular resistance of 836 ± 264 dyne-sec/cm^5, cardiac index of 3.0 ± 0.5 L/min/m^2, and exogenous norepinephrine requirement of 15.1 ± 13.8 μg/min. AVP infusions were instituted from 10 to 240 minutes after weaning from bypass, and hemodynamic responses are summarized in Table 2. Patients receiving AVP showed dramatic increases in mean arterial pressure (from 60 ± 15 to 86 ± 10 mm Hg; $P<0.0001$) and systemic vascular resistance (from 836 ± 264 to 1556 ± 493 dyne-sec/cm^5; $P<0.0001$) within 1 hour. Notably, these increases in blood pressure and vascular tone were accompanied by a reduction in mean norepinephrine doses (from 15.1 ± 13.8 to 5.2 ± 5.6 μg/min; $P<0.05$), with 7 of 20 (35%) patients tapered completely off norepinephrine within 15 minutes.

Etiology of Vasodilatory Shock and Mechanism of Action of AVP

Although CPB is typically associated with a marked increase in plasma vasopressin concentrations, a few authors have documented cases of post-bypass vasopressin

Table 2

Summary the Effects of AVP in Heart Transplant Patients with Vasodilatory Hypotension

Parameter	Pre-AVP	1 hour post-AVP	2 hours post-AVP
Hemodynamics			
MAP (mm Hg)	60 ± 15	85.5 ± 10.2*	84.9 ± 6.7*
CVP (mm Hg)	8.4 ± 5.9	14.8 ± 4.0†	13.7 ± 5.6‡
SVR (dyne-sec/cm^5)	836 ± 264	1556 ± 493*	1656 ± 706*
CI (L/min/m^2)	3.0 ± 0.5	2.5 ± 0.6‡	2.4 ± 0.8‡
Norepinephrine support			
number of patients	20	13	11
μg/min	15.1 ± 13.8	5.2 ± 5.6†	5.9 ± 8.7

AVP = arginine vasopressin; MAP = mean arterial pressure; CVP = central venous pressure; SVR = systemic vascular resistance; CI = cardiac index
* $P <0.0001$ versus pre-AVP value; † $P <0.01$ versus pre-AVP value; ‡ $P <0.05$ versus pre-AVP value.

deficiency manifesting as diabetes insipidus,[28,29] and others have described a post-bypass vasodilatory syndrome that is responsive to agents such as angiotensin II[30] and octreotide.[31] Our LVAD and heart transplant recipients with post-bypass vasodi-latory shock were exquisitely sensitive to the pressor effect of vasopressin. The dose of vasopressin administered to these patients, 0.1 U/min, is one fourth to one ninth that administered to cirrhotics for the control of bleeding esophageal varices with minimal (<15 mm Hg) effect on arterial pressure.[32] This dose provides a steady state plasma concentration of greater than 150 pg/mL,[25] comparable to levels previously reported after CPB.[23] We observed rapid hemodynamic responses despite the absence of a loading dose, and in several patients vasopressin administration could be subsequently decreased to 0.01 U/min with maintenance of blood pressure without catecholamine pressor support. The high sensitivity to low doses of vasopressin suggested a deficiency of the hormone, and we in fact found that plasma levels were inappropriately low for the degree of hypotension in the majority of our LVAD patients, consistent with a defect in baroreflex-mediated secretion (Fig. 1). However, subjects with moderately elevated levels also responded to the hormone (Fig. 2), suggesting a relative deficiency in this group as well.

The mechanism(s) contributing to vasopressin deficiency in LVAD and heart transplant recipients are the subject of speculation. First, autonomic failure is well known to cause vasopressin deficiency[33] and hypersensitivity.[11] Sympathetic function appears to be impaired in some patients after CPB,[34,35] and congestive heart failure may contribute to this dysfunction by down-regulating adrenergic receptors. Second, strong vasopressin secretogogues, such as extreme hyperosmolality, are known to deplete hypothalamic and neurohypophyseal stores of the hormone.[36,37] CPB is a potent stimulus to vasopressin secretion, and patients with end-stage heart failure and excessive preoperative baroreflex-mediated release of vasopressin could be at greater risk for exhaustion of hormone stores.

The mechanism(s) by which AVP acts as a pressor in patients resistant to catecholamines are not clear, but a number of intriguing possibilities exist. Vasodilatory shock after CPB is likely due to pathologic activation of several vasodilator mechanisms. Interleukin-1–dependent nitric oxide is elevated in inflammatory states and atrial natriuretic peptide (ANP) is increased after CPB, and both promote vasodilation through increased levels of intracellular cyclic guanine monophosphate (cGMP).[38,39] Also, K_{ATP} channels of vascular smooth muscle are activated by tissue hypoxia and hypoperfusion (and presumably by CPB), and this activation causes vasodilation by inducing cellular hyperpolarization and inhibiting voltage-gated calcium channels.[40] Both catecholamines and AVP affect vasoconstriction by increasing intracellular calcium levels in vascular smooth muscle through activation of voltage-gated calcium channels, and the activation of vasodilator pathways could impair this calcium-dependent mechanism. However, in contrast to catecholamines, AVP also inhibits the production of cGMP by interleukin-1 and by ANP,[41,42] and inhibits the K_{ATP} channel of vascular smooth muscle.[40] Thus, the efficacy of AVP as a pressor in a variety of clinical scenarios in which catecholamines are ineffective may rest on its ability to specifically counteract pathologically activated vasodilatory mechanisms. This hypothesis may also explain the restoration of catecholamine sensitivity, which we have frequently observed after AVP administration.

Summary

Vasodilatory hypotension is a frequent complication of CPB in patients with end-stage heart failure who are undergoing LVAD insertion or heart transplantation.

An increased risk of post-bypass vasodilatory hypotension has also been observed in patients with heart failure who are not undergoing cardiac replacement therapy. Although the pathogenetic mechanisms are not completely understood, relative or absolute vasopressin deficiency appears to be an important characteristic of this condition. We have found that physiologic replacement doses of AVP are effective in reversing this pathologic vasodilatory state, in restoring mean arterial pressure, and in reducing the requirement for catecholamine pressor agents. Although compelling, our results must be considered preliminary in the absence of a clinical outcome trial. Accordingly, a large-scale controlled trial of AVP for the treatment of vasodilatory shock after CPB is currently under way.

References

1. Moat NE, Shore DF, Evans TW. Organ dysfunction and cardiopulmonary bypass: The role of complement and complement regulatory proteins. *Eur J Cardiothorac Surg* 1993; 7(11):563–573.
2. Yiu P, Robin J, Pattison CW. Reversal of refractory hypotension with single-dose methylene blue after coronary artery bypass surgery. *J Thorac Cardiovasc Surg* 1999;118:195–197.
3. Kirklin JK. Prospects for understanding and eliminating the deleterious effects of cardiopulmonary bypass. *Ann Thorac Surg* 1991;51:529–531.
4. Cowley AW Jr, Monos E, Guyton AC. Interaction of vasopressin and the baroreceptor reflex system in the regulation of arterial blood pressure in the dog. *Circ Res* 1974;34: 505–514.
5. Brooks V. Vasopressin and ANG II in the control of ACTH secretion and arterial and atrial pressures. *Am J Physiol* 1989;256:R339-R347.
6. Bertelstone HJ, Nasmyth PA. Vasopressin potentiation of catecholamine actions in the dog, rat, cat, and rat aortic strip. *Am J Physiol* 1965;208:754–762.
7. Monos E, Koltay E, Kovach AGB. Adrenal blood flow and corticosteroid secretion: Effect of vasopressin on blood circulation and corticosteroid secretion in the dog before and after acute hypophysectomy. *Acta Physiol Hung* 1967;31:149–157.
8. Aylward PE, Floras JS, Leimbach WN, Abboud FM. Effects of vasopressin on the circulation and its baroreflex control in healthy men. *Circulation* 1986;73:1145–1154.
9. Rocha E, Silva M Jr, Rosenberg M. Release of vasopressin in response to hemorrhage and its role in the mechanism of blood pressure regulation. *J Physiol (Lond)* 1969;202:535–557.
10. Carp H, Vadhera R, Jayaram A, Garvey D. Endogenous vasopressin and renin-angiotensin systems support blood pressure after epidural block in humans. *Anesthesiology* 1994;80: 1000–1007.
11. Wagner HN Jr, Braunwald E. The pressor effect of the antidiuretic principle of the posterior pituitary in orthostatic hypotension. *J Clin Invest* 1956;35:1412–1418.
12. Puritz R, Lightman SL, Wilcox CS, et al. Blood pressure and vasopressin in progressive autonomic failure. *Brain* 1983;106:503–511.
13. Landry DW, Levin HR, Gallant EM. Vasopressin deficiency contributes to the vasodilatation of septic shock. *Circulation* 1997;95:1122–1125.
14. Landry DW, Levin HR, Gallant EM, et al. Vasopressin pressor hypersensitivity in vasodilatory shock. *Crit Care Med* 1997;25:1279–1282.
15. Argenziano M, Choudhri AF, Moazami N, et al. A prospective randomized trial of arginine vasopressin in the treatment of vasodilatory shock after left ventricular assist device placement. *Circulation* 1997;96(suppl):II286-II290.
16. Argenziano M, Choudhri AF, Landry DW. A novel approach to the treatment of vasodilatory shock after cardiac transplantation. *Circulation* 1997;96(suppl):I371.
17. Argenziano M, Chen JM, Choudhri AF, et al. Management of vasodilatory shock after cardiac surgery: Identification of predisposing factors and use of a novel pressor agent. *J Thorac Cardiovasc Surg* 1998;116:973–980.
18. Nambi P, Whitman M. Vascular vasopressin receptors mediate inhibition of beta adrenergic receptor-induced cyclic AMP accumulation. *J Pharmacol Exp Ther* 1986;237:143–146.

19. Philbin DM, Coggins CH. Plasma vasopressin levels during cardiopulmonary bypass with and without profound haemodilution. *Can Anaesth Soc* 1978;25:282–285.
20. Philbin DM, Coggins CH. Plasma antidiuretic hormone levels in cardiac surgical patients during morphine and halothane anaesthesia. *Anaesthesiology* 1978;48:95–98.
21. Wu W-H, Zbuzek VK, Bellevue G. Vasopressin release during cardiac operation. *J Thorac Cardiovasc Surg* 1980;79:83–90.
22. Levine FH, Philbin DN, Kono K, et al. Plasma vasopressin levels and urinary sodium excretion during cardiopulmonary bypass with and without pulsatile flow. *Ann Thorac Surg* 1981;32:63–67.
23. Feddersen K, Aurell M, Delin K, et al. Effects of cardiopulmonary bypass and prostacyclin on plasma catecholamines, angiotensin II and arginine vasopressin. *Acta Anaesthesiol Scand* 1985;29:224–230.
24. Agnoletti G, Scotti C, Panzali AF, et al. Plasma levels of atrial natriuretic factor (ANF) and urinary excretion on ANF, arginine vasopressin and catecholamines in children with congenital heart disease: Effect of cardiac surgery. *Eur J Cardiothorac Surg* 1993;7:533–539.
25. Mohring J, Glanzer K, Maciel JA Jr, et al. Greatly enhanced pressor response to antidiuretic hormone in patients with impaired cardiovascular reflexes due to idiopathic orthostatic hypotension. *J Cardiovasc Pharmacol* 1980;2:367–376.
26. Lindner KH, Prengel AW, Brinkmann A, et al. Vasopressin administration in refractory cardiac arrest. *Ann Intern Med* 1996;124:1061–1064.
27. Argenziano M, Chen JC, Cullinane S, et al. Arginine vasopressin in the management of vasodilatory shock after cardiac transplantation. *J Heart Lung Transplant* 1999;18:814–817.
28. Kuan P, Messenger JC, Ellestad MH. Transient central diabetes insipidus after aortocoronary bypass operations. *Am J Cardiol* 1983;52:1181–1183.
29. Robinson RO, Pagliero KM. Polyuria after cardiac surgery. *Br Med J* 1970;3:265–266.
30. Egener TH, Comunale ME, Leckie RS. The use of a somatostatin analog in the treatment of refractory hypotension after cardiopulmonary bypass. *J Cardiothorac Vasc Anesth* 1992; 6:458–460.
31. Thaker U, Geary V, Chalmers P, Sheikh F. Low systemic vascular resistance during cardiac surgery: Case reports, brief review, and management with angiotensin II. *J Cardiothorac Vasc Anesth* 1990;4:360–363.
32. Moreau R, Hadengue A, Soupisonechin T, et al. Abnormal pressor response to vasopressin in patients with cirrhosis: Evidence for impaired buffering mechanisms. *Hepatology* 1990; 12:7–12.
33. Zerbe RL, Henry DP, Robertson GL. Vasopressin response to orthostatic hypotension. Etiologic and clinical implications. *Am J Med* 1983;74:265–271.
34. Zeitlhofer J, Asenbaum S, Spiss C, et al. Central nervous system function after cardiopulmonary bypass. *Eur Heart J* 1993;14:885–890.
35. Murphy DA, Armour JA. Influences of cardiopulmonary bypass, temperature, cardioplegia, and topical hypothermia on cardiac innervation. *J Thorac Cardiovasc Surg* 1992; 103:1192–1199.
36. Jones CW, Pickering BT. Comparison of the effects of water deprivation and sodium chloride imbibition on the hormone content of the neurohypophysis of the rat. *J Physiol* 1969;203:449–458.
37. Cooke CR, Wall BM, Jones GV, et al. Reversible vasopressin deficiency in severe hypernatremia. *Am J Kidney Dis* 1993;22:44–52.
38. Beasley D, Cohen RA, Levinsky NG. Interleukin-1 inhibits contraction of vascular smooth muscle. *J Clin Invest* 1989;83:331–335.
39. Winquist RJ, Faison EP, Waldman SA, et al. Atrial natriuretic factor elicits an endothelium-independent relaxation and activates particulate guanylate cyclase in vascular smooth muscle. *Proc Natl Acad Sci U S A* 1984;81:7661–7664.
40. Wakatsuki T, Nakaya Y, Inoue I. Vasopressin modulates K-channel activities of cultured smooth muscle cells from porcine coronary artery. *Am J Physiol* 1992;283:H491-H496.
41. Kusano E, Tian S, Umino T, et al. Arginine vasopressin inhibits interleukin-1-beta-stimulated nitric oxide and cyclic guanosine monophosphate production via the V1 receptor in cultured rat vascular smooth muscle cells. *J Hypertens* 1997;15:627–632.
42. Nambi P, Whitman M, Gessner G, et al. Vasopressin-mediated inhibition of atrial natriuretic factor-stimulated cGMP accumulation in an established smooth muscle cell line. *Proc Natl Acad Sci U S A* 1986;83:8492–8495.

Chapter 10

Left Ventricular Recovery During Left Ventricular Assist Device Support

Johannes Mueller, MD and Roland Hetzer, MD, PhD

Mechanical cardiac assist devices are used mainly in patients with end-stage heart failure in order to stabilize the hemodynamic condition of the patients until a cardiac transplantation can be undertaken.[1,2] Depending on the assist device used, a specific mode of operation is programmed and a cannulation approach selected in order to unload the ventricles.

Several centers have reported that, in selected patients, under special conditions, some hearts with severely impaired cardiac function have the ability to normalize or near normalize when supported by a left ventricular assist device (LVAD). Although this observation is not new, the decision to electively remove the pump without cardiac transplantation has only recently been made.[3,4]

This experience gave rise to more questions than answers, and leads us to ask not only why patients with chronic heart failure can be weaned from the device, but also why other patients do not recover and cannot be weaned. Are there any predictive parameters available prior to LVAD implantation or very soon after device placement that will enable us to ascertain whether the hearts might recover? Questions even arose about the pathophysiologic nature of heart failure, its reversibility, the significance of so-called "familial cardiomyopathies," and also about active or chronic myocarditis. Although our experience is insufficient to definitively answer these questions, these issues are the subject of many research projects worldwide.

In reality, patients almost always receive their LVAD as a bridge to transplantation, and only after they have been on the device for several weeks can a decision about weaning be made. Even after LVAD explantation, the uncertainty of how long the improved cardiac performance may last persists.

History of Weaning from Mechanical Cardiac Support

The first patients to be weaned from mechanical cardiac support were those with postcardiotomy shock, acute myocarditis, a short history of cardiac failure, or

From Goldstein DJ and Oz MC (eds). *Cardiac Assist Devices*. Armonk, NY: Futura Publishing Co., Inc.; ©2000.

acute graft failure after cardiac transplantation.[5,6] It seemed plausible that this approach was successful because of appropriate treatment of acute single-organ failure,[7,8] particularly in the patients with myocarditis.

In our experience, every patient with idiopathic dilated cardiomyopathy (IDC) who needs LVAD placement is a potential candidate for weaning from LVAD, since predictive factors that discriminate among patients who might later be weaned are lacking. Numerous factors appear to be important and become apparent throughout the period of LVAD support.

Implantation and Perioperative Management

The inflow cannula of the LVAD is attached to the left ventricular apex with an epicardial sewing ring.[9,10] There is a degree of freedom as to where the suture ring should be placed and how it should be attached; however, a position should be selected that is far enough away from the coronary arteries to avoid injury. In addition, the sutures are placed to minimize damage to myocardial tissue and to avoid the loss of viable myocardium.

Following the placement of LVADs, right heart dysfunction, if present, is managed with use of inotropic support, nitric oxide, and tri-iodothyronine (T_3) to reduce right ventricular afterload and to increase right ventricular performance.[11-16] We routinely administer nitric oxide at 40 ppm and T_3 20 μg as a bolus for approximately 10 minutes before starting the pump, and thereafter 1 μg/h for 3 days independently of body weight and preoperative thyroid hormone level.

Dependent on type of LVAD used and the mode of operation chosen, several degrees of left ventricular unloading can be achieved. The demand for maximal pump output leads to the maximal possible left ventricular unloading with the consequently low intraventricular volume and pressure. Under the condition of elevated central venous pressure and right ventricular volume, an interventricular septum shift into the left ventricle frequently occurs. The physiologic cardiac geometry of a banana-shaped right ventricle is transformed to a banana-shaped left ventricle. Therefore, we try to adjust the LVAD output under echocardiographic control to a level that avoids this deleterious reshaping of the right ventricle. This is in contrast to the usual goal of maximizing the pump output in LVAD patients.

This pump adjustment, together with inotropic support, adequate volume loading, and the administration of nitric oxide and T_3, leads to the optimization of right ventricular performance. All other perioperative measures for treating patients after pump implantation do not differ from the well established and frequently published treatment of these patients.

Medical Therapy

After patients have left the intensive care unit and are hemodynamically and physically stabilized, aggressive medical treatment of heart failure is initiated. This includes β-blockers, angiotensin-converting enzyme (ACE) inhibitors, digitalis, low-dose loop diuretics, electrolytes, trace elements, and a cocktail of antioxidants and enzymes.[17-25] This medical regimen is aimed at attaining afterload reduction, a moderate heart rate, volume restriction, oxidative stress compensation, and increased fibrinolysis. Although the efficacy of antioxidants and enzymes remains unproven, in our early experience this nutritional supplementation reduces the number of infections and possibly the number of thromboembolic events. Furthermore, this approach may support the ability of the heart to recover and to remain stable.

Autoantibodies Directed Against the β_1-Adrenoceptor

Autoantibodies directed against the β_1-adrenoreceptor (A-β_1-AABs) were first detected in patients with Chagas' disease.[26] We have found pathologic ranges of the antibody in approximately 80% of our patients with end-stage IDC and in all patients who required circulatory assistance,[3,27–31] although these levels decrease dramatically while the patient is on device support. Since we hypothesize that the presence of A-β_1-AABs results from an inflammatory myocardial process, the disappearance of the autoantibodies may represent resolution of the inflammation. Indeed, in 23% of mechanically supported LVAD patients, cardiac function recovered to near normal levels concomitant with a gradual disappearance of A-β_1-AABs (Fig. 1).

Although the pathophysiologic role of the A-β_1-AABs for induction, maintenance, or progression of IDC remains unproven, in vitro receptor and animal studies suggest that A-β_1-AABs contribute to the progressive deterioration of cardiac function in patients with IDC. Findings that affinity-purified A-β_1-AABs from sera of IDC patients increased the spontaneous beating rate of isolated cultured cardiomyocytes and that this positive chronotropic effect was selectively blocked by β_1-adrenoceptor antagonists indicate that A-β_1-AABs express their effect via the β_1-adrenoceptor cascade.[32,33] In these experiments, their stimulating effect lasted for an excess of 6 hours, while stimulation with β_1-adrenergic agonists such as isoproterenol induced a down-regulation of the β_1-adrenoceptors within 1 hour.[34] Therefore, a chronic

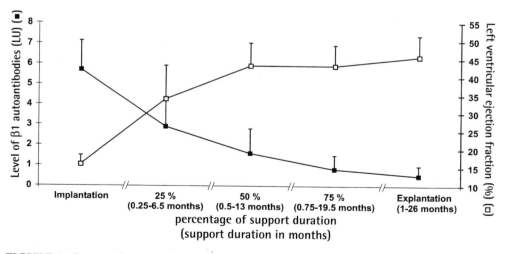

FIGURE 1. Course of autoantibodies directed against the β_1-adrenoceptor and ejection fraction. As the level of antibodies decreases over time (weekly measurements), left ventricular ejection fraction improves.

adrenergic-like stimulation by A-β_1-AABs that may further induce myocardial inflammation can be assumed, such as in the case of high-frequency stimulation by a pacemaker in animal experiments. In contrast to the effect of adrenergic stimulation, which induces a well known reduction of β-adrenoceptor density, the chronic stimulation of the heart by A-β_1-AABs does not lead to a down-regulation of the β_1-adrenoceptors.[35]

Detection of the A-β_1-AABs is performed by a bioassay, the details of which have been previously published. The underlying principle is the measurement of the chronotropic effect of A-β_1-AABs on primary cultures of neonatal rat cardiomyocytes. The increase in the number of contractions after addition of the immunoglobulin G (IgG) fraction prepared from the patients' serum is defined and scaled as LU (laboratory units). Values below 1.5 LU are considered negative, and values above 3.0 LU are positive.[36]

Cardiac Performance Following LVAD Implantation

Echocardiography is selected for the assessment of cardiac performance, as it is a noninvasive, easy, and frequently applicable method. All examinations are performed by the same operator. Left ventricular intracavitary dimensions in diastole (LVIDd) are measured by motion mode, while left ventricular ejection fraction (LVEF) is calculated from two reliable orthogonal views that use the biplanar Simpson's rule approach.[37] Studies are conducted once a week post device implantation. With a regularly running pump, if LVEF and LVIDd reveal normalization of cardiac function (LVEF 40% to 45%) and dimension (LVIDd 55 mm), the pump is set at the lowest possible pumping frequency. Eventually, the pump is stopped in order to evaluate the heart without mechanical support. To prevent thrombus formation inside the pump, 10,000 international units (IU) of heparin is administered before stopping the pump. Additionally, the device is allowed to pump once a minute.[3,38]

Since no completely load-independent index to appropriately measure the contractile state exists, our selected parameters have limitations.[39] LVEF measurements are load-dependent, but they are widely used and reproducible across centers.[40-43] To assess whether the observed increase in LVEF in the treatment group might be caused by afterload reduction instead of an improvement in the contractile state, the meridional end-systolic wall stress is calculated using cuff systolic blood pressure in a generally accepted and invasively validated formula according to Pouseille's law.[44-46]

The impact of preload changes on LVEF is difficult to assess. However, considering the significant reduction in LVIDd as well as an absence of significant changes in transmitral peak E wave velocity and E/A ratio throughout the follow-up period, a significant contribution of preload changes to the increase in LVEF cannot be justifiably assumed either.[47,48] Although echocardiography enables the measurement of innumerable other parameters, including wall motion velocity, which may contribute to a general picture of cardiac performance, LVEF and LVIDd seem sufficient to assess the process of reverse remodeling.

Pump Adjustment Following Improvement

If prolonged unloading of the ventricle leads to enhanced development of myocardial fibrosis, an appropriate adjustment of the pumping mode to the extent allow-

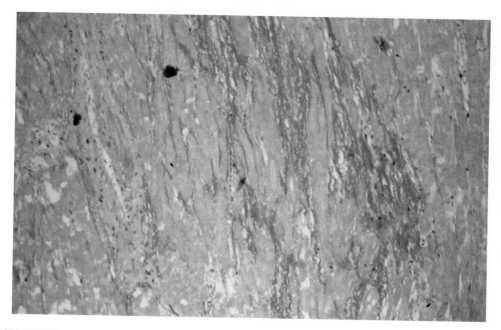

CHAPTER 10, FIGURE 3. Histology of myocardial specimens taken at the time of device placement shows 27% fibrosis (Carstair's fibrosis staining technique ×400).

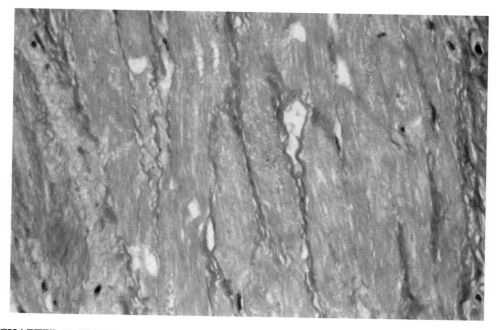

CHAPTER 10, FIGURE 4. Histology of myocardial specimens taken at the time of device removal reveals 19% fibrosis (Carstair's fibrosis staining technique ×400).

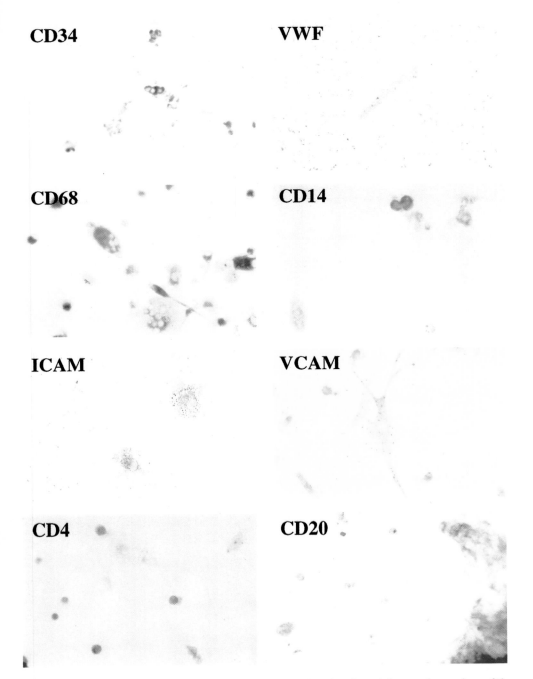

CHAPTER 23, FIGURE 4. Cellular blood elements and molecules arising on the surface of the HeartMate textured surface. CD34 = marker for pluripotent stem cell; CD6 = marker for activated macrophage; VWF = von Willebrand factor; CD14 = marker for monocyte; ICAM = intercellular adhesion molecule; VCAM = vascular cell adhesion molecule; CD4 = marker for T cells; CD20 = marker for activated B cells. Courtesy of Talia Spanier, MD, Columbia University.

able by the individual pump settings seems a valuable adjunct to optimizing the recovery process. Whereas early postoperative maximal unloading of the left ventricle is the goal of every pump, chronically loading the heart may have benefits thereafter. To reach this goal, the Novacor (Baxter Healthcare Corp., Oakland, CA) device must be adjusted to the fill-to-empty or synchronized modes (depending on the volume status of the patient), and the TCI HeartMate VE (Thermo Cardiosystems, Woburn, MA) to the automatic mode.[49] Loading of the heart can be achieved with the Novacor device by installing a longer eject delay or by adjusting the device to a fixed rate mode. The HeartMate device has to be switched to the fixed rate mode.

Running a pump in a fixed rate mode randomly leads to a synchronization of the heart and the pump and, thereby, to ventricular unloading, but in phases of asynchrony between the heart and the device, the heart can be extremely loaded. Our investigations have revealed that an optimal unloaded left ventricle (Novacor, synchronized mode) develops pressure values of between 40 mm Hg and 60 mm Hg. However, a loaded ventricle with a pumping rate of 50 bpm produces various pressure values between 40 mm Hg and 180 mm Hg. The provision of an adjustment choice seems appropriate for patients who are potential candidates for device removal. Thus, a mode switch to fixed rate pumping is instituted and a step-by-step reduction from approximately 90 bpm to the lowest possible rate of 50 bpm by weekly increments of 10 bpm is undertaken. The Novacor device offers the possibility of prolonging step-by-step ejection delay, which also increases the afterload. More sophisticated possibilities of pump adjustment for increasing afterload are desirable but are not available in currently available devices. Of course, a low pumping rate requires the appropriate anticoagulation for the patient.

Device Explantation

The device explantation procedure is an important part of the weaning process and is key to the successful maintenance of long-term cardiac function. Following administration of heparin (10,000 U), the pump is turned off for approximately 30 minutes. During this time, and until the end of the procedure, continuous transesophageal echocardiography is performed. Once hemodynamic stability is confirmed, the explantation begins by opening the pocket that contains the device and ligating both the inflow and outflow conduits from below the diaphragm in patients with a Novacor device, and via an additional left thoracotomy to the inflow cannula in patients with Thermo Cardiosystems devices. With this technique, the rigid apical portion of the inflow cannula remains in the left ventricle and the aortic part of the outflow cannula also remains in place.[3,49,50]

Based on our past (and painful) experience, we have developed strict rules for the treatment of patients during device removal that aim to leave the heart as undisturbed as possible. The underlying concept is that myocytes, during the time of unloading, have developed some degree of atrophy and are extremely sensitive to catecholamines.[51,52] Therefore, the transition from an unloaded heart to a loaded one should proceed as smoothly as possible to avoid myocyte destruction. For this reason, we avoid extracorporeal circulation and refrain from using inotropes. Furthermore, great care is taken in restricting volume loading, aiming for a central venous pressure of between 1 and 4 mm Hg. The same principles are applied to blood pressure control. We accept low blood pressures (50 mm Hg) for a period of 1 hour or even longer, since it has been shown that blood pressure decreases with pump stoppage but recovers without intervention within 1 hour. We sometimes administer ACE inhibitors and β-blockers within hours of surgery to keep blood pressure and heart rate acceptably low.

Follow-Up After Device Removal

As soon as possible after surgery, heart failure medications (which had been administered prior to device removal) are restarted to maintain blood pressure and, hence, left ventricular afterload and heart rate at as low a rate as possible (blood pressure 100 mm Hg, resting heart rate 55 bpm). Transthoracic echocardiography is performed daily or every other day. No exercise testing or myocardial oxygen consumption tests are performed for the first 2 to 3 postoperative months.

Two to 3 weeks after device removal, the patients are discharged home. Thereafter, weekly outpatient visits are used to repeat echocardiographic examination and to adjust heart failure regimen. After the first month, the visits are reduced to once monthly and, thereafter, to four to six visits per year as long as cardiac performance remains stable.

Experiences and Observations

The experiences described in this section are the result of evolving observations made while dealing with an increasing number of patients. In our early experience, we believed that maximal unloading of the left heart over as long a period as possible would result in the most optimal recovery of cardiac function. A detailed analysis of this early data, however, revealed that this approach was not satisfactory.

In early 1995, we first explanted an LVAD from a patient with IDC who had received a device 5 months earlier. During the support time, the patient showed a rapid return to normal echocardiographic values for ventricular dimensions and for ventricular ejection fraction, as demonstrated by repeated short periods of LVAD cessation. In our initial report we referred to this patient and to four others who successively underwent the same procedure.[3] As of this writing, 24 patients have undergone explantation out of a total population of 105 patients who have received implantable devices since 1995. In the weaned patients, the mean left ventricular diastolic diameter decreased from 76 mm at the time of device insertion to 55 mm after removal, and increased again to 58 mm in patients who exhibited long-term stable cardiac function after a cumulative follow-up of 32 patient-years. Two months after device implantation, the diameter had reached a mean of 43 mm. Mean LVEF rose from 16% to 46% after device removal, and remained at that level in the long-term stable patients.

Of the 24 explanted patients, 14 have enjoyed stable cardiac performance without any signs of deterioration of echocardiographic data. Cardiac stability has now been observed for 3 months to 4.5 years and, in four patients, for longer than 3 years. Seven patients suffered a recurrence of heart failure after 4 to 24 months following pump explantation. One patient was supported with a paracorporeal LVAD (Berlin

Heart) as a bridge to transplantation and another five patients underwent transplantation without intervening reinstitution of mechanical support. Four patients succumbed from causes unrelated to heart failure.

Comparison between patients who remained stable and those who developed recurrent heart failure revealed statistically significant differences in the following parameters: 1) duration of heart failure prior to device placement (2 versus 9 years); 2) time required on device support to reach criteria for explantation (120 versus 301 days); 3) left ventricular diastolic diameter (50 versus 59 mm), LVEF (49% versus 40%) at the time of explantation; and 4) LVEF 2 months after explantation (47% versus 36%).[3,49,50]

An interesting finding was the relationship between the duration of cardiac unloading and the improvement of cardiac performance. Improvement of LVEF and diameter advanced stepwise over time until a maximum of performance was reached. This "optimal value" was not improved with further length of mechanical support. On the contrary, the longer the unloading of the ventricle, the more the cardiac performance decreased (Fig. 2). This was most dramatically seen in patients who remained on the device for prolonged periods of time (more than 6 months) and who finally underwent cardiac transplantation. At the time of transplantation, their cardiac performance had approached that seen before LVAD placement even though they had exhibited an intervening period of improvement. Therefore, we believe that long-term unloading is a major contributing factor to myocardial fibrosis (Fig. 3).[51,52] We speculate that a mode of pump operation designed to maximally unload the left ventricle may be the reason for the increased myocardial fibrosis seen

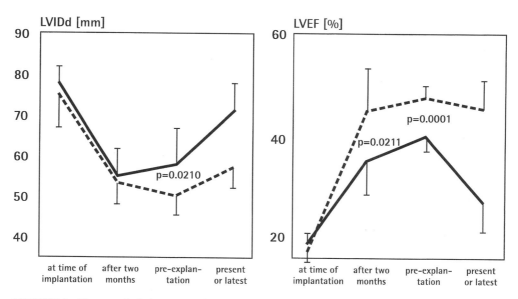

FIGURE 2. Changes in left ventricular internal diameter in diastole (LVIDd) and left ventricular ejection fraction (LVEF) during the time on assist device. The dashed line corresponds to the group of patients who exhibited long-term stable cardiac function and size while the bold line represents the group with recurrent heart failure. Additionally, the described reduction of mean LVEF and increase in mean LVIDd between the 2-month value and the time of device removal is apparent.

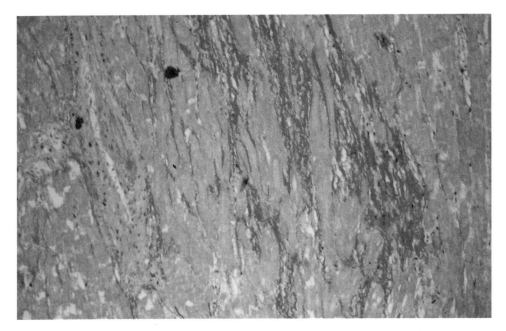

FIGURE 3. Histology of myocardial specimens taken at the time of device placement shows 27% fibrosis (Carstair's fibrosis staining technique ×400). See color plate.

at the time of transplantation. Indeed, in our population of patients, we observed a mean increase in myocardial fibrosis of 7% for patients whose devices were adjusted to maximum unloading (synchronized mode with the Novacor device, maximum left ventricular pressure 60 mm Hg or automatic mode with the Thermo Cardiosystems device). In contrast, patients whose devices were set for maximal loading (lowest possible fixed rate mode for Novacor, and left ventricular pressure between 40 mm Hg and 180 mm Hg for the Thermo Cardiosystems device), a mean decrease of 11% in myocardial fibrosis was documented (Fig. 4). The fact that a certain degree of intraventricular pressure is necessary for a balanced myocardial metabolism has been described.[53]

Timing of Device Explantation

Based on our findings, two periods in the post-implantation phase appear to be critical for successful device explantation. The first period, which must not be missed, is the moment when maximal left ventricular decompression should be abandoned for an increase in cardiac loading. According to our experience, this occurs approximately 2 to 3 months after LVAD placement, at which time echocardiographic examinations reveal a sufficient degree of improvement or when A-β_1-AABs are no longer detectable in the LVAD recipient's serum. Figure 2 shows the relationship between antibody titers and improvement in LVEF over time, as well as the mean moment of disappearance of these antibodies in the 24 weaned patients.

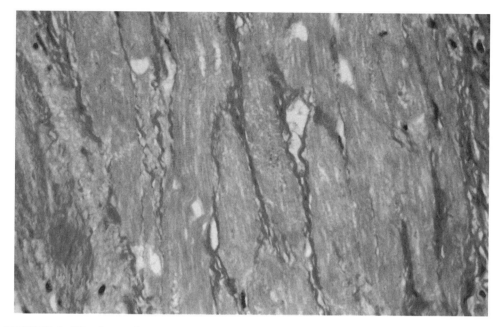

FIGURE 4. Histology of myocardial specimens taken at the time of device removal reveals 19% fibrosis (Carstair's fibrosis staining technique ×400). See color plate.

While optimal coronary perfusion and unloading of the left ventricle are of paramount importance in the early postoperative period, to reduce myocardial inflammation and ischemia, the later disappearance of A-β_1-AABs signals the disappearance of the inflammatory process. From this moment on, optimization of cardiac function by gradual loading should be pursued if myocardial fibrosis is to be averted and device explantation is desired. The pump should be switched to a mode of low loading with the aim of reaching maximum loading within 3 to 4 weeks.

The second critical period is marked by device removal, which should be entertained only if the above mentioned criteria are reached while the device is set to maximal loading. Our experience demonstrates that if criteria for explantation are not reached at the time of maximum loading, then the likelihood of reaching them thereafter is very low.

A distinct example of this approach was seen in a patient with familial dilated cardiomyopathy, a condition that was not thought to be amenable to device weaning. The patient in question is a 43-year-old man with a 6-year history of heart failure who underwent Novacor implantation in 1997. His brother had undergone cardiac transplantation at the age of 25 years. At the time of implantation, echocardiography revealed an LVEF of 15% and an LVIDd of 83 mm. He was documented to have a pathologic level of A-β_1-AABs (6.4 LU). After 60 days of mechanical support, A-β_1-AABs became undetectable, and 80 days after device placement he underwent device removal. His LVEF had increased to 49% and LVIDd had shrunken to 55 mm. Since that time, he has enjoyed stable cardiac function (LVEF 42%, LVIDd 59 mm) and has returned to work.

Are There Any Predictive Parameters for Successful Weaning?

Although many groups worldwide are involved in the search for reliable, reproducible, and easily measurable parameters that will make possible the classification of those patients who will be eligible for weaning prior to implantation of an assist device, to date there are no convincing data that will enable such a prediction. We have revealed that younger patients with shorter histories of heart failure, with a low degree of myocardial fibrosis, and with a faster recovery on mechanical support have a higher probability of successful weaning. This information, however, is difficult to translate into clinical practice when trying to make a decision regarding implantation. In our view, all patients who undergo device placement as a bridge to transplantation are potential candidates for weaning without any certainty of reaching this goal.

Many serum markers have been shown to be pathologically altered at the time of device implantation, and are subsequently improved or normalized at the time of device removal. These include tumor necrosis factor-α, metalloproteinases II and IX, metallothionine, β-receptor density and responsiveness, apoptosis, atrial natriuretic factor, nitric oxide synthase, interleukin-6, and annexin I, II, IV, and VI.[54–72] However, all these parameters are not predictive in determining the reversibility of cardiac malfunction pre-implantation. Rather, they are markers of chronic overload, sympathetic nervous system hyperactivity, and, most likely, secondary phenomena of the disease. These parameters can, however, discriminate patients with reverse remodeling from those who remain dilated, even after mechanical decompression has been instituted.

Conclusions

In contrast to other groups who are more skeptical with regard to the possibility and success of weaning patients from mechanical support, we strongly believe that weaning patients from an assist device will be part of a general concept for the progressive treatment of heart failure. According to our findings, overcoming the inflammatory state associated with end-stage dilated cardiomyopathy is a precondition for reverse remodeling of cardiac dilation. To achieve this state, we have treated patients who have dilated cardiomyopathy with immunoadsorption to remove the inflammatory autoantibodies.[73] Success with this approach has led us to incorporate immunoadsorption into an evolving concept for the treatment of IDC, which should begin with optimal medical management (Fig. 5). If the medical treatment fails to improve cardiac status, we institute immunoadsorption if pathologic levels of A-β_1-AABs are demonstrated. If cardiac function cannot be stabilized and if criteria for heart transplantation are met, the patient is placed on the waiting list for transplantation. If further deterioration occurs before a donor becomes available, then mechanical support is instituted with the hope of reversing the ongoing cardiac impairment. If improvement does not supervene, the assist system remains a valuable bridge to transplantation.

Our approach to the patient with end-stage IDC can be summarized as follows: 1) if the decision to insert an LVAD is made, the implantation should be undertaken

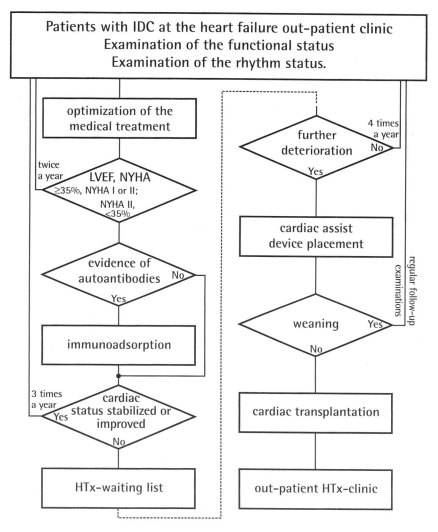

FIGURE 5. Scheme for the progressive treatment of patients with end-stage idiopathic dilated cardiomyopathy.

as early as possible; the probability of inducing reverse remodeling after device placement decreases with increasing impairment of the preoperative cardiac status; 2) aggressive medical and antioxidative treatment of heart failure should be pursued to enhance the chance of reverse remodeling; 3) to entertain the possibility of explantation, echocardiographic studies performed by two independent operators with the pump off should document LVEF and LVIDd of at least 50% and 55 mm, respectively; 4) after a loading period of the left ventricle by gradual device adjustment, explantation should be done as early as possible once the above criteria have been met; further unloading does not contribute to additional improvement and may, in fact, be deleterious; 5) the explantation procedure should be done without inotropic support or cardioplegia, and with a minimum volume load; 6) an antifailure medical regimen should be continued soon after device removal; 7) exercise testing should be postponed for the first 2 to 3 months after device removal; and 8) thorough routine outpatient monitoring including echocardiographic studies should be undertaken.

Summary

This chapter documents our experience with a cohort of 24 patients with IDC who underwent successful LVAD explantation. We have described how to identify potentially suitable patients for the weaning procedure, how to optimize ventricular recovery, assess recovery, institute the weaning process, perform the explantation procedure, and manage the patients after explantation.

The patients reported here were all implanted as a rescue therapy and with the initial intention of bridging to cardiac transplantation. Our experience suggests that reverse remodeling and bridge to recovery are promising options for the treatment of advanced heart failure. Although the approach was not successful in the long term in all weaned patients, the waiting time on the transplant list was bridged with a low risk for unexpected events, which, in contrast, may happen in patients who are mechanically supported for extended periods prior to transplantation (ie, thromboembolism, infection, device malfunction). The time saved for patients after device explantation and before heart failure recurs is a gain in life time.

Having demonstrated that LVAD support is capable of reversing the cardiomyopathic disease in some patients, our next goal is to define the subgroup of patients with IDC that is most likely to be successfully weaned. While some parameters can be identified to play a role in the worsening process of cardiac dilation, they appear to be markers rather than causative factors for the disease. It is therefore not surprising that during the process of reverse remodeling, these parameters improved or normalized. Although a better understanding of the prospect of myocardial recovery from IDC has been gained and some clinical success has been achieved with chronic ventricular unloading, no reliable predictors have been discerned to foretell long-lasting cardiac recovery.

References

1. Hunt S, Frazier OH, Myers TJ, et al. Mechanical circulatory support and cardiac transplantation. *Circulation* 1998;97:2079–2090.
2. Goldstein DJ, Oz MC, Rose EA. Implantable left ventricular assist devices. *N Engl J Med* 1998;339:1522–1533.
3. Müller J, Wallukat G, Weng YG, et al. Weaning from mechanical cardiac support in patients with idiopathic dilated cardiomyopathy. *Circulation* 1997;96(2):542–549.
4. Nakatani T, Sasako Y, Kumon K, et al. Long-term circulatory support to promote recovery from profound heart failure. *ASAIO J* 1995;41:M526-M530.
5. DeBakey ME. Left ventricular bypass for cardiac assistance. *Am J Cardiol* 1971;27:3–10.
6. Pennington DG, Samuels LD, Williams G, et al. Experience with the Pierce-Donachy ventricular assist device in postcardiotomy patients in cardiogenic shock. *World J Surg* 1985; 9:37–46.
7. Marelli D, Laks H, Amsel B, et al. Temporary mechanical support with the BVS 5000 assist device during treatment of acute myocarditis. *J Card Surg* 1997;12:55–58.

8. Parillo JE. Myocarditis: How should we treat in 1998? *J Heart Lung Transplant* 1998,17:941–944.
9. McCarthy PM, Sabik JE. Implantable circulatory support devices as a bridge to heart transplantation. *Semin Thorac Cardiovasc Surg* 1994;6:174–180.
10. Frazier OH. The development of an implantable, portable, electrically powered left ventricular assist device. *Semin Thorac Cardiovasc Surg* 1994;6:181–187.
11. Salamonsen RF, Kaye D, Esmore DS. Inhalation of nitric oxide provides selective pulmonary vasodilation, aiding mechanical cardiac assist with the Thoratec left ventricular assist device. *Anaesth Intensive Care* 1994;22:209–210.
12. Argenziano M, Choudhri AF, Moazami N, et al. Randomized, double blind trial of inhaled nitric oxide in LVAD recipients with pulmonary hypertension. *Ann Thorac Surg* 1998;65:340–345.
13. Wagner F, Dandel M, Gunther G. Nitric oxide inhalation in the treatment of right ventricular dysfunction following left ventricular assist device implantation. *Circulation* 1997;96(suppl):II291-II296.
14. Timek T, Bonz A, Dillmann R, et al. The effect of triiodothyronine on myocardial contractile performance after epinephrine exposure: Implications for donor heart management. *J Heart Lung Transplant* 1998;17:931–940.
15. Gomberg-Maitland M, Frishman WH. Thyroid hormone and cardiovascular disease. *Am Heart J* 1998;135:187–196.
16. Malik FS, Mehra MR, Uber PA, et al. Intravenous thyroid hormone supplementation in heart failure with cardiogenic shock. *J Card Fail* 1999;5:31–37.
17. The SOLVD Investigators. Effect of enalapril on survival in patients with reduced left ventricular ejection fractions and congestive heart failure. *N Engl J Med* 1991;325:293–302.
18. Packer M. Effects of beta adrenergic blockade on survival of patients with chronic heart failure. *Am J Cardiol* 1997;80:46L-54L.
19. Waagstein F. Efficacy of beta blockers in idiopathic cardiomyopathy and ischemic cardiomyopathy. *Am J Cardiol* 1997;80:45J-49J.
20. Kukin M, Kalman J, Charney RH, et al. Prospective randomized comparison of effect of long-term treatment with metoprolol or carvedilol on symptoms, exercise, ejection fraction, and oxidative stress in heart failure. *Circulation* 1999;99:2645–2651.
21. Bali AM, Sole MJ. Oxidative stress and the pathogenesis of heart failure. *Cardiol Clin* 1998;16:665–675.
22. Sawyer DB, Colucci WS. Nitric oxide and the failing myocardium. *Cardiol Clin* 1998;16:657–664.
23. Ito K, Akita H, Kanazawa K, et al. Comparison of effects of ascorbic acid on endothelium-dependent vasodilation in patients with chronic congestive heart failure secondary to idiopathic cardiomyopathy versus patients with effort angina pectoris secondary to coronary artery disease. *Am J Cardiol* 1998;82:762–767.
24. Givertz MM, Colucci WS. New targets for heart failure therapy: Endothelin, inflammatory cytokines, and oxidative stress. *Lancet* 1998;352(suppl):S134-S138.
25. Keith M, Geranmayegan A, Sole MJ, et al. Increased oxidative stress in patients with congestive heart failure. *J Am Coll Cardiol* 1998;31:1352–1356.
26. Borda ES, Pascual J, Cossio PM, et al. Circulating IgG in Chagas disease which binds to β adrenoreceptor of myocardium and modulates its activity. *Clin Exp Immunol* 1984;57:679–686.
27. Podlowski S, Luther HP, Morwinski R, et al. Agonistic anti-β1-adrenergic receptor autoantibodies from cardiomyopathy patients reduce the β1-adrenergic receptor expression in neonatal rat cardiomyocytes. *Circulation* 1998;98:2470–2476.
28. Wallukat G, Wollenberger A. Effects of serum gamma globulin fractions of patients with allergic asthma and dilated cardiomyopathy on chronotropic β-adrenoreceptor function in cultured neonatal rat heart myocytes. *Biomed Biochem Acta* 1987;46:634–639.
29. Limas CJ, Goldenberg IF, Limas C. Autoantibodies against beta adrenoreceptors in human dilated cardiomyopathy. *Circ Res* 1989;64:97–103.
30. Krause EG, Bartel S, Beyerdorfer I, Wallukat G. Activation of cyclic-AMP-dependent protein kinase in cardiomyocytes by anti-β1-adrenoreceptor autoantibodies from patients with idiopathic dilated cardiomyopathy. *Blood Press Suppl* 1996;3:37–40.
31. Wallukat G, Kayser A, Wollenberger A. The β1-adrenoreceptor as antigen: Functional aspects. *Eur Heart J* 1995;16:85–88.

32. Magnusson Y, Wallukat G, Waagstein F, et al. Autoimmunity in idiopathic dilated cardiomyopathy. Characterization of antibodies against the beta-1-adrenoreceptor with positive chronotropic effect. *Circulation* 1994;89:2760–2767.

33. Jahns R, Boivin V, Siegmund C, et al. Autoantibodies activating human beta-1-adrenergic receptors in the failing human heart. *Circulation* 1993;87:454–463.

34. Ungerer M, Bohm M, Elce JS, et al. Altered expression of beta-adrenergic receptor kinase and beta1-adrenergic receptors in the failing human heart. *Circulation* 1993;87:454–463.

35. Matsui S, Fu ML, Katsuda S, et al. Peptides derived from cardiovascular G-protein coupled receptors induce morphological cardiomyopathic changes in immunized rabbits. *J Mol Cell Cardiol* 1997;29:641–655.

36. Wallukat G, Wollenberger A, Morwinski R, Pitschner HF. Anti-beta1-adrenoreceptor antibodies with chronotropic activity from serum of patients with dilated cardiomyopathy: Mapping of epitopes in the first and second extracellular loops. *J Mol Cell Cardiol* 1995; 27:397–406.

37. Feigenbaum H. Echocardiographic evaluation of cardiac chambers. In Feigenbaum H (ed): *Echocardiography*. Philadelphia: Lea & Febiger; 1994:134–180.

38. Loebe M, Mueller J, Hetzer R. Ventricular assistance for recovery of heart failure. *Curr Opin Cardiol* 1999;14:234–248.

39. Ross J Jr. Assessment of cardiac function and myocardial contractility. In Alexander RW, Schlant RC, Fuster V (eds): *Hurst's The Heart*. 9th ed. New York: McGraw-Hill; 1998: 727–743.

40. Lejemtel TH, Sonnenblick EH, Frishmann W. Diagnosis and management of heart failure. In Alexander RW, Schlant RC, Fuster V (eds): *Hurst's The Heart*. 9th ed. New York: McGraw-Hill; 1998:745–781.

41. Feigenbaum H. Echocardiographic examination of the left ventricle. *Circulation* 1975;51: 1–7.

42. Feigenbaum H. Echocardiography. In Braunwald E (ed): *Heart Disease*. 4th ed. Philadelphia: W.B. Saunders Co.; 1992:64–115.

43. Vuille C, Weyman AE. Left ventricle I: General considerations, assessment of chamber size and function. In Weyman AE (ed): *Principles and Practice of Echocardiography*. 2nd ed. Philadelphia: Lea & Febiger; 1994:557–624.

44. De Simone G, Devereux RB, Roman MJ, et al. Assessment of left ventricular function by the midwall fractional shortening/end-systolic stress relation in human hypertension. *J Am Coll Cardiol* 1994;23:1444–1451.

45. Reichek N, Wilson J, St. John Sutton M, et al. Noninvasive determination of left ventricular end-systolic stress: Validation of the method and initial application. *Circulation* 1982;65: 99–108.

46. Aurigemma GP, Douglass PS, Gaasch WH. Quantitative evaluation of left ventricular structure, wall stress and systolic function. In Otto CM (ed): *The Practice of Clinical Echocardiography*. Philadelphia: W.B. Saunders Co.; 1997:1–24.

47. Hurrell DG, Nishimura RA, Istrup DM, Appleton CP. Utility of preload alteration in assessment of left ventricular filling pressure by Doppler echocardiography: A simultaneous characterization and Doppler echocardiographic study. *J Am Coll Cardiol* 1997;30: 459–467.

48. Lewis JF. Doppler and two-dimensional echocardiographic evaluation in acute and long-term management of the heart failure patient. In Otto CM (ed): *The Practice of Clinical Echocardiography*. Philadelphia: W.B. Saunders Co.; 1997:433–448.

49. Hetzer R, Mueller J, Weng Y, et al. Cardiac recovery in dilated cardiomyopathy by unloading with a left ventricular assist device. *Ann Thorac Surg* 1999;68:742–749.

50. Hetzer R, Mueller J. Midterm follow-up of patients who had LVAD removal following recovery in end-stage dilated cardiomyopathy. *J Thorac Cardiovasc Surg* 1999. In press.

51. Kinoshita M, Takano H, Taenaka Y, et al. Cardiac disuse atrophy during LVAD pumping. *ASAIO Trans* 1988;34:208–212.

52. Kinoshita M, Takano H, Takaichi S, et al. Influence of prolonged ventricular assistance on myocardial histopathology in the intact heart. *Ann Thorac Surg* 1996;61:640–645.

53. Tomantek RJ, Cooper G. Morphological changes in the mechanically unloaded myocardial cell. *Anat Rec* 1981;200:271–280.

54. Nakatani S, McCarthy PM, Kottke-Marchant K, et al. Left ventricular echocardiographic and histologic changes: Impact of chronic unloading by an implantable ventricular assist device. *J Am Coll Cardiol* 1996;27:894–901.

55. McCarthy PM, Nakatani S, Vargo R, et al. Structural and left ventricular histological changes after implantable LVAD insertion. *Ann Thorac Surg* 1995;59:609–613.

56. Schenin SA, Capek P, Radovancevic B, et al. The effect of prolonged left ventricular support on myocardial histopathology in patients with end-stage cardiomyopathy. *ASAIO J* 1992; 38:M271-M274.

57. Lee SH, Doliba N, Osbakken M, et al. Improvement of myocardial mitochondrial function after hemodynamic support with left ventricular assist devices in patients with heart failure. *J Thorac Cardiovasc Surg* 1998;116:344–349.

58. James KB, McCarthy PM, Thomas JD, et al. Effect of the implantable left ventricular assist device on neuroendocrine activation in heart failure. *Circulation* 1995;92(suppl):II191-II195.

59. James KB, Rodkey S, McCarthy PM, et al. Exercise performance and chronotropic response in heart failure patients with implantable left ventricular assist devices. *Am J Cardiol* 1998; 81:1230–1232.

60. Milting H, Bartling B, Schumann H, et al. Altered levels of mRNA of apoptosis-mediating genes after midterm mechanical ventricular support in dilative cardiomyopathy—first results of the Halle Assist Induced Recovery Study (HAIR). *Thorac Cardiovasc Surg* 1999; 47:48–50.

61. Belland SE, Grunstei R, Jeevanandam V, Eisen HJ. The effect of sustained mechanical support with left ventricular assist devices on myocardial apoptosis in patients with severe dilated cardiomyopathy. *J Heart Lung Transplant* 1998;17:83–84.

62. Dipla K, Mattiello JA, Jeevanandam V, et al. Myocyte recovery after mechanical circulatory support in humans with end-stage heart failure. *Circulation* 1998;97:2316–2322.

63. Hummel M, Czerlinski S, Friedel N, et al. Interleukin-6 and interleukin-8 as predictors of outcome in ventricular assist device patients before heart transplantation. *Crit Care Med* 1994;22:448–454.

64. Goldstein DJ, Moazami N, Seldomridge JA, et al. Circulatory resuscitation with left ventricular assist device support reduces interleukins-6 and 8 levels. *Ann Thorac Surg* 1997;63: 971–974.

65. Mancini D, Beniaminovitz A, Levin HR, et al. Low incidence of myocardial recovery after left ventricular assist device implantation in patients with chronic heart failure. *Circulation* 1998;98:2383–2389.

66. Termuhlen DF, Swartz MT, Pennington DG, et al. Predictors for weaning patients from ventricular assist devices. *ASAIO Trans* 1988;34:131–139.

67. Fujimura M, Komamura K, Sasaki T, et al. Experience of weaning from left ventricular assist system in an acutely ill patient with dilated cardiomyopathy and severe left ventricular dysfunction: A case report. *J Cardiol* 1998;31:31–36.

68. Nakatani T, Sasako Y, Kobayashi J, et al. Recovery of cardiac function by long-term left ventricular support in patients with end-stage cardiomyopathy. *ASAIO J* 1998;44:M516-M520.

69. Altermose GT, Gritsus V, Jeevanandam V, et al. Altered myocardial phenotype after mechanical support in human beings with advanced cardiomyopathy. *J Heart Lung Transplant* 1997;16:756–773.

70. Baba HA, Tjan TDT, August C, et al. Metallothionine is involved in reverse remodeling after prolonged left ventricular assist device support. *J Heart Lung Transplant* 1999;18:20. Abstract.

71. Ogletree-Hughes ML, Barrett-Stull L, Smedira PM, et al. Mechanical unloading restores beta adrenergic responsiveness in the failing human heart. *J Heart Lung Transplant* 1999; 18:22. Abstract.

72. Li YY, Feldman AM, Sun Y, McTiernan CF. Differential expression of tissue inhibitors of metalloproteinases in the failing human heart. *Circulation* 1998;98:1728–1734.

73. Mueller J, Wallukat G, Dandel M, et al. Immunoglobulin adsorption in patients with idiopathic dilated cardiomyopathy. *Circulation* 1999. In press.

Chapter 11

Exercise Performance in Patients with Left Ventricular Assist Devices

Donna Mancini, MD and Ainat Beniaminovitz, MD

Introduction

Physical exercise requires the interaction of the pulmonary, cardiac, vascular, and skeletal muscle systems to meet an increased metabolic demand. Each system, in turn, can limit maximal exercise performance. In normal humans, exercise capacity is primarily limited by the cardiac output response. The metabolic capacity of skeletal muscle and minute ventilation at peak exercise are well below maximal levels.[1,2] In patients with congestive heart failure (CHF), changes occur in the muscles, blood vessels, and lungs that have an impact on exercise performance such that cardiac output is not the sole determinant of peak exercise capacity. This chapter reviews the pathophysiology of exercise in patients with heart failure, and discusses how it is impacted by the insertion of a left ventricular assist device (LVAD).

Measurement of Exercise Capacity

Exercise capacity is best quantified by the measurement of oxygen consumption during exercise using metabolic carts that contain rapidly responding CO_2 and O_2 analyzers. Patients breathe through a specially constructed valve that captures all of the exhaled air and directs it into the metabolic cart. A variety of ventilatory parameters are measured from standard equations. Among these, peak oxygen consumption (VO_2) is the most critical measurement. It provides not only an objective assessment of functional capacity in patients with heart failure but also an indirect assessment of cardiovascular reserve. Oxygen consumption equals the difference between oxygen delivery and oxygen extraction. Oxygen delivery is dependent on cardiac output, pulmonary function, and hemoglobin content. Oxygen extraction relies primarily on the metabolic capacity of skeletal muscle and its ability to vasodilate and to extract oxygen. If patients with normal hemoglobin and lung function

From Goldstein DJ and Oz MC (eds). *Cardiac Assist Devices*. Armonk, NY: Futura Publishing Co., Inc.; ©2000.

exercise maximally, VO_2 will primarily reflect their ability to increase cardiac output.[1,2]

Pathophysiology of Exercise Performance in Heart Failure

Decreased exercise capacity in patients with heart failure has been traditionally attributed to a reduced cardiac output response to exercise that leads to skeletal muscle underperfusion and intramuscular lactic acidosis. In 1981, Weber et al[3] performed exercise hemodynamic measurements and ventilatory gas measurements during progressive treadmill exercise in 40 patients with heart failure. They classified patients into four groups. Class A comprised the least limited patients while the most limited patients were those in Class D. A correlation between worsening heart failure and cardiac output response to exercise became evident. During exercise, a patient with Class D heart failure could increase his or her cardiac output twofold, whereas a normal individual could increase his or her cardiac output response fivefold. Skeletal muscle perfusion during exercise is also reduced, and the reduction parallels the severity of heart failure.

Although peak VO_2 is clearly dependent on the cardiac output response to exercise, patients with similarly reduced left ventricular ejection fractions may display a wide range of exercise capacities. Moreover, acute therapeutic interventions, including the use of positive inotropic agents, acutely enhance exercise hemodynamic measurements yet do not increase exercise capacity.[4,5]

Changes in Arteriolar Vasodilation

Reduced exercise capacity in patients with heart failure may be due to an abnormality in arteriolar vasodilation. Indeed, Zelis et al[6-8] demonstrated that fluid and sodium retention can impair arteriolar vasodilation in humans. Rhythmic handgrip exercises were performed in patients with heart failure (due to rheumatic heart disease) and in control subjects, with measurement of forearm blood flow.[6] In the former, forearm blood flow was reduced at rest and at each level of exercise. Forearm oxygen extraction was increased in heart failure patients as compared to control subjects. As this small muscle mass exercise would not require an increase in cardiac output, it was inferred that the difference in forearm perfusion could not be related to central hemodynamic factors but to changes in local arteriolar vasodilation.

Zelis and colleagues[7] measured the arterial sodium content in the aorta and femoral artery in normal dogs and in a canine model of heart failure produced by rapid ventricular pacing. A significant increase in the arterial sodium content in the heart failure animals was demonstrated. These investigators postulated that arteriolar stiffness from increased salt and water content resulted in an abnormal vasodilatory response in heart failure.

Abnormalities in vasodilation may also result from changes in the vascular endothelium. Endothelial cells produce nitric oxide, which promotes local relaxation of vascular smooth muscle, a process that is attenuated in patients with heart failure.[9,10] Forearm blood flow was measured at rest and during intra-arterial infusions of methacholine in normal subjects and in patients with heart failure. Methacholine releases endothelium-derived relaxing factor through stimulation of muscarinic receptors. Forearm blood flow responses to methacholine were attenuated in heart failure subjects compared to normal subjects. Interestingly, vascular remodeling can occur with chronic heart failure therapy; we and others have demonstrated that the use of angiotensin-converting enzyme (ACE) inhibitors can improve leg blood flow and exercise capacity.[11,12]

Metabolic Abnormalities and Intrinsic Muscle Changes

Intrinsic skeletal muscle changes also contribute to exercise intolerance in heart failure patients.[13–20] Metabolic abnormalities have been described during exercise, by use of phosphorus-31 nuclear magnetic resonance imaging, a technique that permits noninvasive monitoring of phosphocreatine, inorganic phosphate, adenosine triphosphate, and pH in working muscle. During exercise, adenosine diphosphate (ADP) is a key stimulant to mitochondrial oxidative phosphorylation. The inorganic phosphorous-to-phosphocreatine (Pi/PCr) ratio correlates closely with ADP concentration. By monitoring changes in the Pi/PCr ratio at different work levels, alterations in the control of oxidative phosphorylation can be detected. Exercise also activates glycolysis, producing an increase in intracellular lactate concentration and a decrease in intracellular pH. By monitoring changes in muscle pH during exercise, changes in glycolytic activity can be detected. With use of this technology, the metabolic behavior of both the forearm and calf muscle during exercise in patients with heart failure has been examined. Patients with heart failure have a more pronounced increase in the Pi/PCr ratio and a more rapid drop in local pH than do normal subjects performing comparable workloads. These metabolic abnormalities appear to be independent of skeletal muscle ischemia.[14,15]

Muscle biopsy studies in patients with heart failure have also demonstrated histochemical abnormalities including fiber atrophy, a shift in fiber composition with an increase in easily fatigable glycolytic type IIb fibers and a decrease in the fatigue-resistant oxidative type I fibers, reduced oxidative enzymes, and mitochondrial changes.[17–20] A majority of patients with mild to severe heart failure also exhibit generalized muscle atrophy as demonstrated by anthropomorphic measurements and magnetic resonance imaging.[21]

The observation that aerobic training can improve maximal exercise capacity by 15% to 30% in patients with heart failure[22,23] has led to the belief that these intrinsic muscle changes are most likely due to deconditioning. Indeed, exercise training in heart failure patients has resulted in significant elevations in peak cardiac output, peak arteriovenous O_2 difference, and peak leg blood flow. Moreover, heart rate at rest and throughout exercise has been shown to decrease, as has leg lactate production. Notably, leg blood flow during submaximal exercise did not increase, suggesting that the major benefit derived from training was a result of enhanced oxygen extraction by skeletal muscle.[22] Analogously, in a rat infarct model of heart failure, the major benefit derived from training was not from an increase in oxygen delivery, but rather from an increased capacity of the skeletal muscle to extract oxygen.[24] Despite the indisputable benefits of training, the metabolic abnormalities observed with exercise in patients with heart failure, while improved, are not normalized.[25,26]

Additional factors, including caloric protein malnutrition, perturbances in the neuro-hormonal milieu, and chronic skeletal muscle underperfusion, may be implicated in the development of the intrinsic muscle changes typically seen in heart failure patients.

Mechanisms of Dyspnea in Heart Failure

During exercise, patients with heart failure clearly experience a greater sense of dyspnea than do normal subjects at any given workload. Potential mechanisms for dyspnea in heart failure include decreased lung compliance, increased airway resistance, increased ventilatory drive from ventilation/perfusion mismatch and increased CO_2 production, respiratory muscle dysfunction from respiratory weakness and/or ischemia, and intrinsic skeletal muscle changes.

Pulmonary limitations to exercise performance may exist in some heart failure patients. Airflow obstruction may contribute to reduced exercise performance. Bronchial hyper-responsiveness has been described in patients with severely impaired left ventricular function following inhalation of the cholinergic agonist methacholine.[27] The inhalation of the vasoconstrictor agent methoxamine (Vasoxyl, Glaxo Wellcome Inc., Research Triangle Park, NC), which prevents the methacholine-induced bronchial obstruction, significantly improved submaximal and maximal exercise performance in these patients.[28]

An excessive ventilatory response to exercise has consistently been described in patients with heart failure.[1,2] This exaggerated response parallels the increasing severity of CHF and does not appear to be related to acute increases in intrapulmonary pressure.[29] No significant correlation is observed between the ventilatory response to exercise expressed as ventilation normalized by CO_2 production versus peak exercise pulmonary capillary wedge pressure. Moreover, acute therapeutic interventions designed to lower resting and exercise pulmonary capillary wedge pressures do not affect the ventilatory response to exercise.

An increase in pulmonary dead space ventilation appears to be a major factor contributing to the excess ventilatory response observed in heart failure patients. Pulmonary dead space/breath nearly doubles during exercise in patients with heart failure but remains unchanged in normal subjects.[30] The increase in exercise ventilation may result partially from metabolic changes that occur in the working skeletal muscle. Early release of lactic acid will result in an increase in CO_2 production and will thus stimulate ventilation. Aerobic training can delay the onset of the anaerobic threshold and has been successfully used to improve the ventilatory response in these patients.

Dyspnea may be closely related to the neural drive to the respiratory muscles. Increased work of breathing and/or respiratory muscle weakness can cause an increased neural drive, resulting in worsening dyspnea. Recent studies have described an increase in diaphragmatic work with exercise in patients with heart failure, at rest and throughout exercise.[31] Reduced maximal inspiratory and expiratory mouth pressures consistent with respiratory muscle weakness have also been demonstrated.[32]

During exercise, the respiratory muscles may become ischemic.[33] With use of near infrared spectroscopy, a noninvasive technique that is able to quantify muscle oxygenation, accessory respiratory muscle deoxygenation was demonstrated in patients with heart failure, but not in normal subjects. Furthermore, respiratory muscle endurance has also been shown to be reduced in heart failure patients.[34] Therefore, the sensation of dyspnea may be exacerbated in patients with heart failure, as the increased work of breathing has to be performed by weak and underperfused muscles. Selective respiratory muscle training can ameliorate dyspnea and improve exercise performance in these patients.[35]

Use of LVADs in Patients with End-Stage Heart Failure

With the increased referral of patients with end-stage heart failure for cardiac transplantation, and the relatively fixed donor pool, greater numbers of patients with refractory heart failure are undergoing insertion of LVADs as a bridge to transplant.[36–38] This patient population has enabled us to learn about the impact of these devices on exercise capacity in heart failure, both acutely and over time. Later chapters of this text describe in detail the structure, placement, and function of the two most common types of portable (or wearable) LVADs in current use: the HeartMate (Thermo Cardiosystems Inc., Woburn, MA) and Novacor (Baxter Healthcare Corp., Oakland, CA) devices. This discussion focuses on the former device. The pump is implanted preperitoneally. The inflow cannula is inserted into the apex of the left ventricle and the outflow cannula is anastomosed to the ascending aorta. The pump uses a pusher-plate mechanism that can be driven pneumatically or electrically. The chamber capacity is approximately 83 mL. For the pneumatic device, the rate of cycling ranges from 20 to 140 strokes/min. In the electric device, the rate range is from 50 to 120 strokes/min. Maximum device output is approximately 10 L/min. The device can be set at a fixed rate or programmed into an auto mode. This mode is dependent on the function of an internal sensor, which senses blood volume on a beat-to-beat basis. In the auto mode, LVAD filling is dependent on left ventricular preload and, thus, right ventricular function. Native heart rate and LVAD rates are dissociated at rest and with exercise, as the mechanisms driving these two rates are different.

LVAD filling and emptying can occur either in series or in parallel to native cardiac function.[39] If the native left ventricle is not generating adequate pressure to open the native aortic valve, then the circulation of the heart and the device are in series. In this situation, the aortic valve remains closed and cardiac output is derived exclusively from the mechanical device. Indeed, Fick or thermodilution cardiac outputs will equal the measurements derived from the LVAD sensor. If there is some recovery of native left ventricular function such that adequate pressure can be generated to open the native aortic valve, then the circulations become parallel. In this instance, cardiac output is determined from the combined output of the two circulations and, hence, Fick or thermodilution cardiac outputs will exceed the device output.

If sufficient myocardial recovery occurs, the timing of native and device ejection may become more important. The native heart will have a significant increase in afterload if its ejection occurs immediately after device ejection. With the HeartMate device there is no system that allows for synchronous filling and emptying. The

Novacor system has a timing mechanism that uses the electrocardiogram such that synchronous performance of the two pumps can be achieved. Whether synchronous performance can aid in myocardial recovery is unknown at this time. Mueller et al have used a weaning protocol in their LVAD patients that permits synchronous filling and ejecting.[40] In their experience, the rate of recovery of left ventricular function and explantation is higher than we have observed.

Maximal Exercise Capacity in LVAD Patients

Few studies have used measurement of oxygen consumption to examine peak exercise performance in LVAD recipients.[39,41–43] In a preliminary report, Murali et al[42] described peak VO_2 in seven patients who received the Novacor system. Peak VO_2 averaged 16 mL/kg/min. More recently, Jaski et al[41] reported the results of exercise hemodynamic measurements in 10 LVAD patients during supine bicycle exercise; oxygen consumption during supine exercise was 8.2 mL/kg/min, and averaged 14.1 mL/kg/min during upright exercise. Submaximal and maximal exercise performance in 14 patients with the HeartMate device at our institution was compared with that in 20 patients with mild, moderate, and severe heart failure.[43] In LVAD recipients, peak VO_2 averaged 17 mL/kg/min.

Most recently, we compared the hemodynamic response to exercise in 65 patients with moderate to severe heart failure and in 20 LVAD patients.[44] Table 1 shows the rest and exercise hemodynamics for the heart failure and LVAD groups. Peak VO_2 was significantly higher in the LVAD patients than in the heart failure patients, as was the VO_2 at the anaerobic threshold. Hemodynamic measurements at rest and during exercise were significantly improved in patients with devices compared with ambulatory patients with severe heart failure. Exercise capacity, as measured by

Table 1
Rest and Peak Exercise Measurements in CHF and LVAD Patients

	Heart Failure		LVAD	
	Rest	Peak	Rest	Peak
VO_2, mL/kg/min	3.9 ± 0.7	12.1 ± 3.0	4.1 ± 0.5	16.0 ± 3.8*
Heart Rate, bpm	86 ± 16	125 ± 24	95 ± 15	148 ± 24*
MAP, mm Hg	87 ± 1	87 ± 14	94 ± 9*	96 ± 12*
RAP, mm Hg	4 ± 5	11 ± 8	3 ± 3	8 ± 4
PAP, mm Hg	28 ± 11	48 ± 12	18 ± 4*	30 ± 5*
PCWP, mm Hg	16 ± 10	31 ± 11	5 ± 3*	14 ± 6*
Pulmonary artery O_2 saturation, %	53 ± 8	27 ± 9	59 ± 4*	35 ± 6*
Cardiac output, L/min	4.04 ± 1.02	7.58 ± 2.15	4.9 ± 0.9*	11.2 ± 2.6*
Cardiac index, L/min/m²	2.06 ± 0.47	3.8 ± 1.31	2.6 ± 0.4*	5.8 ± 1.1*
Lactate, mmol/L	1.0 ± 0.5	5.2 ± 1.7	0.9 ± 0.5	5.0 ± 2.5

MAP = mean arterial pressure; RAP = right atrial pressure; PAP = pulmonary artery pressure; PCWP = pulmonary capillary wedge pressure LVAD = left ventricular assist device.
* $P < 0.01$ LVAD vs heart failure
Adapted with permission from Reference 44.

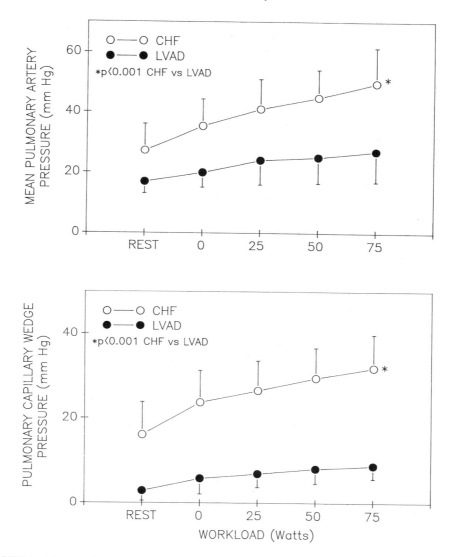

FIGURE 1. Mean pulmonary artery pressure and pulmonary capillary wedge pressure at rest and throughout exercise in heart failure (CHF) and left ventricular assist device (LVAD) patients.

peak VO_2, was also significantly better in the device patients. Figures 1 and 2 demonstrate the remarkable reduction in pulmonary pressures and the improvement in cardiac output throughout exercise in the LVAD patients. In this study, medical treatment of LVAD patients was not optimized. Indeed, only 15% of patients in this group were receiving ACE inhibitors; therefore their level of exercise performance was achieved almost exclusively from device therapy. We speculate that maximal medical therapy would have improved the exercise performance of the device patients, particularly those patients with significant right ventricular dysfunction.

A peak VO_2 in the range of 15 to 20 mL/kg/min, as described in these studies, is suggestive of considerable functional impairment. However, prior to implantation of the device, all of these patients had been bedridden and inotropic-dependent.

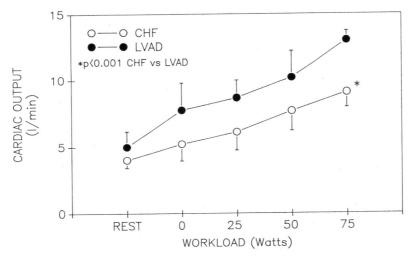

FIGURE 2. Cardiac output at rest and throughout exercise in heart failure (CHF) and left ventricular assist device (LVAD) patients.

Moreover, a fraction of these patients required temporary mechanical support with a balloon pump or a short-term assist device. The pre-implant VO_2 of these patients was essentially equivalent to the resting oxygen consumption (ie, approximately 3.5 mL/kg/min). The increment in peak VO_2 afforded by the device was much greater than that described with any single heart failure medication, and similar to that observed following cardiac transplantation.[45,46] Following transplantation, exercise performance remains reduced, resulting perhaps from chronotropic incompetence, chronic irreversible changes in the peripheral muscles and vasculature, donor-recipient size mismatch, and the effect of chronic immunosuppressive drugs.

The measured peak VO_2 in LVAD patients is lower than that predicted on the basis of maximum device output. For example, if the maximum device output is 10 L/min, the peak VO_2 for a 70-kg man should approach 25 mL/kg/min. Inability to achieve maximal performance may be the result of peripheral abnormalities and/ or right ventricular dysfunction that is not treated with LVAD support. Abnormalities in the vasculature and/or skeletal muscle described in patients with heart failure may be irreversible. Vasodilatory capacity of the LVAD patients is improved over time but is not normalized. No studies have yet evaluated intrinsic skeletal muscle changes in these patients.

Several studies have focused on acute right heart function after LVAD insertion (see Chapter 7), yet none have described the effect of extended LVAD support on right ventricular function. We surmise that right ventricular dysfunction may be the limiting factor to exercise capacity in some patients. A particularly illustrative case is that of a 47-year-old man with a dilated cardiomyopathy who required an LVAD as a bridge to transplant. His medical regimen prior to transplant included LVAD support, ACE inhibition (enalapril [Vasotec], Merck & Co. Inc., West Point, PA), and calcium channel blockade (amlodipine [Norvasc], Pfizer Inc., New York, NY). On his exercise test 3 months following device insertion, peak VO_2 was only 12.6 mL/ kg/min. Flow through the device at peak exercise was 7.4 L/min with a Fick cardiac output of 10.7 L/min. Echocardiogram at peak exercise demonstrated native aortic valve opening with only mildly reduced left ventricular function. The Fick cardiac output and echocardiogram suggested some degree of myocardial recovery. As will be discussed later in the chapter, exercise was repeated with minimal device support. With the device fixed to provide a flow of only 1.6 L/min, peak VO_2 was 9.6 mL/kg/min with a Fick cardiac output of 9.9 L/min. Echocardiogram demonstrated an ejection fraction of approximately 40%. Measurement of nuclear ejection fraction 2 days prior to the exercise study showed a first-pass right ventricular ejection fraction of only 14% and a left ventricular ejection fraction of 44%. In this particular patient, exercise was most probably limited by right ventricular dysfunction. At the time of transplant, direct observation of the heart revealed almost normal left ventricular function with a dilated right ventricle. We opted to proceed with transplant rather than LVAD explant alone, due to the right ventricular dysfunction. In the future, optimization of medical therapy may permit full recovery and explantation of the device without transplant.

Submaximal Exercise Capacity in LVAD Patients

Assessment of submaximal exercise capacity using the 6-minute walk test has been shown to be a valid and reproducible measure in patients with chronic heart failure.[47,48] Indeed, the performance of a patient during a submaximal test may be more reflective of his or her ability to manage the physically stressful activities of daily living. Submaximal exercise capacity is generally quantified by a variety of walk tests. The most commonly used test is the 6-minute walk test. Briefly, patients are instructed to walk as much as possible for a 6-minute period. A quiet, empty corridor at least 20 meters long comprises the typical course. Distance markers and chairs are provided along the route. Encouragement delivered during the test is standardized, as it has been shown to improve performance.[47] The significance of the 6-minute test is underscored by the results of the Study of Left Ventricular Dysfunction (SOLVD),[48] in which distance walked was found to be an independent predictor of mortality comparable to left ventricular ejection fraction. Patients with the lowest (<300 m) performance levels had a significantly greater mortality as well as a greater hospitalization rate for heart failure than did those with the highest (>450 m) performance levels.

The improvement in maximal exercise performance in LVAD patients suggests a concomitant improvement in submaximal exercise and endurance. We compared the submaximal exercise capacity of LVAD patients to that of normal subjects and patients with heart failure. An encouraged 6-minute walk test with metabolic measurements was performed in 14 patients with LVADs, in 20 patients with mild to moderate CHF, and in 14 patients with severe heart failure dependent on dobutamine.[43] Distance walked was significantly greater for LVAD patients than for dobutamine-dependent patients and similar to patients with mild heart failure (Fig. 3). The performance level of the patients with LVAD would be categorized into the SOLVD group with the best survival. In contrast, the dobutamine-dependent patients would be classified with the worst prognostic group.

Although the quality of life was not measured in this study, functional capacity is an integral component of one's overall sense of well-being and satisfaction. The

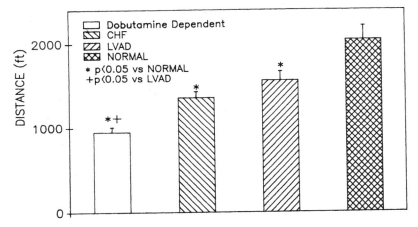

FIGURE 3. Histograms showing submaximal exercise performance in patients with moderate heart failure, patients dependent on dobutamine, left ventricular assist device (LVAD) patients, and normal subjects.

results of this study suggest that the quality of life is better in LVAD-supported patients than in their dobutamine counterparts.

Serial Assessment of Exercise Capacity in LVAD Patients

Serial assessment of submaximal exercise capacity in LVAD recipients was performed to evaluate for changes over time and, if present, to determine whether they were related to improvements in the cardiac output response. Sustained improvement of submaximal exercise capacity in LVAD patients was demonstrated while LVAD flows remained unchanged (Fig. 4).[43] These findings suggest that peripheral

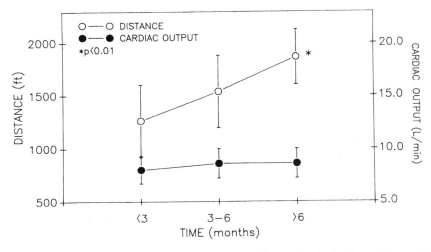

FIGURE 4. Six-minute walk distance and left ventricular assist device flows in patients with assist devices for different durations.

mechanisms such as muscle conditioning and/or reversal of neurohormonal activation—rather than central mechanisms—underlie this improvement. Indeed, all of our LVAD patients participated in a progressive physical therapy program.[49] Our findings are in agreement with those of Kahn et al,[50] who described a delayed and incomplete reversal of impaired metabolic vasodilatation in patients with heart failure following device implantation. Whether the improvement seen in the endurance is due to continued reversal of the abnormal metabolic vasodilatation, reversal of intrinsic skeletal muscle abnormalities, recovery of the native heart cannot be determined from this study.

Only one prior study examined changes in peak exercise performance over time in LVAD patients. In 10 LVAD recipients, peak VO_2 was measured 2 months after implantation. In four patients, measurements were again repeated 5 months following implantation. Peak VO_2 increased from 12.5 to 15.4 mL/kg/min.[51]

Use of Exercise Testing to Assess Myocardial Recovery

One frequent finding in LVAD patients is that the Fick cardiac output is greater than the LVAD sensor measurements. As discussed earlier in this chapter, this discrepancy becomes evident when the native left ventricle also contributes to the cardiac output, creating a circulation parallel to that of the LVAD. Echocardiographic studies demonstrate that the aortic valve is mostly closed at rest. With stress, the aortic valve opens and the native heart contributes to total cardiac output. The increase in Fick cardiac output over the device output may be a useful parameter to evaluate myocardial recovery. Conversely, a reduction in the Fick cardiac output versus the LVAD flow suggests either device malfunction or native aortic insufficiency. Figure 5 demonstrates the differences in Fick and LVAD sensor flow at peak exercise in 20 LVAD patients.

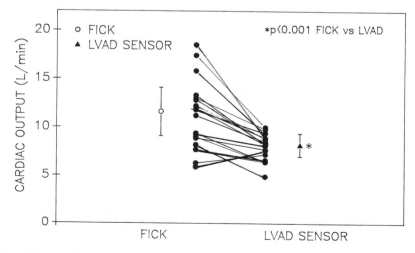

FIGURE 5. Fick and left ventricular assist device (LVAD) sensor cardiac outputs at maximal exercise in LVAD patients.

Profound ventricular pressure and volume unloading provided by LVAD support may lead to reverse remodeling at the genetic, biochemical, histologic, and functional levels. Other mechanisms that have been implicated in the reversal of the remodeling process include decrease in myocardial fibrosis and reduction in myocardial matrix metalloprotease expression, decrease in stretch, increased myocardial perfusion, normalization of neurohormonal disturbances, reduction in cytokine release, and decline in myocardial cell apoptosis.[52–62]

A recent report by Mueller et al[40] identified 5 of 17 patients with dilated cardiomyopathy who were supported by an LVAD for greater than 160 days and who were successfully explanted and maintained normal cardiac function. All of these patients presumably had irreversible end-stage heart failure; despite this, however, left ventricular function could be dramatically modified and almost returned to normal for short periods. A retrospective review of patients who received a mechanical bridge to transplant at our institution was performed to determine the incidence of patients who were successfully explanted.[63] Only 5 of 111 LVAD recipients were identified. The clinical characteristics of these patients are listed in Table 2. The first patient was an 18-year-old male with a cardiomyopathy who was supported with the device for 186 days. At operation for transplantation his cardiac function appeared satisfactory by hemodynamic and echocardiographic criteria with the device turned off and, hence, device explantation rather than cardiac transplantation was performed. Despite early adequate cardiac function, he experienced a rapid decrease in ejection fraction from 72% to 20%, and expired from heart failure 3 months after explantation. The second patient was a 47-year-old man with ischemic heart disease who underwent coronary artery bypass grafting complicated by heart failure and ventricular tachycardia. He underwent LVAD placement and was supported for 101 days prior to explant due to device infection. He remained in New York Heart Association Class II heart failure with stable ejection fraction until he died suddenly 2 years later. The third patient is a 30-year-old man who underwent LVAD placement for dilated cardiomyopathy complicated by atrial tachyarrhythmias. After 66 days of uninterrupted mechanical support, the LVAD was removed. Twenty-two months later, he was readmitted with severe CHF requiring inotropic support. His ejection fraction had slowly deteriorated from 45% to 28% over 18 months. He suffered a cardiac arrest and required reimplantation of the LVAD 684 days after explant. Sixty days after the second device had been implanted, the LVAD failed and was removed.

Table 2

Clinical Characteristics and Outcomes of Five LVAD Recipients who Underwent Device Explanation Without Transplantation

Patient	Age (yrs)	Sex	Etiology of Heart Failure	Duration of Implant (days)	Outcome
1	18	M	Idiopathic CMP	186	Expired from CHF, 3 month f/up
2	47	M	Ischemic CMP	101	Sudden death, 27 month f/up
3	30	M	Idiopathic CMP	66	LVAD, 24 month f/up
4	47	M	Idiopathic CMP	58	Alive, 15 month f/up
5	14	F	Idiopathic CMP	380	LVAD, 6 month f/up

CMP = Cardiomyopathy; CHF = congestive heart failure; LVAD = left ventricular assist device; f/up = follow-up. Adapted with permission from Reference 63.

Unsupported left ventricular ejection fraction had again risen to 50%. The fourth patient is a 47-year-old man with cardiomyopathy who was supported for 58 days prior to explant for device infection. He remains in Class I heart failure 22 months after device explant. His ejection fraction has remained stable. The last patient is a 14-year-old female with idiopathic cardiomyopathy who underwent device removal after 380 days of support because of recurrent device infection. Despite treatment with diuretics, digoxin, ACE inhibition, and carvedilol, she experienced a rapid decline in left ventricular function and required reimplantation of the device at 170 days. She subsequently underwent successful transplantation.

For the past 3 years we have prospectively attempted to identify potential explant candidates by the use of exercise testing.[63] Approximately 3 months after device implantation, a maximal exercise test with hemodynamic monitoring and respiratory gas analysis is performed with the LVAD in the auto mode. The electric device is interfaced with a pneumatic console such that the rate can be decreased to 20 cycles/min. This enables us to fix device output at approximately 1.5 L/min. The patients are acutely heparinized to prevent device thrombus in the setting of low flows. Hemodynamic measurements are recorded as the device rate is decreased. A repeat exercise test is then performed if the patient remains hemodynamically stable.

Of the 15 patients who were exercised with maximal device support, only seven remained normotensive and could exercise with a fixed rate of 20 cycles/min. In these patients, peak VO_2 declined from 17.3 ± 3.9 to 13.0 ± 6.1 mL/kg/min.[63] The increment in Fick cardiac output over the device during exercise in the auto mode ranged from 0 to 10.3 L/min. One of these patients was explanted. In one patient where Fick cardiac output was over 10 L/min higher than the LVAD sensor, myocardial recovery at the time of transplant could not be evaluated due to surgical difficulties. Although the incidence of full myocardial recovery is low, the frequency of partial recovery is in the order of 50%. All of the patients who are able to exercise with minimal device support exhibit partial degrees of myocardial recovery.

In our experience, the use of LVAD support has been associated with full and sustained myocardial recovery in 29% of patients with dilated cardiomyopathy who received the device. Differences between our experience and that of Mueller et al[40] may be due to differences in the severity of the heart failure, baseline medical therapy, or in the rate and mode of weaning of the device. Another important distinction between our experience and that of Mueller et al[40] is that normalization of left ventricular function in our explanted patients has not been sustained despite aggressive medical therapy. Three of our five patients have experienced redilation of the left ventricle with decrease in ejection fraction and recurrence of symptoms following device removal.

Summary

Exercise performance in patients with heart failure is limited by changes that occur in central cardiac function and by peripheral mechanisms that affect the muscular, vascular, and pulmonary systems. Insertion of an LVAD can significantly improve, albeit not normalize, exercise performance in patients with severe heart failure. Exercise performance remains reduced due to several different mechanisms including persistent right ventricular dysfunction and chronic peripheral changes.

With chronic LVAD support, submaximal and peak exercise performance improves, due to slow reversal of these peripheral changes as well as restoration of native right and left ventricular function. Exercise testing can be used as a means of quantifying cardiac recovery and determining if LVAD explantation is feasible. Much information remains to be elicited about the impact of LVADs on exercise performance of patients with heart failure. Hopefully, the knowledge gained from the study of these unique patients will provide insights that can be extrapolated to improve the exercise tolerance in the much larger pool of patients with all degrees of heart failure.

References

1. Wasserman K, Hansen J, Sue D, Whipp B. The physiology of exercise. In *Principles of Exercise Testing and Interpretation*. Philadelphia: Lea and Febiger; 1987:1–45.
2. Weber K, Janicki J. Chronic cardiac failure. In *Cardiopulmonary Exercise Testing: Physiologic Principles and Clinical Applications*. Philadelphia: W.B. Saunders; 1986:168–196.
3. Weber K, Kinasewitz G, Janicki J, Fishman A. Oxygen utilization and ventilation during exercise in patients with chronic cardiac failure. *Circulation* 1982;65:1213–1223.
4. Maskin C, Forman R, Sonnenblick E, LeJemtel T. Failure of dobutamine to increase exercise capacity despite hemodynamic improvement in severe chronic heart failure. *Am J Cardiol* 1983;51:177–182.
5. Wilson J, Martin J, Schwartz D, Ferraro N. Exercise tolerance in patients with heart failure: Role of impaired nutritive flow to skeletal muscle. *Circulation* 1984;69:1079–1087.
6. Zelis R, Mason D, Braunwald E, et al. A comparison of the effects of vasodilator stimuli on peripheral resistance vessels in normal subjects and in patients with congestive heart failure. *J Clin Invest* 1968;47:960–970.
7. Zelis R, Delea C, Coleman H, Mason D. Arterial sodium content in experimental congestive heart failure. *Circulation* 1970;61:213–216.
8. Zelis R, Flaim S. Alterations in vasomotor tone in congestive heart failure. *Prog Cardiovasc Dis* 1982;24:437–459.
9. Kubo S, Rector T, Bank A, et al. Endothelium-dependent vasodilation is attenuated in patients with heart failure. *Circulation* 1991;84:1589–1596.
10. Katz S, Biasucci L, Sabba C, et al. Impaired endothelium-mediated vasodilation in the peripheral vasculature of patients with congestive heart failure. *J Am Coll Cardiol* 1992;19:918–925.
11. Mancini D, Davis L, Wexler JP, et al. Dependence of enhanced maximal exercise performance on increased peak skeletal muscle perfusion during long-term captopril therapy in heart failure. *J Am Coll Cardiol* 1987;10:845–850.
12. Drexler H, Banhardt U, Meinhertz T, et al. Contrasting peripheral short-term and long term effects of converting enzyme inhibition in patients with congestive heart failure: A double-blind, placebo controlled trial. *Circulation* 1989;79:491–502.
13. Wilson J, Fink L, Maris J, et al. Evaluation of energy metabolism in skeletal muscle of patients with heart failure with gated phosphorus-31 nuclear magnetic resonance. *Circulation* 1985;71:57–62.
14. Weiner D, Fink L, Maris J, et al. Abnormal skeletal muscle bioenergetics during exercise in patients with heart failure: Role of reduced muscle blood flow. *Circulation* 1986;73:1127–1136.
15. Massie B, Conway M, Rajagopalan B, et al. Skeletal muscle metabolism during exercise under ischemic conditions in congestive heart failure: Evidence for abnormalities unrelated to blood flow. *Circulation* 1988;78:320–326.
16. Mancini DM, Wilson JR, Bolinger L, et al. In vivo magnetic resonance spectroscopy measurement of deoxymyoglobin during exercise in patients with heart failure: Demonstration of abnormal muscle metabolism despite adequate oxygenation. *Circulation* 1994;90:500–508.
17. Lipkin D, Jones D, Round J, Poole-Wilson P. Abnormalities of skeletal muscle in patients with chronic heart failure. *Int J Cardiol* 1988;18:187–195.

18. Mancini DM, Coyle E, Coggan A, et al. Contribution of intrinsic skeletal muscle changes to 31P NMR skeletal muscle metabolic abnormalities in patients with heart failure. *Circulation* 1989;80:1338–1346.

19. Sullivan M, Green H, Cobb F. Skeletal muscle biochemistry and histology in ambulatory patients with long-term heart failure. *Circulation* 1990;81:518–527.

20. Drexler H, Riede U, Munzel T, et al. Alterations of skeletal muscle in chronic heart failure. *Circulation* 1992;85:1751–1759.

21. Mancini DM, Walter G, Reichek N, et al. Contribution of skeletal muscle atrophy to exercise intolerance and altered muscle metabolism in heart failure. *Circulation* 1992;85:1364–1373.

22. Sullivan M, Higginbotham M, Cobb F. Exercise training in patients with severe left ventricular dysfunction: Hemodynamic and metabolic effects. *Circulation* 1988;78:506–515.

23. Coats A, Adamopoulos S, Radaelli A, et al. Controlled trial of physical training in chronic heart failure. *Circulation* 1992;85:2119–2131.

24. Musch T, Moore R, Leathers D, et al. Endurance training in rats with chronic heart failure induced by myocardial infarction. *Circulation* 1986;74:431–441.

25. Minotti J, Johnson E, Hudson T, et al. Skeletal muscle response to exercise training in congestive heart failure. *J Clin Invest* 1990;86:751–758.

26. Adamopoulos S, Coats A, Arnolda L, et al. Effects of physical training on skeletal muscle metabolism in chronic heart failure: 31P NMR spectroscopy study. *Circulation* 1991;84(suppl II):II74.

27. Cabanes L, Weber S, Matran R, et al. Bronchial hyperresponsiveness to methacholine in patients with impaired left ventricular function. *N Engl J Med* 1989;320:1317–1322.

28. Cabanes L, Costes F, Weber S, et al. Improvement in exercise performance by inhalation of methoxamine in patients with impaired left ventricular function. *N Engl J Med* 1992;326:1661–1665.

29. Fink L, Wilson JR, Ferraro N. Exercise ventilation and pulmonary artery wedge pressure in chronic stable congestive heart failure. *Am J Cardiol* 1986;57:249–253.

30. Sullivan M, Higginbotham M, Cobb F. Increased exercise ventilation in patients with chronic heart failure. Intact ventilatory control despite hemodynamic and pulmonary abnormalities. *Circulation* 1988;77:552–559.

31. Mancini DM, Henson D, LaManca J, Levine S. Respiratory muscle function and dyspnea in patients with chronic congestive heart failure. *Circulation* 1992;86:909–918.

32. Hammond M, Bauer K, Sharp J, Rocha R. Respiratory muscle strength in congestive heart failure. *Chest* 1990;98:1091–1094.

33. Mancini D, Nazzaro D, Ferraro N, et al. Demonstration of respiratory muscle deoxygenation during exercise in patients with heart failure. *J Am Coll Cardiol* 1991;18:492–498.

34. Mancini DM, Henson D, LaManca J, Levine S. Evidence of reduced respiratory muscle endurance in patients with heart failure. *J Am Coll Cardiol* 1994;24:972–981.

35. Mancini DM, Henson D, La Manca J, et al. Benefit of selective respiratory muscle training on exercise capacity in patients with chronic congestive heart failure. *Circulation* 1995;91:320–329.

36. Frazier OH, Duncan M, Radovancevic B, et al. Successful bridge to heart transplantation with a new left ventricular assist device. *J Heart Lung Transplant* 1992;11:530–537.

37. Frazier OH, Rose E, MacManus Q, et al. Multicenter clinical evaluation of the HeartMate 1000 IP left ventricular assist device. *Ann Thorac Surg* 1992;53:1080–1090.

38. McCarthy P, Portner P, Tobler H, et al. Clinical experience with the Novacor ventricular assist system. *J Thorac Cardiovasc Surg* 1991;102:578–587.

39. Branch K, Dembilsky W, Peterson K, et al. Physiology of the native heart and Thermo-Cardiosystems left ventricular assist device complex at rest and during exercise: Implications for chronic support. *J Heart Lung Transplant* 1994;13:641–651.

40. Mueller J, Wallukat G, Weng Y, et al. Weaning from mechanical support in patients with dilated cardiomyopathy. *Circulation* 1997;96:542–549.

41. Jaski B, Branch K, Adamson R, et al. Exercise hemodynamics during long-term implantation of a left ventricular assist device in patients awaiting heart transplantation. *J Am Coll Cardiol* 1993;22:1574–1580.

42. Murali S, Uretsky B, Estrada-Quintero T, et al. Metabolic and ventilatory responses to exercise in heart failure patients on a left ventricular assist system support. *Circulation* 1991;84:II354A.

43. Foray A, Williams D, Reemtsma K, et al. Assessment of submaximal exercise capacity in patients with left ventricular assist devices. *Circulation* 1996;94(suppl I):222–226.
44. Mancini D, Goldsmith R, Levin H, et al. Comparison of exercise performance in patients with severe heart failure versus left ventricular assist devices. *Circulation* 1998;98:1178–1183.
45. Mandak J, Aaronson K, Mancini D. Serial assessment of exercise capacity post cardiac transplant. *J Heart Lung Transplant* 1995;14:468–478.
46. Marzo KP, Wilson JR, Mancini DM. Effects of cardiac transplantation on ventilatory response to exercise. *Am J Cardiol* 1992;69:547–553.
47. Guyatt G. Use of the six-minute walk test as an outcome measure in clinical trials in chronic heart failure. *Heart Failure* 1987;7:211–217.
48. Bittner V, Weiner D, Yusuf S, et al. for the SOLVD Investigators. Prediction of mortality and morbidity with a 6-minute walk test in patients with left ventricular dysfunction. *JAMA* 1993;270:1702–1707.
49. Morrone T, Buck L, Catanese K, et al. Early progressive mobilization of patients with left ventricular assist devices is safe and optimizes recovery before heart transplantation. *J Heart Lung Transplant* 1996;15:423–429.
50. Kahn ST, Levin H, Oz M, Katz S. Delayed reversal of impaired metabolic vasodilation in patients with end-stage heart failure during long-term circulatory support with a left ventricular assist device. *J Heart Lung Transplant* 1997;16:449–453.
51. Nishmura M, Radovancevic B, Odegaard P, et al. Exercise capacity recovers slowly but fully in patients with left ventricular assist device. *ASAIO J* 1996;42:M568-M570.
52. Rose E, Frazier OH. Resurrection after mechanical support. *Circulation* 1997;96:393–395.
53. Levin H, Oz M, Chen J, et al. Reversal of chronic ventricular dilation in patients with end stage cardiomyopathy by prolonged mechanical unloading. *Circulation* 1995;91:2717–2720.
54. Levin H, Oz M, Catanese K, et al. Transient normalization of systolic and diastolic function after support with a left ventricular assist device in a patient with dilated cardiomyopathy. *J Heart Lung Transplant* 1996;15:840–842.
55. Frazier OH, Benedict C, Radovancevic B, et al. Improved left ventricular function after chronic left ventricular unloading. *Ann Thorac Surg* 1996;62:675–682.
56. Holman W, Bourge B, Kirklin J. Case report: Circulatory support for 70 days with resolution of acute heart failure. *J Thorac Cardiovasc Surg* 1991;102:932–934.
57. Schenin S, Capek P, Radovancevic B, et al. The effect of prolonged left ventricular assist support on myocardial histopathology in patients with end stage cardiomyopathy. *ASAIO* 1992;38:M271-M274.
58. Lee S, Oskbakken M, Doliba N, et al. LVAD therapy improves myocardial mitochondrial metabolism in patients with heart failure. *Circulation* 1996;94(8):294I.
59. Dipla K, Mattiello J, Jeevanandam V, et al. Myocyte recovery after mechanical circulatory support in humans with end-stage heart failure. *Circulation* 1998;97:2316–2322.
60. Zafeiridis A, Jeevanandam V, Houser S, Margulies K. Regression of cellular hypertrophy after left ventricular assist device support. *Circulation* 1998;98:656–662.
61. Belland S, Grunstein R, Jeevanandam V, Eisen H. The effect of sustained mechanical support with left ventricular assist devices on myocardial apoptosis in patients with severe dilated cardiomyopathy. *J Heart Lung Transplant* 1998;17:83A.
62. Belland S, Jeevanandam V, Eisen H. Reduced myocardial matrix metalloproteinase expression as a result of sustained mechanical support with left ventricular assist devices in patients with severe dilated cardiomyopathy. *J Heart Lung Transplant* 1998;17:84A.
63. Mancini D, Beniaminovitz A, Levin H, et al. Low incidence of myocardial recovery following left ventricular assist device implantation in patients with chronic heart failure. *Circulation* 1998;98:2383–2389.

Chapter 12

Outpatient Left Ventricular Assist Therapy

Katharine A. Catanese, MSN and David L.S. Morales, MD

In the current economic environment for cost containment, discharge of left ventricular assist device (LVAD) recipients home to await transplantation has become essential as the population of patients with end-stage heart failure has increased and the wait for a donor heart has grown longer. Fortunately, for the following reasons, the creation of mechanical assist outpatient programs has become possible: 1) confidence in the reliability of these devices has allowed patients and physicians to be more comfortable with outpatient therapy; 2) the simplification and improved durability of these devices has allowed for extended duration of support; and 3) there has been a change in the perception of the LVAD from a last-effort therapeutic option to a safe and reliable bridge to recovery and transplant.[1] In addition to evaluating the usual measures of treatment success (ie, improved hemodynamics, morbidity, and mortality), programs are now being asked to evaluate patient outcomes such as satisfaction, functional capabilities, and quality-of-life issues.[2–7] It has become evident that for mechanical assist programs to survive, patients will have to be managed on an outpatient basis.

Early efforts to discharge LVAD patients were relegated to medically run housing.[3] Successful experiences with these early practices have resulted in the establishment of numerous outpatient programs.[8–10] Despite these successes, the perception of the LVAD as a reliable device to support a patient at home is not well recognized by the medical community. The largest reported multicenter experience consisted of 21 patients from the four most experienced LVAD programs.[8] The largest single outpatient program consists of 19 patients.[1] The literature documenting the safety and reliability of outpatient LVADs is therefore sparse.

The efficacy of LVAD support was recognized by the Food and Drug Administration's (FDA) approval in 1998 of two portable LVADs for outpatient use: the TCI Vented Electric (VE) HeartMate (Thermo Cardiosystems, Inc., Woburn, MA) and the Novacor 100 LVAS (Novacor, Baxter Healthcare Corp., Oakland CA). These "wearable" devices are described in detail in Chapters 23 and 24. A third device, the Thoratec

From Goldstein DJ and Oz MC (eds). *Cardiac Assist Devices*. Armonk, NY: Futura Publishing Co., Inc.; ©2000.

Table 1

World Experience with Outpatient LVAD Support

Device	Total # Patients Discharged US/Non-US	Outpatient Support Days	Outpatient Mortality
Novacor 100	71/134[2]	32,157 (88.1 yrs)	0
Thermo Cardiosystems VE LVAD	141/120	28,981 (79.4 yrs)	2
Thoratec TLC II	0/5	100 (0.27 yrs)	0
TOTAL	471	61,237 (167.8 yrs)	2 (0.012/patient-yr)

Data exclude overnight or day trips. [2] Includes patients discharged to outpatient housing. LVAD = left ventricular assist device. Table derived from data from the following sources: G. Marchesani, Thoratec Laboratories, November 1998; D. Jacobs, Novacor Division, Baxter Healthcare Corporation, December 1998; and T. Krauskopf, Thermo Cardiosystems, November 1998.

TLC-II (Thoratec Laboratories, Berkeley, CA) (see Chapter 19) is currently available for outpatient use in Canada and Europe, and can serve as a uni- or biventricular assist device. This device has received approval for an investigational device exemption from the FDA and has begun clinical trials in the United States (J. Reedy, Director Clinical Services/International Sales, personal communication, November 1998). The total worldwide LVAD outpatient experience consists of 471 patients representing a total of 61,237 patient-support days (167.8 years). Table 1 summarizes the total worldwide outpatient experience through December 1998. The mortality for LVAD recipients supported in the outpatient setting is 0.012 per outpatient-year. This compares favorably with Status I Class IV heart failure patients (66% 1-year mortality) and the general mortality of patients on the heart transplant list (up to 30% die per year awaiting an organ).[11]

Creating an Outpatient LVAD Program

Program Structure

The infrastructure of the LVAD outpatient program evolves to resemble the inpatient service. A multidisciplinary team that includes a cardiac surgeon, nurses, cardiologists, bioengineers, physician assistants, social workers, physical therapists, and a financial manager is necessary to maintain an outpatient LVAD program. At the center of this structure is a core team composed of advanced practice nurses who are responsible for the day-to-day operation of the outpatient program.

Vital to this infrastructure is: 1) a modern and well organized communication system through which questions can be efficiently addressed; 2) a 24-hour on-call emergency system; 3) team members who are knowledgeable of specific emergency protocols and guidelines; and 4) maintenance of the necessary back-up equipment and resources to support patients out of the hospital.

Another important aspect to this infrastructure is the creation of an outpatient consult service that comprises specialists who are involved in the inpatient management of these unique patients and who can be called upon whenever the need arises in the outpatient setting.

Initiation of Outpatient Therapy

Our approach to outpatient therapy is to prepare patients and families for discharge prior to LVAD implantation. This practice allows outpatient therapy to be viewed as a natural progression of care. Discharge planning begins at the time of initial contact with the LVAD coordinator. This method allows for early identification of potential obstacles to outpatient therapy. In addition to the standard physical and psychological assessments, information is gathered regarding the home environment, functional status, and coping and support mechanisms that are available to the patient. Solutions to barriers for patient release are then explored with additional members of the LVAD team. Possible resolutions to these barriers are then discussed with the patient and their families. The social worker plays a key role; he or she assists patients and families with home care services, financial matters, and housing, and provide much needed emotional support.

The screening process is modified on an individual basis depending upon the patient's age, condition, knowledge deficit, educational needs, and coping mechanisms. Initially, these critically ill patients have limited attention span and functional reserve. Consideration must be given to whether the patient is a child, adolescent, or adult, as well as to the associated variation in learning styles. The way these patients and caregivers respond to the idea of LVAD placement can be highly variable. Education practices are adapted to meet these variances.[5]

Preoperative Patient Education

In the nonemergent setting, preoperative education of the patient and his/her family is undertaken. General information regarding the device is provided and sufficient time is allotted to answer questions. Educational information in the form of booklets and pictures is used to supplement verbal instruction.

Postoperative Education

Depending on the patient's preoperative condition, this may be the first time patients have the capacity to understand and communicate. Instruction usually begins with very basic information, such as how to make battery connections and change power sources. Often this instruction is provided by a physical therapist who begins early mobilization. Responsibility for day-to-day management of the device is gradually shifted to the patient and primary caregiver. As proficiency increases, more details regarding advisory warnings and alarms are incorporated. Repetitive demonstrations ensure that LVAD patients and their primary caregivers receive adequate training. Recipients must be able to independently maintain their devices in the outpatient setting. Postoperative education includes instructions for monitoring LVAD parameters, medications, showering, wound care management, and emergency procedures.

Fail-Safe Rescues

Several fail-safe mechanisms exist for patients supported with LVADs. First, the program provides training in device self-management for patients and their companions. Patients are taught how to operate and troubleshoot the system, as well as procedures to follow during an emergency. Second, external control devices allow for components to be exchanged in the event of malfunction. Finally, in the very rare event of catastrophic LVAD failure, the patient's native heart has usually recovered enough function to keep patients alive; moreover, the patient or caregiver may actuate the device pneumatically with a hand pump until the LVAD team is contacted.

Home Environment

Safety assessment of the home environment is ascertained prior to discharge. Generally, this information can be obtained by discussion with the patient and caregivers. In particular, patients' homes are checked for properly grounded outlets. Some centers check wall outlets for reverse polarization, using a standard circuit tester. Power base units are usually placed so that they are not on wall switches. Patients are cautioned to avoid static electricity (ie, TV, computer screens) because it can change the LVAD to an asynchronous pumping mode at 40 bpm. Some institutions routinely make a home visit as part of the discharge assessment. In addition, the need for home care services such as equipment requirements, nursing care, and physical therapy is determined during the rehabilitative phase. Visiting nursing services are often used to aid in the transition from hospital to home. Visiting nursing provides reinforcement of hospital training regarding the LVAD, emergency procedures, medications, and wound care management. Table 2 lists our institutional discharge checklist.

Notification of the presence of life support equipment in the home is given to power and electrical companies prior to discharge. Most outpatient devices have enough back-up power to deem generators unnecessary. Instructions are given to patients to keep a flashlight near the power base unit to allow them to connect to alternate power sources in the event of total power failure in the home. Procedures to be followed in the event of power outages are clearly outlined for patients and caregivers.

Emergency Resources

Patients participating in outpatient therapy should have access to a dedicated 24-hour emergency phone line. In addition, patients carry wallet-sized identification cards with emergency telephone numbers and contact information. Most patients awaiting heart transplantation carry beepers to respond to possible organ transplantation. Some programs may require primary caregivers to be certified in basic cardiac life support.[12] In addition, centers may notify any in-service local emergency room personnel about the LVAD patient in their area.

Emergency first-response systems vary from state to state. Training of local emergency medical service teams facilitates safety during first response. Plans for

---

Table 2

Columbia Presbyterian LVAD Discharge Checklist

Trained LVAD recipient on the following:
1. Change batteries
2. Switch from battery to power base unit support
3. How and when to hand pump
4. How and when to change controller
5. How to use shower kit

Trained the LVAD recipient's companion on the following:
1. Change batteries
2. Switch from battery to power base unit support
3. How and when to hand pump
4. How and when to change controller
5. How to use shower kit
6. How to clean surgical site
7. How to change dressing using sterile technique

Informed the LVAD recipient on the following:
1. What to do in an emergency situation
2. When to call 911 and when to contact LVAD team
3. Medications
4. Return for follow-up visit

Patient sent home with the following:
1. Power base unit
2. Eight batteries with two battery clips
3. One 24-hour emergency pack
4. One hand pump
5. One controller
6. One back-up controller
7. One hoister

LVAD = left ventricular assist device.

---

transporting the patient to the cardiac center after initial stabilization are clearly delineated.

Community Services

Some LVAD programs have elected to have the patient's primary care physician follow the patient on a routine basis due to distance from the cardiac center. These patients obtain routine follow-up locally and return to the cardiac center at 4- to 6-week intervals or as needed. In addition, some LVAD programs make home visits part of their ongoing assessment. Home evaluation includes physical, neurologic, and psychological assessment, as well as wound inspection.[13] Communication is key between the local health care provider and the LVAD center.

Patient Discharge

General Release Protocol

With the FDA approval of both long-term devices, an opportunity has been created to base the decision of patient discharge on medical condition and clinical judgment rather than on governmental requirements.

A patient release protocol includes a stepwise program to ensure safe release of LVAD recipients. Generally, patients are released for short day trips with a companion, until they are accustomed to being away from the hospital. Criteria for discharge may vary between institutions and devices but guidelines for release may include the following: 1) the patient is clinically stable with no medical contraindications to release, such as active infection or significant end organ dysfunction; 2) the recipient and caregiver have undergone training in the care and management of their devices; 3) the patient and primary caregiver have demonstrated the ability to successfully maintain the device as an outpatient; 4) the primary caregiver adequately demonstrates proper wound care management; and 5) the patient has completed the designated number of day trips away from the hospital.

Depending on institutional policies and the type of device implanted, some patients may be released into transitional or intermediate care facilities prior to formal discharge. Transitional facilities may include inpatient rehabilitation centers and/or an out-of-hospital type residence.[3] These facilities range from hotel-type rooms to institutions staffed with full-time bioengineering support.

Specific protocols for patient discharge suggested by the different LVAD manufacturers have been previously described.[5,10,13]

Outpatient Costs

With the improvement in technologies and treatments for end-stage heart failure, there are new opportunities to treat patients in their home environment; this raises questions about the cost of inpatient care compared to outpatient care. Some investigators believe that reallocation of spending from the inpatient to the outpatient setting would greatly alleviate the most costly component of heart failure treatment.[14] Critically ill patients with end-stage congestive heart failure generally await transplantation in an intensive care unit.[15] Outpatient mechanical support for these patients may be one option in defraying hospital costs. While the initial cost of mechanical circulatory support is considerable, the ability to streamline patients to discharge and to maintain them on an out-of-hospital basis may lessen the $35 billion burden heart failure places on society.[14]

Few analyses of the long-term costs associated with mechanical assist technology exist. Evaluation of costs associated with outpatient therapy is even more sparse (see Chapter 15). One study estimated the cost of 1 week of outpatient support to be $352 (including professional fees, medications, and laboratory tests).[16] Daily outpatient expenditures for medication and medical supplies have been reported to be as low as $27 per day.[17] Outpatient costs were estimated using the International Classification of Disease codes,[18] a random sampling of local pharmacies, and *Drug Topics Redbook*.[19] We estimated the cost of outpatient services (clinic visits, medications, laboratory tests) to be $429.80 per month (Table 3).[17] While these costs are not all inclusive (ie, they do not include transportation, visiting nursing, etc.), when compared to the hospital cost of room and board for a nonacute bed ($1608/day), they may represent substantial savings.

In the absence of FDA requirements for the discharge of LVAD patients, associated costs of this type of treatment should continue to decrease. Additionally, reduction in manufacturing cost and increased competition among manufacturers will

Table 3

Outpatient LVAD Costs

Item	Unit Cost ($)	First Month Cost ($)	Monthly Cost ($)
Professional fee CPT 99221 (patient seen by nurse only)	100	300	100
Venipuncture CPT 36415/001	10	30	10
Weekly laboratory fees	Coagulation profile - 24.00 Hepatic profile - 20.00 Chemistry profile - 8.00 Complete blood count - 14.00	198	66
Dressing supplies	4×4 gauze (6) - 0.18 ea Sterile gloves - 1.14 Nonsterile gloves - 1.40 Op-site - 1.55	155.1	155.1
Medications	Iron replacement (2) - 0.32 ea Pepcid AC 10 mg (1) - 0.28 Multivitamin (1) - 0.13 Enteric aspirin (1) - 0.2 Captopril 25 mg (3) - 0.68 ea	19.2 8.4 3.9 6 61.2 Total 133.8	19.2 8.4 3.9 6 61.2 Total 133.8
	Totals	781.8	429.8

LVAD = left ventricular assist device.

likely decrease the cost of the devices themselves. The broader economic benefit of successful LVAD outpatient treatment is the return of patients as productive members of their families and society.

The Columbia Presbyterian Outpatient Experience

From February 1, 1993 through December 25, 1998, a total of 86 patients underwent implantation of a TCI VE HeartMate LVAD at Columbia Presbyterian Medical Center. Fifty-three (62%) of these LVAD patients were released from the hospital. Nine patients made only day trips and 44 patients (51%) were totally discharged. Our results will focus on the 44 patients who were fully discharged, which better reflect the outpatient experience. This group consisted of 40 male and 4 female patients with a mean age of 46 ± 16 years. The etiology of heart failure was ischemic cardiomyopathy in 17 patients (39%), idiopathic cardiomyopathy in 22 patients (50%), alcoholic cardiomyopathy in 3 patients (7%), familial cardiomyopathy in 1 patient (2%), and viral cardiomyopathy in 1 patient (2%). These patients were at home a total of 4546 days, with a mean of 105 ± 16 days of outpatient support. The cohort averaged $62 \pm 25\%$ of their LVAD support time as outpatients. All but two of these patients were sent home before the FDA approval of the TCI VE LVAD. Sixteen

Table 4

Thermo Cardiosystems VE LVAD Patient Outcomes at Columbia Presbyterian

Patient Status	# Patients	Transplanted	Expired	Explanted	Ongoing
LVAD patients discharged	44	42	0	2	0
LVAD patients not discharged	42	17	18	2	5
Total VE LVAD patients	86	59	18	4	5

VE LVAD = vented electric left ventricular assist device.

patients required hospitalization for a minimum of 30 days before discharge secondary to FDA restrictions. Minimal length of stay criteria were later lowered to 14 days until final FDA approval of the TCI device in September 1998.

The outcomes of all 44 outpatients are depicted in Table 4. There were no deaths in the outpatient group. All outpatients were successfully bridged to transplant or recovery.

The average wait for a donor heart in those patients who underwent transplantation was 148 ± 130 days. The average length of stay post transplantation for LVAD outpatients was 18 ± 8 days.

Outpatient Adverse Clinical Events

None of the patients experienced complications while out of the hospital on day trips. There were, however, several adverse events noted in the outpatient experience.

Bleeding

Bleeding was defined as blood loss that required hospital admission or surgical intervention, or that which caused death. In our outpatient experience, three patients (7%) experienced bleeding events. Two of these patients required reoperation. The first patient had a tear in the outflow graft on the 352nd day of support. This patient presented to the outpatient clinic with vague symptoms and was found to have a decreased hematocrit on routine lab work. Further investigation revealed a large collection around the LVAD device. This patient was taken to the operating room and the outflow graft was replaced. He was discharged on postoperative day 13 without further complications and was later transplanted after an additional 252 days of outpatient support.

The second patient presented to the outpatient clinic complaining of weakness, and was noted to have a hematocrit of 25%. After imaging studies revealed a peri-LVAD collection, he was taken to the operating room for primary repair of a small hole in the outflow graft and was discharged on postoperative day five. The patient was supported for an additional 237 days prior to undergoing successful transplantation.

The third patient had a self-limited bleed from the drive line tract after vigorous sexual activity on the 64th day of LVAD support. The patient was admitted for

3 days of observation and was discharged without intervention. The incidence of outpatient bleeding events in this cohort was 0.020 events per patient-month.

Neurologic Events

One patient (2%) experienced a retinal microembolization that caused loss of lateral vision in the left eye 83 days after implantation. This patient was admitted for 3 days for observation. He was not anticoagulated and although no source of emboli was found, it was believed to be device-related. This loss of lateral vision did not impair this patient from returning to school or from snowboarding during his remaining outpatient LVAD support. The patient was successfully transplanted after an additional 125 days of uneventful outpatient support. The incidence of thromboembolic events in this outpatient cohort was 0.0066 per patient-month.

Infections

Non–Device-Related Infections Non–device-related infections were defined as fever and/or leukocytosis with a positive culture (ie, blood, catheters, urine, stool, etc.) requiring antimicrobial treatment, not directly related to the device. Detailed records were kept prospectively and we reviewed infections that developed after the patients entered into the release protocol. Four (9%) patients developed non–device-related clinical infections, all bacterial in nature. Two patients had central line infections. The patients' infections developed while they were receiving intravenous gamma globulin therapy for an elevated panel reactive antibody test. All catheter-related infections resolved with intravenous antibiotics and removal of the lines. None of the outpatients developed pneumonias but one patient was treated for a urinary tract infection. One patient developed a positive throat/sputum culture for *Streptococcus A* and was treated with Penicillin VK for 10 days as an outpatient. The incidence of non–device-related infection was 0.040 per outpatient-month. Our experience suggests that infection does not impact mortality or preclude successful transplantation in the outpatient group.[20]

Device-Related Infections Device-related infections were defined as positive culture in the presence of leukocytosis, and/or fever requiring medical or surgical intervention. Eight (18%) patients developed a device-related infection while participating in the release program. Five patients had only drive line infections. Drive line infections were characterized as erythema, drainage, or purulence at the exit site in the presence of positive culture. An infection of the surfaces of the LVAD device itself was defined as "LVAD endocarditis." Three of the five patients with drive line infections experienced fevers with elevated white cell counts on oral antibiotics. Two of these patients resumed outpatient therapy after treatment with intravenous antibiotics. The third patient underwent transplantation. The additional two patients were successfully treated with oral antibiotics on an outpatient basis. The sixth patient experienced fever and chills, with a purulent draining wound on the 71st day of LVAD support. The patient was readmitted for intravenous antibiotic therapy. The seventh patient experienced a device infection and underwent explantation of the LVAD on day 389 of support. Unfortunately, she developed progressive heart failure and on post-explant day 178, underwent placement of a second LVAD. This patient was successfully transplanted 89 days later. A total of 75 days out of these 89 days (84%) were at home. The eighth patient had LVAD endocarditis. The incidence of device-related infection was 0.053 per outpatient-month.

Device Malfunction

Several mechanical malfunctions occurred in the outpatient experience. A major malfunction is defined as one in which the pump itself is not functioning properly, causing hemodynamic compromise, and/or requiring immediate intervention or LVAD replacement. A minor malfunction requires replacement of one of the extracorporeal components (ie, controller, battery system).

There were 66 minor malfunctions affecting 20 patients (45%). These included batteries not fully charging, continuous advisory warnings, and controller malfunctions. The majority of these events were corrected by the patients themselves or in the outpatient clinic. Only one of these events required admission to the hospital, and this was for 3 days to ensure proper function of the new controller. The incidence of a minor controller malfunction was 0.44 per outpatient-month.

There were three major malfunctions. The first patient presented to a local hospital with the LVAD operating at a basal rate of 40 bpm. The patient was clinically stable and was transferred to our institution. After troubleshooting of the device, the patient underwent LVAD replacement that day. Upon explantation of the device, it was discovered that the cam slope had broken loose, thus inhibiting the pusher-plate from fully compressing the blood chamber. The patient recovered without complication, was discharged, and was successfully transplanted 112 days later. The second patient presented with a controller alarm secondary to high motor current. Further investigation attributed the alarm to the excessive wearing of the ball bearings. The patient remained clinically stable with adequate LVAD outputs. The patient was discharged home and continued to work but was closely followed. Progressive deterioration of the device occurred and the LVAD was changed on the 270th support day in order to avoid clinical complications. As expected, the LVAD ball bearings had worn, making the resistance too great for the motor to work efficiently. The patient was subsequently discharged home and successfully transplanted 335 days later. The third patient presented to the LVAD clinic for routine follow-up. The patient complained of intermittent controller alarming. Investigation revealed a controller malfunction and during controller exchange, it was thought that a static discharge sent the controller into a basal rate of 40 bpm. Repeated controller changes failed to correct the situation. The patient was placed on a pneumatic back-up at 80 bpm. On the fourth day of admission, however, the patient began to exhibit symptoms of congestive heart failure and the decision was made to replace the device on the 124th day of support. Upon interrogation of the explanted LVAD, damage to the power conductor was discovered and thought to be the main cause of failure. Following LVAD replacement, the patient was discharged home and underwent successful transplant after 70 days of support with her second LVAD. The incidence of major LVAD dysfunction was 0.020 per outpatient-month.

A major concern for outpatient therapy is that the device will malfunction or stop pumping, causing immediate hemodynamic instability. It is therefore important to note that all of the major malfunctions in our experience were recognized in the outpatient setting, early, and were addressed in an efficient manner before any clinical ramifications occurred. Strict physiologic criteria for discharge and safety nets (ie, patient and companion training) allowed for this early identification of LVAD problems. A 24-hour emergency access system assured that these problems were handled in a safe, systematic, and timely fashion.

There were 18 unscheduled hospitalizations affecting 12 of 44 outpatients (27%), with a median hospital stay of 7 days (range 3 to 5 days) for a total of 171 readmission days. These days were not included in the total number of outpatient LVAD support days. The reasons for these readmissions were due to the complications discussed above. There were eight scheduled admissions, ranging from 1 to 3 days, for intravenous gamma globulin therapy for a positive panel reactive antibody test. All of the patients who were readmitted were discharged. The 18 unscheduled readmissions resulted in discharge (n = 15), transplant (n = 2), or explant (n = 1). None of the unscheduled hospitalizations resulted in death. The frequency for readmission is quite low, considering most LVAD recipients were status I patients on inotropic therapy and/or in the intensive care unit, and would never have been discharged home originally. Even if they did improve and were sent home, an average group of 44 Class III to IV heart failure patients is admitted 50 times per year (4 per patient-year).[21] The incidence of unscheduled admissions per outpatient was 0.27 and the incidence of the event per outpatient month was 0.12.

Summary

Our experience with LVAD outpatient therapy has been rewarding. Initial concerns of complications occurring in the absence of medical supervision, device failure in particular, were allayed for three main reasons. First, complications outside of the hospital were infrequent. Second, if they did occur, the safety systems set up by the program allowed early detection followed by a rapid and seamless plan of action. This system has contributed to a zero mortality in the outpatient experience. Third, no complications occurred as a result of the outpatient status; all complications could have occurred in the hospital. Thus, whether the patients were in or out of the hospital made no difference in regard to safety. However, being an outpatient did have several benefits in terms of cost and quality of life.

The economic benefit is more concrete, as the cost of caring for an outpatient LVAD is inexpensive. As can be gathered from Table 3, the weekly cost for supplies/medicines for an outpatient is $63.45 and the cost for outpatient clinic visits depends on how often the patient is seen. If readmissions are excluded, the cost of caring for a "healthy" LVAD outpatient for the first month is $781.80, even with weekly clinic visits, and, hence, is less than half the charge of 1 day of boarding on our nonacute hospital floor ($1608). This is important because LVAD outpatients are at home for 62% of the time. Therefore, the economic benefit of treating an LVAD patient on an outpatient basis can be considerable.

Another major benefit of outpatient therapy may be the enhancement in the quality of life for these patients.[22] Previous data demonstrated that prior to LVAD implantation patients often experience difficulties in physical and psychosocial well-being.[10] In addition, data show that as early as 4 weeks after LVAD insertion, patients show minimal dysfunction in most areas of quality of life. All 44 LVAD outpatients performed activities of daily living and none required home attendants. Activities included bicycling, fishing, driving, attending movies, spending time with friends and families, caring for children, and exercising. Thirty percent of patients were able to resume work and/or school, 33% resumed sexual activity, and 44% resumed driving. Notably, several adults did not resume working (despite being able to do so) because of issues regarding insurance and disability policies.

The above observations and conclusions are convincing; however, they are based on the perceptions and opinions of a third party, the caregivers. Dew et al[22] performed a formal quality-of-life study on LVAD outpatients (n = 10), comparing them to themselves as inpatients, to a different LVAD inpatient cohort (n = 25), to recipients 7 months post-transplant (n = 97), and to patients awaiting transplant at home (n = 38). Using the Sickness Impact Profile subclasses for physical function, LVAD outpatients significantly improved in sleep/rest, body care/movement, mobility, and ambulation when compared to transplant candidates at home or to LVAD inpatients.[2,22] LVAD outpatients closely resembled the transplant recipients in physical functional status. Overall, it is clear that LVAD outpatients experience improvement in the physical, psychological, and social aspects of their life when discharged, and these are significantly better than those seen in transplant candidates at home or LVAD inpatients.

We feel that an outpatient program is safe and economical while being socially, physically, and psychologically beneficial to the patient. We have discharged 51% of our LVAD recipients home. A low complication rate and demonstrable confidence in our patients' abilities to handle these minor complications have led to these successes. This certitude, together with the economic and quality-of-life benefits, make outpatient LVAD care a necessity for an LVAD program to thrive.

References

1. DeRose JJ Jr, Umana JP, Argenziano M, et al. Implantable left ventricular assist devices provide an excellent outpatient bridge to transplantation and recovery. *J Am Coll Cardiol* 1997;30(7):1773–1777.
2. Dew MA, Kormos RL, Roth LH, et al. Life quality in the era of bridging to cardiac transplantation. Bridge patients in an outpatient setting. *ASAIO J* 1993;39:145–152.
3. Kormos RL, Murali S, Dew MA, et al. Chronic mechanical circulatory support: Rehabilitation, low morbidity, and superior survival. *Ann Thorac Surg* 1994;57:1051–1057.
4. Moskowitz AJ, Weinberg AD, Oz MC, Williams DL. Quality of life with an implanted left ventricular assist device. *Ann Thorac Surg* 1997;64(6):1764–1769.
5. Moroney DA, Powers K. Outpatient use of left ventricular assist devices: Nursing, technical, and educational considerations. *Am J Crit Care* 1997;6(5):355–362.
6. Arabia FA, Smith RG, Jaffe C, et al. Cost analysis of the Novacor left ventricular assist system as an outpatient bridge to heart transplantation. *ASAIO J* 1996;42(5):M546-M549.
7. Mehta SM, Aufiero TX, Pae WE Jr, et al. Mechanical ventricular assistance: An economical and effective means of treating end-stage heart disease. *Ann Thorac Surg* 1995;60(2): 284–290.
8. Myers TJ, Catanese KA, Vargo RL, Dressler DK. Extended cardiac support with a portable left ventricular assist system in the home. *ASAIO J* 1996;42(5):M576-M579.

9. DeRose JJ, Argenziano M, Sun BC, et al. Implantable left ventricular assist devices: An evolving long-term cardiac replacement therapy. *Ann Surg* 1997;226:461–468.
10. Catanese KA, Goldstein DJ, Williams DL, et al. Outpatient left ventricular assist device support: A destination rather than a bridge. *Ann Thorac Surg* 1996;62(3):646–652.
11. Evans RW. Cardiac replacement: Estimation of need, demand, and supply. In Rose EA, Stevenson LW (eds): *Management of End-Stage Heart Disease*. Philadelphia, PA: Lippincott-Raven Publishers; 1998:13–24.
12. Mundinger, MO. Sounding board advanced-practice nursing: Good medicine for physicians? *N Engl J Med* 1994;330:211–214.
13. Pristas JM, Winowich S, Nastala CJ, et al. Protocol for releasing Novacor left ventricular assist system patients out-of-hospital. *ASAIO J* 1995;41(3):M539-M543.
14. Robbins MA, O'Connell JB. Economic impact of heart failure. In Rose EA Stevenson LW (eds): *Management of End-Stage Heart Disease*. Philadelphia, PA: Lippincott-Raven Publishers; 1998:3–11.
15. Fey O, El-Banayosy A, Arosuglu L, et al. Out-of-hospital experience in patients with implantable mechanical circulatory support: Present and future trends. *Eur J Cardiothorac Surg* 1997;11(suppl):851–853.
16. Cloy MF, Myers TJ, Stutts LA, et al. Hospital charges for conventional therapy versus left ventricular assist system therapy in heart transplant patients. *ASAIO J* 1995;41:M535-M539.
17. Gelijns AC, Richards AF, Williams DL, et al. Evolving costs of long-term left ventricular assist device implantation. *Ann Thorac Surg* 1997;64(5):1312–1319.
18. *International Classification of Diseases*. 9th Revision 1999. Los Angeles, California: Practice Management Information Corporation; 1998.
19. *Drug Topics Redbook*. Montevale, New Jersey: Medical Economics Company, Inc. 1998
20. Argenziano M, Catanese KA, Moazami N, et al. The influence of infection on survival and successful transplantation in patients with left ventricular assist devices. *J Heart Lung Transplant* 1997;16(8):822–831.
21. Pina IL, Zimmer R, Gil V. End-points for evaluation of therapies. In Rose EA, Stevenson LW (eds): *Management of End-Stage Heart Disease*. Philadelphia, PA: Lippincott-Raven Publishers; 1998:25–35.
22. Dew MA, Kormos RL, Winowich BB, et al. Quality of life outcomes in left ventricular assist system inpatients and outpatients. *ASAIO J* 1999;45:218–225.

Chapter 13

Rehabilitation of the Ventricular Assist Device Recipient

Theresa M. Morrone, MS, PT, C.C.S. and Lori A. Buck, MS, PT, C.C.S.

Introduction

The success of left ventricular assist devices (LVADs) in achieving superior survival rates to transplantation has been attributed to two key factors. First, these devices restore perfusion to chronically starved end organs, resulting in improved physiologic status. Second, the attainment of effective circulatory support provides an opportunity for aggressive physical rehabilitation, which is of paramount importance in converting the wasted and bedbound end-stage heart failure patient into an ambulating reconditioned heart transplant candidate. The significance of the latter has been underscored by Frazier et al,[1] who reported a 91% post-transplantation survival rate among 75 LVAD recipients who were aggressively rehabilitated pre-transplantation versus a 67% post-transplantation survival rate among 33 nonrehabilitated control patients. The length of mechanical support and physical rehabilitation following LVAD placement also appears to play a role in the success of transplantation. In a series of 133 patients, Ashton et al[2] found a threefold increase in transplant perioperative mortality in patients who were supported for less than 30 days when compared with the cohort of patients who were mechanically supported for more than 30 days. The authors attributed the observed differences to the longer time available for normalization of end organ function and for aggressive physical rehabilitation.

End-stage heart failure patients who undergo implantation of an LVAD have typically been hospitalized and bedbound for several days, if not weeks. Their mobility and general physical status is limited by the frequent need for intravenous catheters, cardiac monitors, and endotracheal and bladder tubes. In addition, these patients commonly reside in intensive care units (ICUs), where priority is given to the hemodynamic status and end organ function whereas measures to maintain physical conditioning are rarely, if at all, instituted. The above considerations often result in

From Goldstein DJ and Oz MC (eds). *Cardiac Assist Devices*. Armonk, NY: Futura Publishing Co., Inc.; ©2000.

167

the institution of mechanical support in debilitated patients with muscle atrophy, respiratory compromise, bone demineralization, and loss of skin integrity.[3,4]

The following discussion is mostly relevant to recipients of implantable LVADs, as these are the patients who eventually are ambulated, exercised, and, in most instances, discharged home to await transplantation. For recipients of short-term mechanical support, most of the physical therapy sessions are focused on the prevention of the debilitating effects of bed rest and immobilization.

Patient Evaluation

Optimal rehabilitation is contingent upon a thorough evaluation performed for the purpose of identifying patient problems, establishing realistic goals, and formulating an individualized plan of care. Ideally, the end-stage heart failure patient should be examined preoperatively to establish baseline measures of physical functioning and to educate the patient and family about the rehabilitation process that is to ensue. Because ventricular assist device implantation often occurs on an emergent basis, a preoperative physical therapy evaluation is not always feasible; however, some information in this regard can be gathered from family members. Postoperatively, the patient is best served when examined within the first 48 hours following surgery.

The evaluation begins with a detailed review of the medical record. The etiology of heart failure, duration of illness, presence of dysrhythmias, and status of end organ function are noted. The medical history is reviewed for identification of comorbid disease that could affect physical function. The social history is gathered, including available social supports and prior functional status, work, and leisure habits. Because the type of device implanted (ie, intracorporeal versus extracorporeal) will have a significant impact on the extent of physical activity that the patient will be able to undertake, information regarding precautions and activity limitations is collected from the ventricular assist device team. The perioperative course is reviewed with special attention paid to complications that may impact on rehabilitation. Finally, current medications and laboratory data are noted.

The physical examination starts with an assessment of mental status, including level of consciousness, orientation, and ability to follow commands. General observations are made regarding the presenting position of the patient, vital signs, presence and location of intravascular and transcutaneous lines and tubes, and mechanical ventilation settings. The ventricular assist device rate, volume, flow, and mode (fixed versus automatic) are noted.

A detailed examination of the skin integrity is performed; particular attention is paid to common sites of pressure ulceration including the occiput, sacrum, heels, and malleoli. The extremities are assessed for presence of edema and signs of peripheral circulatory compromise, which are frequently found in patients receiving vasoactive medications. Examination of the chest includes observation of chest shape and symmetry, breathing pattern, auscultation for breath sounds, and evaluation of cough effectiveness. Rhythm interpretation is noted. Of note, the peripheral pulse reflects device rate and not native heart rate. A gross assessment of sensation, range of motion, and muscle strength is performed in an attempt to find limitations that might impair function. A more detailed examination is carried out if any deficits are found. The patient's functional status is evaluated, including bed mobility, transfers, and, eventually, ambulatory status. The gait pattern is examined for deficits that could compromise safety and/or endurance. Subtle gait impairments may not be readily observable at slow speeds during the acute postoperative period but may appear as the rehabilitation process progresses and the speed of ambulation increases.

Finally, a 6-minute walk test and/or a low-level bicycle or treadmill exercise tolerance test are used to evaluate functional capacity. A symptom-limited cardiopulmonary exercise test with blood gas analysis is the most accurate measure of oxygen consumption.[5] We do not carry out this measurement until at least 4 to 6 weeks after surgery, to allow for postoperative healing and return of end organ function to baseline.

Treatment

The ICU

Patients meeting criteria for ventricular assist device implantation often require a prolonged recovery period that includes several days in the ICU. Indeed, our group reported a mean ICU stay of 8 ± 5 days.[6] The ventricular assist device recipient is usually seen within 48 hours of the operation. Initially, hemodynamic instability, use of extracorporeal mechanical support, or use of continuous hemofiltration may limit or preclude mobilization of the patient. The goal of physical therapy in these early postoperative days is to prevent the deleterious effects of immobilization and bed rest.

While sedated, treatment strategies include 1) chest physical therapy with suctioning; 2) positioning with use of a 2-hour turning schedule as feasible while maintaining hemodynamic stability; 3) use of towel rolls, pillows, and bolsters to relieve pressure over bony prominence; 4) elevation of edematous extremities; 5) splinting of the distal lower extremities with ankle-foot orthoses to prevent ankle plantarflexion contractures and heel skin breakdown; and 6) placement of the patient on a pressure-relief mattress until he or she can stand out of bed to a chair with regularity.

As sedation is weaned, treatment is advanced to enhance the mechanics of breathing, including deep breathing and splinted coughing; also, active assistive and active range-of-motion exercises, in-bed mobility activities, and positioning out of bed to a chair are instituted. If the patient is unable to shift his or her body weight, a pressure-relieving cushion is provided in order to prevent sacral and ischial decubitus ulcers. As condition improves, transfer training is initiated. Ambulation can begin once the pulmonary artery catheter is removed and adequate muscle strength is regained. Safe ambulation requires a minimum strength of 3/5 in selective lower extremity muscles. Native heart rate and rhythm, blood pressure, oxygen saturation, device rate, volume and flow, and symptoms are all monitored throughout the rehabilitation sessions. A specific mobilization method is outlined in Table 1.[7]

Step-Down Unit/Regular Floor Care

The patient is reevaluated on a daily basis. The goals following transfer out of the ICU include independence in 1) device management including battery operation

---

Table 1

Mobilization of the LVAD Recipient

1. Note resting supine heart rate, blood pressure, LVAD rate, flow and volume.
2. Note all drips and location of lines and tubes.
3. Withhold treatment if:
   a. LVAD rate <50 bpm
   b. LVAD volume <30 mL
   c. LVAD flow <3.0 L/min
   d. Systolic blood pressure <80 mm Hg
   e. Heart rate >150 bpm
   f. Sustained ventricular tachycardia or fibrillation
4. Assist supine patient to sit, being certain not to kink or apply torque to the device drive line.
5. Dangle legs 3 to 5 minutes.
6. Assess for orthostasis.
7. Proceed to lower extremity active range of motion or,
8. Prepare to ambulate. For:
   a. Pneumatic LVAD recipients–position the console in front of the patient as if a rolling walker; however, the console handle should not be used to bear weight.
   b. Electric LVAD recipients–attach fully charged batteries one at a time. Apply holster and insert batteries. Clip controller to waist belt or holster.
9. Assist sitting patient to stand and begin ambulation as quickly as possible to prevent orthostasis. Secure the assistance of another healthcare worker when ambulating for the first time. There is a high incidence of orthostasis and the sequelae of falling includes LVAD dislodgment, hemorrhage, and death.
10. Reassess blood pressure, heart rate (if telemetry available), LVAD rate, flow, volume and symptoms.

LVAD = left ventricular assist device.
Reprinted with permission from Reference 7.

and hand cranking (Fig. 1); 2) activities of daily living; 3) transfers; 4) hallway ambulation (Fig. 2); and 5) bedside therapeutic exercise program. The physical therapy plan of care includes continuation of airway clearing techniques, education in device management and exercise regimens, transfer training, and gait training. Assistive devices such as long handle reachers and sock aids should be considered. As the patient becomes independent in ambulation, gentle stretching, lower extremity strengthening, and aerobic conditioning on bicycle or treadmill are started in the gym facilities (Figs. 3 and 4). The Borg Scale of Perceived Exertion[8] can be used to guide the intensity of exercise, aiming for a rating of 11 to 13 on the scale of 6 to 20. Upper extremity resistive exercise is delayed until 6 to 8 weeks postoperatively to allow for sternal healing.

Device rate, blood pressure, and symptomatology are routinely monitored in all patients regardless of device type. Implantable pneumatic LVADs (Thermo Cardiosystems HeartMate 1000IP, Woburn, MA) display continuous measurers of volume and flow. For recipients of an electric LVAD (Thermo Cardiosystems HeartMate 1205 VE), connection of the portable device to the power base unit allows for the gathering of this information, particularly when exercise intolerance develops. Native heart rate and rhythm are monitored with portable telemetry during physical therapy only in those patients who have demonstrated arrhythmias in the early postoperative period, and then, only until the dysrhythmia is controlled. All patients are exercised in the more physiologic auto or empty-to-fill modes.

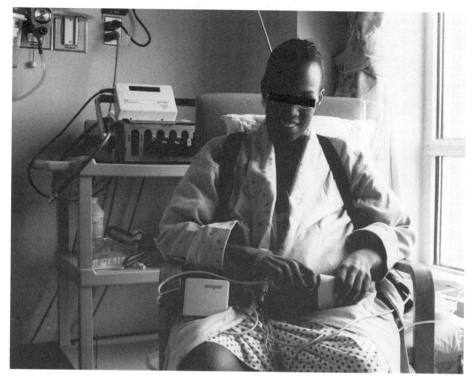

FIGURE 1. Left ventricular assist device recipient troubleshooting device.

An exercise session is terminated when any of the following occurs: 1) subjective intolerance; 2) drop in systolic blood pressure greater than 20 mm Hg or to below 80 mm Hg; and 3) LVAD flow drops below 3 L/min and patient is symptomatic. Immediate intervention under any of these circumstances includes placing the patient in the supine position, obtaining cardiac rhythm, assessing the status of the electric vent, venting the pneumatic console, and contacting the LVAD team. Etiologies of exercise intolerance include hypovolemia, vasodilation with prolonged exercise, decreased drive line air volume, arrhythmia, and sensor failure.[6,9]

Of the first 53 patients who survived LVAD implantation at our institution, 45 (85%) participated in progressive mobilization therapy, 27 (60%) initiated ambulation within 10 days, and 47 (89%) tolerated treadmill exercise for 20 to 30 minutes at a mean workload of 3.2 metabolic equivalents or the equivalent of 2 mph with a 2% grade. In 2571 physical therapy sessions lasting 1814 hours, only 8 minor incidents (all involving decreases in pump flow) occurred, representing 4.4 incidents per 1000 patient-hours.[6,9] There was no resultant morbidity or mortality.

Inpatient Rehabilitation Unit

Patients who are medically stable for discharge home but are not yet functionally independent benefit from transfer to an inpatient rehabilitation unit. In this setting,

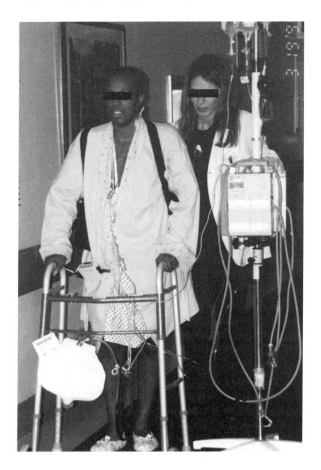

FIGURE 2. Left ventricular assist device recipient ambulating in hallway.

patients can more quickly attain their rehabilitation goals, as physical and occupational therapy are provided twice daily. Furthermore, speech and recreational therapy are available as needed. Transfer into this clinical setting decreases acute care length of stay, helping to contain the costs associated with the care of these patients.

Outpatient Management

The transition to home can be facilitated by participation in an outpatient cardiac rehabilitation program to maximize the patient's strength, flexibility, and aerobic capacity, as well as to gain independence. Patients who do not live near the LVAD center can be referred to a local cardiac rehabilitation program.

The outpatient interview provides an opportunity to ask the LVAD recipient how he or she is functioning at home and in the community. Are there any tasks that he or she finds difficult or impossible to perform? Which of these are most important for his or her quality of life? Specific problems may include stair climbing, bending to reach something on the floor, or getting up from the floor or any low surface. Is the patient ambulating daily? What is the distance he or she has walked? What stops the patient from ambulating further? The treatment goals are individually

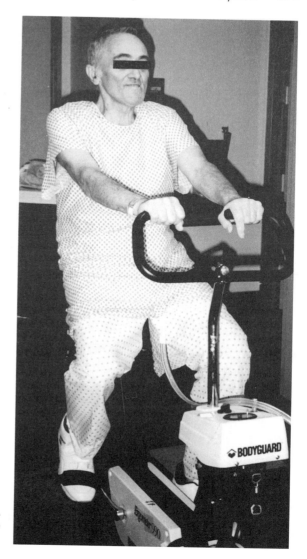

FIGURE 3. Left ventricular assist device recipient exercising on stationary bicycle.

tailored for each patient based on the problems identified in the patient interview and the initial evaluation described above. These goals may include optimization of function by 1) increasing aerobic capacity, strength, and flexibility; 2) preventing postural deformities imposed by the device and the need to carry the battery weight; 3) restoring ideal body weight; 4) gaining independence in a home exercise program; 5) returning to school, work, and/or leisure activities; and 6) psychosocial adjustment.

Aerobic Training

The exercise prescription is described in terms of mode, intensity, duration, and frequency. The exercise mode can include any activity that uses large muscle groups

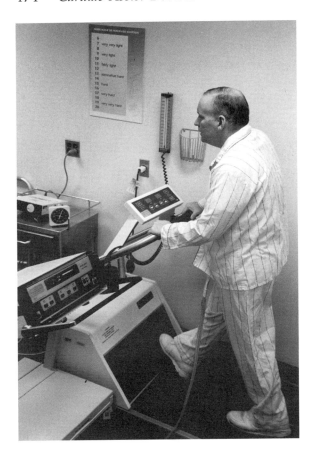

FIGURE 4. Left ventricular assist device recipient exercising on treadmill.

for prolonged periods. It is suggested to this patient population to walk outdoors or on the treadmill or to use a bicycle ergometer. Due to the weight of the LVAD, running and jumping are prohibited and, for air vent precautions, swimming is proscribed, although showering is possible.

Flexibility

Normal function depends on adequate joint range of motion and muscle length. LVAD patients may have limitations in forward bending and trunk rotation due to the presence of the LVAD pump within the abdominal wall. Stretching exercises normally prescribed include exertion of the hamstrings, hip adductors and flexors, and gastrocnemius. As with all patients who have undergone median sternotomy, active shoulder forward elevation should be included in the program. Stretching exercises should be conducted in static positions (without bounce) for 20 to 30 seconds per position, and repeated 3 to 5 times as suggested by the American College of Sports Medicine.[10]

Strengthening

These debilitated patients can benefit from a generalized strengthening program with emphasis placed on areas of focal weakness. Typical plans include the use of free weights, elastic bands, or exercises that use the patient's body weight, such as in modified squats or progressive step heights. Ten to 15 repetitions are recommended for maximal gains in muscular strength and endurance.[10]

The effort expended in the strengthening exercises should not exceed that of the aerobic component of the session. Care should be taken to coordinate exhalation with exertion and to avoid musculoskeletal injury.

Future Directions

The subset of patients who undergo LVAD implantation as a long-term means of mechanical support is faced with great rehabilitation challenges. These patients are prone to complications such as renal dysfunction, cerebrovascular accidents, critical illness neuropathy, and infections that can limit the rehabilitation process. By minimizing the deleterious effects of bed rest, achieving functional independence, and maximizing strength and endurance, physical therapy and rehabilitation play an integral role in the preparation of the LVAD recipient for the rigors of future transplantation.

With the recent Food and Drug Administration approval of LVADs and current trends suggesting longer waiting times for donor organs, an increasing number of patients are being discharged home to await transplantation. Therefore, outside cardiac rehabilitation centers should be able to manage these patients, and they should be given the opportunity to learn about the device and to familiarize themselves with emergent procedures. Indeed, we foresee that these patients will be referred to therapists across regions, settings, and specialties for cardiopulmonary, musculoskeletal, and neuromuscular rehabilitation. Ongoing efforts to educate the physical therapy community will ensure that these patients receive optimal rehabilitation prior to transplantation.

References

1. Frazier OH, Rose EA, McCarthy P, et al. Improved mortality and rehabilitation of transplant candidates treated with a long-term implantable left ventricular assist system. *Ann Surg* 1995;222:327–338.
2. Ashton RC, Goldstein DJ, Rose EA, et al. Duration of LVAD support affects transplant survival. *J Heart Lung Transplant* 1996;15:1151–1157.
3. Kottke FJ. The effects of limitation of activity upon the human body. *JAMA* 1966;196: 825–830.
4. Dean E. Bedrest and deconditioning. *Neurol Report* 1993;17:6–9.
5. Weber KT, Janicki JS. Cardiopulmonary testing for the evaluation of chronic heart failure. *Am J Cardiol* 1985;55:22A-31A.
6. Morrone T, Buck L, Catanes K, et al. Early progressive mobilization of patients with left ventricular assist devices is safe and optimizes recovery before heart transplantation. *J Heart Lung Transplant* 1996;15:423–429.

7. Humphrey R, Buck L, Cahalin L, Morrone T. Physical therapy assessment and intervention for patients with left ventricular assist devices. *Cardiopulm Phys Ther* 1998;9:3–7.
8. Borg G, Linderholm H. Perceived exertion and pulse rate during graded exercise in various age groups. *Acta Med Scand* 1967;472(suppl):194–206.
9. Oz MC, Argenziano M, Catanese KA, et al. Bridge to transplant experience with long-term implantable left ventricular assist devices: Are they an alternative to transplantation? *Circulation* 1997;95:1844–1852.
10. American College of Sports Medicine. *ACSM's Guideline for Exercise Training and Prescription.* Fifth ed. Philadelphia: Williams and Wilkins; 1995:153–193.

Chapter 14

Quality of Life Issues Associated with the Use of Left Ventricular Assist Devices

Peter A. Shapiro, MD

Left ventricular assist systems such as those reviewed elsewhere in this book have demonstrated substantial success in ameliorating the hemodynamic and end organ dysfunction associated with severe impairment of left ventricular function. Demonstration of these effects, however, is not tantamount to proof of improved survival or quality of life (QoL); in fact, evidence supporting claims of such effects is extremely limited. The purpose of this chapter is to review the effects of left ventricular assist device (LVAD) support on QoL in order to gain an understanding of the impact of this revolutionary technology on the psychosocial and emotional well-being of patients with LVADs.

Dramatic anecdotal evidence of the efficacy of these devices is furnished by examples of patients rescued from the verge of death by device implantation. There is no question that some patients recover from otherwise refractory circulatory failure and are able to leave the hospital after LVAD implantation. Some have returned to school and work and have enjoyed substantial physical activity. Beyond anecdotes, more systematic assessment is needed.

Evaluation of QoL, however, is not straightforward. There is no single universally applicable definition or measure of QoL, and subjectivity is inherent in the concept. Quadriplegia, aphasia, dementia, and unremitting pain are examples of conditions believed to often preclude an acceptable QoL, yet many patients affected by these conditions continue to experience living as worthwhile, and judge their QoL to be adequate. Most investigators have stressed that study of QoL should be multidimensional and should incorporate the subjective feelings of the patient. Other investigators have used proxy measures such as return to work, functional status, or days in or out of the hospital to estimate QoL. These and other measures such as costs and medical and psychological complications may fail to incorporate the patient's subjective evaluation of the impact of these aspects of his or her condition into a rating of QoL. Despite this, the published literature on QoL in LVAD recipients is largely limited to such measures.

From Goldstein DJ and Oz MC (eds). *Cardiac Assist Devices*. Armonk, NY: Futura Publishing Co., Inc.; ©2000.

While multiple series have now described the achievement of very desirable medical outcomes, only one has reviewed neuropsychiatric outcomes that have an impact on QoL.[1] In this study, family distress, major depressive disorder, organic mental disorders (ie, delirium, cognitive disorders), and mood and anxiety problems were found to be frequent complications in a cohort of 30 patients, most of whom received pneumatic devices (and were hence unable to leave the hospital to await transplantation). Occult cerebrovascular disease was identified as a significant risk factor for post-implantation neuropsychiatric impairment, including clinical stroke.

A very small number of investigators have actually asked for the subjective assessment of their patients. Dew and colleagues[2] found that outpatient status led to improvement in QoL for two patients compared to their status as inpatients and the status of other patients awaiting transplantation; once in the out-of-hospital setting, their ratings of QoL were comparable to those of transplant recipients. The study was based on a cohort of 24 patients who received the Novacor LVAD system (Baxter Healthcare Corp., Oakland, CA) between 1987 and 1991; of these, 18 patients survived to receive a heart transplant. Domains of QoL evaluated included physical capabilities and limitations, emotional function, social activities, and relationships with others.

Subsequently, the same authors reported on the QoL of LVAD patients who went on to receive heart transplants.[3] There were 163 transplant recipients in a 6-year period, 24 of whom had received LVAD support as a bridge to transplantation for periods ranging from 2 to 226 days. Patients were interviewed 2, 7, and 12 months after transplant. Assessment included measures of self-reported physical functional well-being, psychiatric status, and social adjustment. At 2 months after transplantation, physical functional limitations were reported by 86% of pretransplant LVAD-supported patients compared with 70% of non–LVAD-supported transplant recipients. By 12 months after transplantation, fewer patients in the LVAD cohort (30%) reported limitations than the non-LVAD counterparts (50%), and health perceptions were similar for the two groups. There were more psychological symptoms in the LVAD group throughout the period of study. There was a higher prevalence of cognitive impairment in the LVAD group at 2 months (31% versus 23%), but this difference was not documented at 12 months. Psychiatric disorders occurred in 33% of non-LVAD recipients compared with none of the LVAD patients. Approximately 20% of both groups returned to at least part time employment by 12 months. There were no differences in social adjustment.

In another study by these authors,[4] the status of five Novacor LVAD patients was compared, after transfer from an inpatient to an outpatient halfway house setting, with that of medically managed transplant candidates waiting at home, LVAD patients in the hospital (including the five patients subsequently moved to the outpatient setting), and transplant recipients. Physical function measures (sleep and rest, body care, mobility, and ambulation) in outpatient LVAD patients was almost as good as that in transplant recipients, and substantially better than that in either LVAD inpatients or medically treated transplant candidates at home. For the five LVAD patients evaluated both before and after discharge from the hospital, all measures except sleep and rest improved in the outpatient setting. Sleep seems to be a particular problem because of the difficulty in maintaining a comfortable position in bed due to the position of the transcutaneous drive line, and fear of pulling on it. Among measures of emotional status, depression, anxiety, and anger tended to be lower in LVAD recipients than in medically treated heart transplant candidates at home and better in LVAD outpatients and LVAD inpatients. Overall indices of happiness and life satisfaction in the five LVAD outpatients were high, resembling those of heart transplant recipients. The LVAD outpatients also reported significantly more social activity and interaction than did the LVAD inpatient cohort.

In a study of similar design, Williams and colleagues[5] studied 29 LVAD and transplant recipients, comparing them with patients awaiting transplant without assist devices, and also comparing the experience of the caregivers of each patient group. The authors found improvement in the capacity to perform social roles without limitations, due to physical health, better physical functioning, and improved energy in LVAD patients and transplant recipients compared with transplant candidates, whether waiting at home or inotrope-dependent in-hospital. LVAD patients and transplant recipients scored comparably on all measures. Burden on family members, however, was greater for outpatients with LVADs than for LVAD inpatients or transplant recipients, and greater still for family members of inotrope-dependent hospitalized transplant candidates. While improved hemodynamic/functional status of the patients tended to correlate with lower caregiver burden, outpatient LVAD care added to caregiver responsibilities and perceptions of burden. Cited concerns of caregivers included: 1) feelings of being trapped and inability to sleep due to a perceived need to monitor the LVAD; 2) fear of harming the patient through mistakes in providing LVAD care (eg, risk of causing drive line infections during dressing changes); and 3) fear of inability to intervene properly in the event of LVAD malfunction.

Most recently, Dew and associates[6] conducted a larger study evaluating QoL in LVAD outpatients compared with LVAD inpatients, other heart transplant candidates, and other heart transplant recipients. Of 35 LVAD patients, 18 received the Novacor device and 17 the Thoratec device (Thoratec Laboratories Corp., Berkely, CA). Ten patients were discharged to outpatient care and were reassessed in that setting. Initial assessment took place at an average of 32 days postoperatively, and reassessment after hospital discharge occurred at an average of 59 days after implantation. The remaining 25 LVAD patients, who were not discharged from the hospital to await transplant, comprised the second group. In this latter cohort, seven patients remained in the hospital due to medical complications or unstable coagulation parameters while the other 17 were hospital-bound for reasons unrelated to their medical status. These patients therefore do not represent a true control group, even though they provide a natural comparison group. Comparison groups of transplant recipients (n = 97) and nonhospitalized heart transplant candidates (n = 38) were selected from their respective pools of such patients to match age, sex, and education level of the LVAD patient groups. Transplant recipients were interviewed 7 months after surgery. Patients were assessed with respect to four aspects of functioning: physical functional status, emotional well-being, social functioning, and overall perception of QoL. Caregivers were asked to evaluate their perceived burden of responsibilities and duties. Transplant candidates at home and LVAD inpatients reported more marked limitation of physical function than did LVAD outpatients or transplant recipients. LVAD outpatients reported significant improvement compared with their previous status as inpatients. Similar findings occurred with respect to measures of emotional well-being and social function. Overall perceptions of QoL were similar among LVAD patients in and out of hospital and nonhospitalized transplant candidates, and were inferior to those of transplant recipients. As had been found by Williams et al,[5] caregiver burden was highest for the family members of LVAD outpatients compared with the other three groups.

An innovative approach to QoL assessment further supports the conclusion that

QoL of outpatients with wearable electric LVADs surpasses that of heart failure patients awaiting transplant in or out of hospital on medical therapy, or that of inpatients with LVADs, but is not as good as that of transplant recipients. "Standard gamble" techniques ask patients to make hypothetical trade-offs of potential years of life in return for improvement in their current condition. Such trade-offs result in calculation of the "utility" or preference assigned to various states of health, with a range of zero (poor) to one (best possible). Moskowitz et al[7] evaluated patient preferences using this technique in a small sample of patients before and after LVAD implantation and following subsequent heart transplantation. Utility scores improved from 0.55 before LVAD placement, to 0.81 while on device support, to 0.96 after heart transplantation (only a subgroup of patients was evaluated at all three stages of care). These findings suggest that perceived QoL during LVAD support is not as good as that following heart transplantation, but is good enough to encourage further use of ventricular assist devices.

What factors currently most strongly affect patients' perceptions of QoL with LVADs? Identification of these issues provides an opportunity to target new development efforts with respect to preparation of patients and families as well as to device modification. In a study of 37 patients who received ventricular assist devices between 1996 and 1998 as a bridge to transplantation, most patients reported favorable perceptions of their device.[8] The authors noted that patients' concerns about their devices tended to increase with longer duration of use; interestingly, caregivers had more negative perceptions of device care than the patients did. Risks of stroke, device malfunction, and infection were prominent concerns for family caregivers. Roughly 20% of patients were disturbed by device noise, 35% had concerns about device malfunction, more than 40% expressed concerns regarding the drive line (pain and inability to sleep), and 50% were worried about infectious complications. Psychosocial factors correlated with more negative views were higher education level, more physical functional limitation, and more psychological distress.

In summary, assessments of survival and QoL in patients with LVADs are thus far almost entirely based on small sample sizes with short follow-ups, and are derived from clinical series, which do not provide valid control groups. QoL is a multidimensional construct, but most domains of function and experience have not been investigated. Early studies suggest that patients have an overall favorable adjustment to LVAD implantation and experience life with an LVAD as preferable to life before implantation; to some degree, their greater ease is offset by greater demand on family caregivers. Of course, these studies tend to omit patients who have died or experienced complications that have rendered them unable to complete self-report instruments. Device-related noise, physical discomfort, interference with sleep, and concerns about potential medical complications are prominent sources of anxiety and dissatisfaction. In addition to device malfunctions, bleeding complications, and infections, other problems of potentially considerable significance in determining QoL outcomes are neurologic, psychiatric, and economic. Randomized trials now planned or in progress will provide important new evidence about potential QoL benefits of LVAD placement for patients with end-stage heart disease.

References

1. Shapiro PA, Levin HR, Oz MC. Left ventricular assist devices: Psychosocial burden and implications for heart transplant programs. *Gen Hosp Psychiatry* 1996;18:30S-35S.

2. Dew MA, Kormos RL, Roth LH, et al. Life quality in the era of bridging to cardiac transplantation: Bridge patients in an outpatient setting. *ASAIO J* 1993;39:145–152.
3. Dew MA, Kormos RL, Nastala CJ, et al. *Life Quality Following Heart Transplantation among Patients who Received LVAD Bridges to Transplant.* Abstract presented at the Annual Meeting of the International Society of Heart and Lung Transplantation. San Francisco: 1995.
4. Dew MA, Kormos RL, Nastala CJ, et al. Psychiatric and psychosocial issues and intervention among ventricular assist device patients. In Albert W, Bittner A, Hetzer R (eds): *Quality of Life and Psychosomatics in Mechanical Circulation and Heart Transplantation.* New York: Springer; 1998:17–27.
5. Williams DL, Shapiro PA, Weinberg AD, et al. Quality of life and caregiver burden in LVAD, heart transplant and heart failure patients. *J Heart Lung Transplant* 1996;15:S54.
6. Dew MA, Kormos RL, Winowich S, et al. Quality of life outcomes in left ventricular assist system inpatients and outpatients. *ASAIO J* 1999;45:218–225.
7. Moskowitz AJ, Weinberg AD, Oz MC, Williams DL. Quality of life with an implanted left ventricular assist device. *Ann Thorac Surg* 1997;64:1764–1769.
8. Dew MA, Kormos RL, Winowich S, et al. *Human Factors in Ventricular Assist Device Recipients and their Family Caregivers.* Abstract presented at the American Society for Artificial Internal Organs. San Diego: 1999.

Chapter 15

Economic Considerations of Left Ventricular Assist Device Implantation

Alan J. Moskowitz, MD, Deborah L. Williams, MPH, Anita Tierney, MPH, Ronald G. Levitan, BS, Joshua Zivin, PhD, and Annetine C. Gelijns, PhD

Introduction

Heart failure is a major public health problem, and its management commands a significant amount of healthcare resources. Population-based studies estimate that heart failure afflicts between 3 and 4 million Americans, with about 400,000 new cases being diagnosed each year.[1,2] The number of hospital admissions has increased 10-fold since 1970, and heart failure is the leading diagnosis-related group (DRG) among elderly patients.[3,4] In fact, Medicare alone paid $2.4 billion to hospitals for approximately 613,000 heart failure hospitalizations in 1991 (DRG 127 for heart failure cases only, excluding shock), whereas total treatment costs (including inpatient and outpatient costs) for this condition were estimated to be more than $10 billion in 1991.[5] With use of other estimation techniques, O'Connell and Birstow[6] estimated this figure to be $38 billion. Regardless of which estimate is closer to the truth, both of these figures represent significant resource expenditures (ie, between 1% and 4% of total healthcare costs).

What are the existing treatment options for end-stage heart failure? Advances in medical therapy have had an important impact on symptomatic status and short-term survival in patients with moderate to severe heart failure. However, existing pharmacologic agents have met only with moderate success in Class IV heart failure, and the 1-year survival rate is only 40% to 50%.[7] For these patients, cardiac replacement therapy in the form of cardiac transplantation is now the only viable treatment option.

Among the new therapeutic interventions that are currently under serious consideration is the left ventricular assist device (LVAD). Since 1986, pneumatically

From Goldstein DJ and Oz MC (eds). *Cardiac Assist Devices*. Armonk, NY: Futura Publishing Co., Inc.; ©2000.

driven LVADs have been used experimentally to sustain the lives of end-stage heart failure patients who have decompensated on maximal medical therapy while awaiting cardiac transplantation.[8] The success of this "bridging" experience led to the approval of the Thermo Cardiosystems Inc. (Woburn, MA) LVAD by the Food and Drug Administration (FDA) in September of 1994. During this period, advances in LVAD technology have resulted in the development of a more compact and portable electric version of this device, which opened up the possibility for long-term, out-of-hospital use. In the fall of 1998, the FDA approved two electric LVADs, developed by Thermo Cardiosystems and the Novacor division of Baxter Healthcare Corp. (Oakland, CA), for use as bridging devices.

Given the limitations of current treatment strategies for end-stage heart failure (both the lack of pharmacologic agents and the unavailability of donor hearts), as well as the favorable experience with LVADs, there are increasing pressures to use these devices as alternatives to cardiac transplantation. In the current economic environment of constrained healthcare resources, this broadening of indications must be guided by rigorous trials of the benefits and costs of this emerging technology. Experience with extended usage of LVADs in bridge patients has been quite positive. Such patients have been able to return home to their families with a comparatively good quality of life. Consequently, many in the field have been giving serious consideration to using these devices as long-term treatments for "nonbridge" patients. With the support of the National Heart, Lung, and Blood Institute of the National Institutes of Health (NIH), we are conducting a randomized trial (the REMATCH trial) of this use compared with medical management in patients who require but are not eligible for cardiac transplantation.[9] This trial will evaluate the survival, quality of life, and cost effectiveness of LVAD treatment.

This chapter reviews the existing literature on the costs of LVAD treatment. This information is then used to make projections about the long-term cost effectiveness of LVAD therapy as compared to standard medical therapy. The chapter ends with some observations about the changing nature of the costs of LVAD treatment and the need to conduct further cost effectiveness research in this area.

Costs of LVAD Implantation

Implantation Hospitalization

Empirical data on the costs associated with LVAD implantation are sparse. Our review of the literature disclosed five papers concerning the costing of this device. One study examined hospital and professional charges between 1987 and 1990, and did so for mechanical assist devices produced by three different manufacturers: Novacor, Thoratec, and Symbion.[10] In 32 patients, the mean total charge for implantation, including professional fees, was $221,716. A French study compared the costs of mechanical support in six patients (3 who received total artificial hearts, 1 who received an LVAD, and 2 who received biventricular assist devices) compared with pharmacologic support in 14 patients.[11] With use of payments, the cost per patient at 1 month was $84,683 for those who received a mechanical assist device, and $38,326 for those on medical therapy alone. This experience included five transplantations (before 2 weeks) and three deaths in the 1-month costing period.

The third study reviews the pre-transplantation cost experience of 43 patients, 12 of whom received the Pierce-Donachy LVAD and 31 of whom remained on pharmacologic support alone.[12] For a mean pre-transplant hospital stay of 123.2 days, which included on average 51.6 days of LVAD support, the average cost was $186,131 (charges $302,048). By comparison, the pharmacologically managed patients remained in the hospital prior to transplantation for 52.6 days at an average cost of $100,115 (charges $165,219). A fourth study compared the hospital charges in six patients receiving conventional therapy with six patients receiving conventional therapy plus Thermo Cardiosystems LVAD support.[13] Partly as a result of FDA regulatory policies, the patients in the LVAD group had a significantly longer hospital stay (185 versus 51 days) and, therefore, higher total charges per patient ($435,133 versus $268,696).

We recently reported on our institutional experience with the electrically driven LVAD in 12 adult patients from 1994 through 1995.[14] The outcomes for this population during the period of study included two deaths, eight transplants, and two transplant candidates with device support. The average duration of LVAD support was 177 days, with a range from 13 (due to perioperative mortality) to 481 days (remaining on LVAD support). The average length of stay (LOS) was 43.5 days. We used the ratio of cost to charges method to calculate hospital costs per resource category (Table 1), market prices for drugs and device, and payments for physician services. The average cost of the initial implant-related hospitalization was $161,627 ± $26,932. The cost breakdown by resource use categories is depicted in Table 2.

These studies have several limitations. The first study uses charges as a proxy for costs. Although analyses have historically used provider charges, charges may differ substantially from costs, which are the resource consumed in delivering care. Moreover, not all of the devices in the first study were implantable and, therefore, not all would generate costs and effectiveness measures that would be appropriate for analyzing the prospects of long-term LVAD use. The second study, which took place in France, uses payments made as a surrogate for actual costs, which are known to be country-specific; that is, not easily translatable to other healthcare systems. In

---

Table 1

Summary of Hospital and Professional Services

Resource Category	Subcategories
Inpatient	Regular floor days, special care days (intensive care unit, cardiac care unit, step down unit)
Operating room	
Diagnostics	Computed tomography scan, echocardiography, electroencephalogram, electrocardiogram radioisotopes, radiology diagnostics, ultrasound
Laboratory	Pathology, other laboratory clinical
Therapeutics	Drugs, blood products
Other	Renal dialysis, respiratory therapy, audiology, brace shop, cardiopulmonary
Professional payments	Anesthesiology, cardiology, cardiothoracic surgery, infectious diseases, nephrology, neurology, psychiatry
Left ventricular assist device	Pump, controller, battery pack

Table 2

Vented Electric Left Ventricular Assist Device Cost Summary for 12 Patients

Resource Category	Average Cost: Actual	Average Cost: Sufficient
Inpatient:		
Regular floor & step-down Unit	$23,569 ± 34,047	$7071 ± 7376
Special care days	$15,094 ± 10,914	$14,765 ± 10,874
Operating room	$10,926 ± 1762	$10,818 ± 1725
Diagnostics	$4307 ± 3505	$3900 ± 3574
Laboratory	$4450 ± 1549	$3407 ± 1767
Blood products	$2955 ± 2509	$2873 ± 2562
Drugs	$3817 ± 3666	$3257 ± 3229
Rehabilitation	$1877 ± 1619	$670 ± 423
Miscellaneous	$3345 ± 1720	$3235 ± 1695
Professional payments	$24,203 ± 10,897	$23,935 ± 10,897
LVAD	$67,085	$67,085

LVAD = left ventricular assist device.

addition, the small sample size and select group of patients for each device are significant limitations for generalizing from these results. None of the comparative studies that we cite adequately adjusted for patient differences in severity of illness, which could significantly affect the observed cost differences. Finally, the environment in which LVADs are being used is undergoing substantial change. In particular, prior to 1995, FDA regulation required all patients with implantable LVADs to remain in the hospital. During 1995, this restriction was eased but patients still had to remain in the hospital for a regulated period. Proof of patient safety had to be established through a series of 1-day trial visits home. These restrictions are reflected in the LOS for this study and several of the others cited above.

Estimating the Current Cost of LVAD Treatment

The length of implantation hospitalization has declined since 1995, paralleling reduction in FDA regulatory requirements for hospital discharge and the broadening of the experience with the outpatient care of these patients. Table 2 also shows the projected costs for hospitalizing our 12 vented electric LVAD recipients had the LOS not been regulated by the FDA. This analysis employed objective criteria to establish a day of discharge—what we refer to as "clinically sufficient hospital stay."

These 12 patients would have remained in the hospital for an average of only 17.5 ± 5.3 days rather than the average of 43.5 days they were actually in the hospital. The mean costs of care over that period would have been $74,202 (excluding the cost of the device) and $141,287 (with the cost of the device).

Figure 1 compares the resource consumption categories for the actual versus the clinically sufficient hospital stay as a percentage of total costs. Note that the average cost per day for the actual hospitalization is much lower than the average cost per day of the clinically sufficient course ($4225, or $8058 with device). As men-

Actual   **Clinically Sufficient**

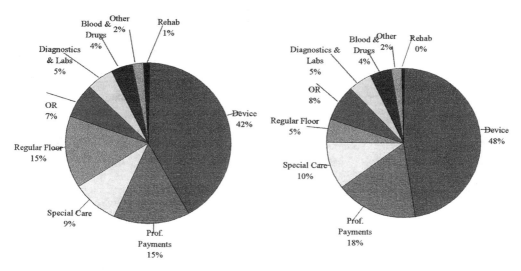

FIGURE 1. Frequency distributions of resource category use for actual and clinically sufficient hospitalizations. Labs = laboratory tests; Prof = professional; OR = operating room; Rehab = rehabilitation.

tioned, this reflects the lack of clinical activities beyond the clinically sufficient hospital stay period. Generally, the only charges listed for patients beyond this period were bed charges, diagnostic and lab tests, and rehabilitation. Given that these diagnostic tests and labs would have been conducted during the weekly outpatient visits if the patients had been discharged, the more than $16,000 difference in bed charges accrued between the clinically sufficient and actual hospitalizations is by far the greatest.

Outpatient and Rehospitalization Costs

Moving beyond the initial hospitalization, we examined outpatient costs and readmissions. The cohort experienced a total of 2012 LVAD support days, of which 1266 days were out of the hospital. This reflects FDA regulations, which, as pointed out previously, until 1995 prohibited the discharge of patients on LVAD support. Looking at the outpatient days for the 1995 implants only, the average was 211 (range 16 to 328 days). The cost of each weekly visit, including professional payments, was $352 (Table 3). The average professional payment per visit was $128. There were a total of 11 readmissions during the period of observation, which involved five patients and 124 hospital days. The total cost of readmissions was $215,093, which corresponds to an average of $43,019 per readmitted patient and $19,554 per readmission. The breakdown of the readmission costs per resource category and the reasons for readmission are depicted in Table 4. Using the 1995 data, we calculated the average actual total cost for an LVAD patient (inpatient and outpatient combined) to be $210,132 over an average period of 9.5 months.

Table 3

Cost of Outpatient LVAD Support for 6 Patients (1995 Implants Only)

Average number of days using device	288.3
Clinically sufficient initial hospital days	17.5
Readmission hospital days (total)	127
Average readmission hospital days (per patient)	21.2
Average total hospital days (per patient)	38.4
Average outpatient days	250
Average weekly professional payments (n = 4)	$128
Cost of weekly laboratory tests and drugs	$224
Total cost of support for 1 week (labs, drugs, and professional payments)	$352

LVAD = left ventricular assist device.

Cost Effectiveness Projections

One objective of an economic evaluation of a clinical intervention is to measure the health resources consumed in relation to the health benefits provided. Cost effectiveness analysis, in particular, looks at how efficiently alternative healthcare interventions use healthcare resources to generate health.[15] The choice of whose costs and whose benefits to include in a cost effectiveness analysis are the factors that give each analysis a particular perspective. The analysis below takes the societal perspective. From this point of view, the constrained resource is the total dollars spent on healthcare by society, and the goal of conducting such an analysis is to establish which interventions the budget should fund to maximize the overall health of society.

The cost effectiveness of a given intervention is measured by the number of dollars consumed for each unit of health being generated, relative to an appropriate standard; the lower this number, the more preferred is the intervention. For patients with end-stage heart failure, who are not eligible for a cardiac transplantation, the therapeutic alternatives include medical therapy, mechanical assistance, left ventricular reduction surgery, and cardiomyoplasty. The first treatment is the standard of care that most patients receive. The latter three are experimental approaches that should be compared with medical therapy.

Table 4

Breakdown of Readmission Days, by Reason

Primary Diagnosis	No. of Readmissions	Average No. of Inpatient Days	Average Cost per Readmission (mean ± SD)
Infection/inflammatory reaction to device	2	14	$23,821 ± $21,262
Congestive heart failure	3	8.3	$8928 ± $11,638
Wound infection	1	12	$20,981 ± $0
Shunt malfunction	1	51	$147,471 ± $0
Aortic outflow graft repair	1	5	$13,059 ± $0
Hypotension	1	2	$1,482 ± $0
Primary cardiomyopathy	1	1	$892 ± $0

The relevant units of health for such a cost effectiveness analysis are survival (ie, years of life) and quality-adjusted survival (ie, years of quality-adjusted life). The latter is the more comprehensive measure of outcome because it takes into consideration both survival and quality of life experienced.

Although there is no absolute criterion by which medical interventions are deemed cost-effective, new interventions such as the LVAD are increasingly compared to the range of health interventions that society currently funds. Thus, calculated cost effectiveness ratios cannot be viewed in isolation, but rather must be viewed with respect to similar healthcare interventions, which, for the LVAD, should include practices such as cardiac transplantation, cardiomyoplasty, and coronary artery bypass surgery.

The first step in calculating incremental cost effectiveness ratios is to gather the average costs and health effects associated with each treatment. The costs of medical management of patients with advanced heart failure have been estimated by a panel of the Institute of Medicine in its report on the Artificial Heart (1990) to be $4800 per month.[16] Adjusting for inflation at 5% per annum, the 1999 annual costs of medical management would be $89,357.

As far as net health benefits are concerned, patients with Class IV heart failure who are on medical management have a 2-year mortality rate of 75% (a life expectancy of approximately 1.44 years). The long-term survival of LVAD recipients remains unknown. A reasonable expectation for such a device is that it will reduce the 2-year mortality of its recipients by one third to one half. In fact, this is underlying hypothesis of the REMATCH trial, an NIH-sponsored evaluation of LVADs in patients with end-stage heart failure, who require, but are not eligible for, cardiac transplantation. Mortality reductions of this magnitude would make the LVAD recipient life expectancy between 2.89 and 4.26 years.

To convert these "unadjusted" life years to quality-adjusted life years (QALY) we must first establish how life with an LVAD is perceived relative to life at full health. We asked this very question to "bridge" patients at our institution.[17] On a scale of zero to 1, where 1 represented full health and zero represented death, the quality of life with an implanted LVAD was rated 0.81, on average. These same patients rated their pre-implant state of health as 0.55, and their post-cardiac-transplantation state of health to be 0.96. If the LVAD is like other heroic interventions, the perceived quality of life will fall off a bit with time. To account for this in our analysis, we use a lower rating (0.75) for the implanted state of health, a value that is closer to that experienced by patients on hemodialysis. When life with an implanted LVAD is worth full health, the average quality-adjusted life expectancy for LVAD recipients would be between 2.16 and 3.19 QALY (depending on whether the LVAD reduced congestive heart failure mortality by one third or one half). In contrast, medical management patients have a quality-adjusted life expectancy of 0.79 QALY. Thus, the expected incremental benefit for LVAD recipients compared to standard medical therapy would be between 1.37 and 2.40 QALY.

Table 5 shows the cost effectiveness calculations using two different estimates for the LOS during implantation (the first is the estimated LOS without FDA regulation, and the second is the actual LOS we observed with bridge patients and FDA regulations in force, regarding discharge). In each case, we give the cost effectiveness ratio under two assumptions of efficacy. The first is that long-term LVAD therapy compared with medical therapy in end-stage heart failure patients will cost, on aver-

Table 5

Incremental Cost-Effectiveness Ratios

Strategy (Implantation LOS 17.5 days)	Incremental Cost	Incremental Effectiveness	Incremental Cost/Effectiveness
LVAD–Low efficacy	$61,938	1.44 years	$46,921
LVAD–High efficacy	$87,013	2.47 years	$37,274

Strategy (Implantation LOS 43.5 days)	Incremental Cost	Incremental Effectiveness	Incremental Cost/Effectiveness
LVAD–Low efficacy	$82,278	1.44 years	$61,762
LVAD–High efficacy	$107,353	2.47 years	$45,756

LOS = length of stay; LVAD = left ventricular assist device.

age, between $37,274 and $46,921 per QALY saved. The second is that the cost per QALY saved for LVAD therapy is between $45,756 and $61,762.

These projections are appropriate for an average population of patients with end-stage heart failure. If the patients in question had another condition that further limited survival (eg, comorbid disease or extreme age), the incremental benefits would be reduced even further, making the intervention less cost-effective. Alternatively, if the LVAD offered an even greater survival benefit, its cost effectiveness ratio would be even more favorable. An important consideration for estimating the cost effectiveness of procedures that increase survival is the future costs of related and unrelated illnesses. Patients with end-stage heart failure, however, have such a short survival, even if the LVAD turns out to be as effective as hypothesized, that future unrelated costs will have little impact on the analysis here.

Conclusions

In the current environment of market-based healthcare reform and cost containment, newly emerging clinical interventions will have to increasingly demonstrate their value, in terms of both benefits and costs. Yet, our review of the literature indicates that the LVAD, a newly emerging, expensive surgical intervention, has not undergone any in-depth analysis of the long-term costs associated with its implantation in heart failure patients.

We reviewed the resource implications of implanting these devices, including the costs of the initial hospitalization, readmissions, and outpatient costs. The projected first year annual cost of LVAD treatment is $204,797, of which the initial hospitalization accounts for approximately 69% ($141,287). Within the initial hospitalization period, the device is by far the single largest cost component. Excluding professional payments, the time spent in the intensive care unit is the next largest contributor to resource consumption, followed by diagnostic tests. As the LVAD is an emerging technology, we can expect that the outcomes, costs, and indications of use will dramatically change over time. The main issue is whether the LVAD will be successful, not as a bridge to transplantation, but as a stand-alone technology.[18]

Table 6

Summary of Cost-Effectiveness Ratios of Selected Heart Disease Treatments

Treatment	Cost Per Life Year Saved or QALYs
CABG surgery left main CAD	$8073
PTCA: severe angina	$8073–$14,859
CABG 3-vessel: severe angina	$16,848
Cardiac transplantation	$37,440
CABG 2 vessel	$39,195
LVAD optimistic	$37,274
LVAD pessimistic	$46,921
PTCA mild angina	$55,224–$119,808
CCU vs intermediate care	
high risk	$81,783
low risk	$344,448

CABG = coronary artery bypass graft; CAD = coronary artery disease; CCU = critical care unit; LVAD = left ventricular assist device; PTCA = percutaneous transluminal coronary angioplasty.
Adapted from the IOM (1991)

Table 6 puts the cost effectiveness of the LVAD into perspective with other cardiac interventions currently funded in most industrialized nations. On the basis of what we are currently willing to pay for, the choice to use LVAD treatment over standard medical therapy offers reasonable value for the expense. This does not mean that LVAD treatment is cost-effective for all potential indications. For instance, cost effectiveness of LVADs as an alternative to transplantation would require a head-to-head comparison of those two strategies. From our preliminary study, transplantation has the advantage of offering a higher quality of life. However, this comparison would also have to weight the benefit of saving a scarce resource (a biologic heart) for another patient who would need it.

In conclusion, we believe that rational decisions concerning the allocation of healthcare resources will increasingly need to depend on research that determines what works and what doesn't work and at what cost. Conducting such research, however, will not eliminate the need to make choices that are exceedingly painful in their nature. That is part of the price that is exacted by scientific and technological progress.

References

1. Ho K, Pinsky J, Kannel W, Levy D. The epidemiology of heart failure: The Framingham Study. *J Am Coll Cardiol* 1993;22:6A-13A.
2. Schocken DD, Arrieta MI, Leaverton PE, Ross EA. Prevalence and mortality rate of congestive heart failure in the United States. *J Am Coll Cardiol* 1992;20:301–306.
3. Yusuf S, Garg R, Held P, Gorlin R. The need for a large randomized trial to evaluate the effects of digitalis on morbidity and mortality in congestive heart failure. *Am J Cardiol* 1992;69:64G-70G.
4. Lorell B. Mortality/incidence/prevalence of heart failure: Current and projected clinical need for mechanical circulatory support. In *The Artificial Heart: Planning for Evolving Technologies*. National Institutes of Health; Bethesda, MD: 1994:9–14.

5. AHCPR. Clinical Practice Guideline #11. *Heart Failure: Evaluation and Care of Patients with Left-Ventricular Systolic Dysfunction*. US Department of Health and Human Services; 1994.
6. O'Connell J, Birstow M. Economic impact of heart failure in the United States: Time for a different approach. *J Heart Lung Transplant* 1994;13:S107-S112.
7. The SOLVD Investigators. Effect of enalapril on survival in patients with reduced left ventricular ejection fractions and congestive heart failure. *N Engl J Med* 1991;325:293-302.
8. Frazier O, Rose E, Macmanus Q, et al. Multicenter clinical evaluation of the HeartMate 1000 IP left ventricular assist device. *Ann Thorac Surg* 1992; 53:1080-1090.
9. Rose E, Moskowitz A, Packer M, et al. The REMATCH trial: Rationale, design, and end points. *Ann Thorac Surg* 1999;67:723-730.
10. Swartz M, Reedy J, Lohmann D, et al. Cost and reimbursement rates for investigational circulatory support. *ASAIO Trans* 1991;37:549-552.
11. Loisance D, Benvenuti C, Lebrun T, et al. Cout, efficacite des strategies therapeutiques chez les candidats a la transplantation cardiaque de savetage. *Arch Mal Coeur Vaiss* 1992; 85:309-314.
12. Mehta S, Aufiero T, Pae W, et al. Mechanical ventricular assistance: An economical and effective means of treating end-stage heart disease. *Ann Thorac Surg* 1995;60:284-291.
13. Cloy M, Myers T, Stutts L, et al. Hospital charges for conventional therapy versus left ventricular assist system therapy in heart transplant patients. *ASAIO Trans* 1995;41:M535-M539.
14. Gelijns A, Richards A, Williams D, et al. Evolving costs of long-term left ventricular assist device implantation. *Ann Thorac Surg* 1997;64:1312-1319.
15. Gold M, Siegel J, Russell L, Weinstein MC. *Cost-Effectiveness in Health and Medicine*. New York: Oxford University Press, Inc.; 1996.
16. Institute of Medicine Committee to Evaluate the Artificial Heart Program of the National Heart, Lung, and Blood Institute. *The Artificial Heart: Prototypes, Policies, and Patients*. Hogness J, Van Antwerp M (eds): Washington, DC: National Academy Press; 1991.
17. Moskowitz A, Weinberg A, Oz M, Williams D. Quality of life with an implanted left ventricular assist device. *Ann Thorac Surg* 1997;64:1764-1769.
18. Catanese K, Goldstein D, Williams D, et al. Outpatient left ventricular assist device support: A destination rather than a bridge. *Ann Thorac Surg* 1996;61:646-653.

Chapter 16

Immunobiology of Left Ventricular Assist Devices

Hendrik-Jan Ankersmit, MD and Silviu Itescu, MD

Introduction

The development of novel materials used for implant surgery and the increasing use of implanted devices has made it evident that no material is biologically inert and that optimal use of biomaterials requires improved knowledge of events that are occurring at the host–implant interface. Biocompatibility may be considered in terms of four separate but inter-related components: 1) the adsorption of proteins and other macromolecules on the material surface; 2) changes in the material induced by the host; 3) local effects of the material on host tissues; and 4) systemic or remote effects of the material on the host. Commonly used biomaterials, including the so-called inert compounds such as titanium, polytetrafluoroethylene, and acrylics, may trigger an array of effects including inflammation, fibrosis, coagulation, and infection. A localized host inflammatory response is a common occurrence irrespective of the material used, and such responses may have an adverse impact on the implant; for example, osteolytic changes around joint implants or fibrosis around mammary implants. In situations in which the biomaterial is in direct contact with the circulation (eg, hemodialysis access), significant changes in systemic immunologic and thrombostatic functions have been described.

Recent advances in the surgical therapy of end-stage heart disease have resulted in the widespread use of left ventricular assist devices (LVADs). Since the biomaterials on the LVAD surface are exposed to the entire host circulation, the biology of the host–LVAD relationship beyond life-sustaining pump and the effects of LVAD implantation on systemic host immunity must be defined. In this chapter, we present an overview of general concepts regarding biomaterial-related host responses, and subsequently delineate our findings on the immunobiologic mechanisms that are triggered in the LVAD patient.

From Goldstein DJ and Oz MC (eds). *Cardiac Assist Devices*. Armonk, NY: Futura Publishing Co., Inc.; ©2000.

Human Immunologic Responses to Implanted Biomaterials

Hemodialysis

The consequences of exposure of the host circulation to the dialysis membrane are a result of two main series of interactions: adsorption of serum proteins onto the membrane and activation of immune pathways by protein or cellular components. Immediately after the start of hemodialysis, serum proteins such as C3b, coagulation factor XII, immunoglobulin G (IgG), albumin, and fibrinogen are adsorbed onto the dialyzer membrane.[1-4] Activation of factor XII results in the release of bradykinin and kininogen, which may induce hypotension and cardiovascular collapse, particularly in the setting of angiotensin-converting enzyme inhibitor use. Binding of C3b results in the generation of the anaphylotoxins C3a and C5a, and is accompanied by an early transient drop in the number of polymorphonuclear leukocytes.[1-4] The transient neutropenia appears to be related to complement-induced changes in the expression of β_2-integrin molecule CD11b/CD18 and the selectin receptor CD62l (L selectin) on the surface of the leukocytes,[5] leading to increased leukocyte adhesiveness and trapping of these cells in the pulmonary vasculature. Moreover, the dialysis membrane induces leukocyte activation and degranulation, as indicated by the release of myeloperoxidase, lactoferrin, and elastase.[6,7]

In addition to its effects on leukocyte number and function, hemodialysis directly affects circulating mononuclear cells. Circulating monocytes become activated, as demonstrated by increase surface expression of various cell markers such as CD11b/CD18, human leukocyte antigen-DR (HLA-DR) and CD14, and heightened production of monocyte-derived proinflammatory cytokines such as interleukins IL-1 and IL-6, and tumor necrosis factor-α (TNF-α).[8-10] However, despite this aberrant state of activation, the circulating monocytes in hemodialysis patients demonstrate a paradoxically decreased functional state marked by reduced phagocytosis, impaired antigen presentation, and reduced cytokine secretion after appropriate stimulation. A similar situation exists with circulating lymphocytes. Despite evidence of T cell and B cell activation accompanying hemodialysis, patients undergoing this procedure demonstrate reductions in CD and CD8 T cell levels,[11,12] and functional T cell and B cell defects.[12,13] These immunologic defects appear to have important consequences, principally by increasing susceptibility to infection.[14] Significantly, infectious diseases represent one of the most important causes of mortality in hemodialysis patients, accounting for 36% of all deaths.[15]

Effects of LVAD–Host Interface on the Immune System

Deposition of Monocytes/Macrophages on the LVAD Surface

The clinical success of LVAD implantation has been accompanied by significant complications, including thromboembolic events in as many as 30% of cases.[16,17] This

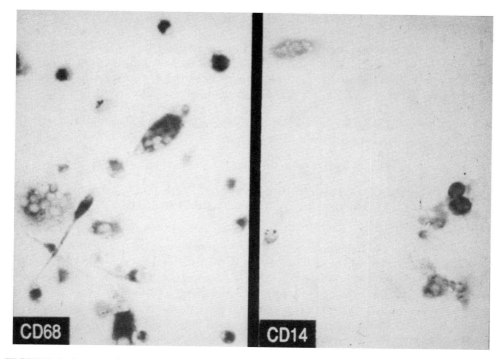

FIGURE 1. Immunohistochemical stain of recipient cells residing on left ventricular assist device surface, demonstrating numerous quiescent, round CD-14–positive monocyte lineage cells and activated CD68-positive monocyte/macrophage lineage cells with cytoplasmic extensions or dendritic-like processes and multinuclear giant cell formation.

complication is reduced to less than 4%[18] in patients who receive textured surface blood contacting surfaces (ie, TCI HeartMate [Thermo Cardiosystems, Woburn, MA]), which support the growth of neointima-type cells.[19,20] Phenotype studies of the cells present on the LVAD surface have revealed that these were mostly of the monocyte/macrophage lineage (Fig. 1). Resting monocytes or activated macrophages were identified as round, quiescent, CD14-positive cells or elongated, often multinucleated, CD68-positive cells with prominent cytoplasmic processes. The macrophage lineage cells were functionally activated, as defined by nuclear factor kappa B (NFkB) expression[21] and augmented production of cytokines and coagulation factors.[22]

Monocyte–T-Cell Interactions on the LVAD Surface

Interspersed among the cells of monocyte/macrophage lineage were T lymphocytes that expressed strong immunoreactivity for CD3, CD4, and CD25 (IL-2 receptors), consistent with activated helper T cells.[23] Moreover, incubation of T cells from the LVAD surface with LVAD material and exogenous IL-2 caused a sevenfold increase in T cell proliferation compared with culture in medium alone, consistent with expansion of in vivo activated T cells. Similarly, T cell aggregates from the

LVAD surface could be sustained in culture for up to 3 weeks in the presence of IL-2 and LVAD material, but not in the absence of either. Finally, with use of the reverse transcriptase-polymerase chain reaction technique to determine the cytokine profile expressed by the neointimal cells on the LVAD surface, all samples studied demonstrated messenger ribonucleic acid (mRNA) for both the Th1 cytokine IL-2 and the Th2 cytokine IL-10, as well as for the monocyte-derived cytokine IL-1.[23] Together, these observations underscore the presence of monocyte–T-cell interactions on the LVAD surface, an event that induces prominent T cell activation via IL-2-receptor–dependent pathways.

Systemic Consequences of Immune Activation Accompanying LVAD Implantation

To determine whether the aberrant T cell activation on the LVAD surface influenced systemic T cell immunity in LVAD recipients, we examined the phenotype and function of *circulating* T cells in LVAD recipients.[24] Circulating T cells from LVAD recipients demonstrated a heightened state of in vivo activation, as defined by surface expression of the activation markers CD95 (Fas), associated with a pathway of cellular apoptosis. CD95 expression was increased in both CD4 and CD8 T cells from LVAD recipients in comparison to controls ($70 \pm 6\%$ versus $22 \pm 4\%$; $P<0.001$, and $69 \pm 7\%$ versus $7 \pm 2\%$; $P<0.001$, respectively). Reflecting this heightened state of in vivo activation, T cells from LVAD recipients had significantly higher spontaneous proliferative activity in comparison to T cells harvested from New York Heart Association (NYHA) Class IV controls.

We next investigated whether this heightened state of T cell activation was associated with increased levels of T cell apoptosis in vivo. Spontaneous T cell apoptosis, defined by binding of annexin V to phosphatidylserine present on T cell membranes undergoing early apoptosis, was significantly higher in both CD4 and CD8 T cells from LVAD recipients when compared with heart failure controls ($39 \pm 5\%$ versus $4 \pm 1\%$; $P<0.001$, and $45 \pm 4\%$ versus $2 \pm 1\%$; $P<0.001$, respectively). Similar abnormalities were observed on T cells from recipients receiving either textured surface (TCI HeartMate) or smooth surface (Novacor, Baxter Healthcare Corp., Oakland, CA) devices. This enhanced state of apoptosis in vivo was further confirmed by analysis of deoxyribonucleic acid (DNA) isolated from freshly obtained T cells. A characteristic fragmentation pattern of apoptosis was observed in DNA from circulating T cells of all LVAD recipients, but not in DNA from T cells derived from control patients.

Despite the high levels of spontaneous proliferation, T cells from LVAD recipients showed defective proliferative responses following activation, specifically via the T cell receptor (TCR) complex (Fig. 2). Following TCR engagement by allogeneic mixed lymphocyte culture, the mean stimulation index (SI) of T cells from LVAD recipients was 74% lower than that of heart failure controls ($P<0.001$). Similarly, following TCR ligation with anti-CD3 monoclonal antibody, the mean SI of T cells from LVAD patients was 83% lower than that of controls ($P<0.001$). In contrast, T cell activation by pathways other than TCR triggering caused similar increases in T cell proliferation in both LVAD recipients and controls.

Since preactivated T cells expressing CD95 (Fas) are susceptible to activation-

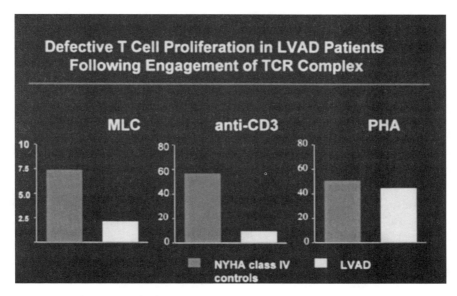

FIGURE 2. Circulating T cells from left ventricular assist device (LVAD) recipients demonstrate defective proliferation following triggering via the T cell receptor (TCR) complex. A. Following TCR engagement by allogeneic mixed lymphocyte culture, the mean stimulation index (SI) of T cells from LVAD recipients was 74% lower than that of T cells from New York Heart Association (NYHA) Class IV controls. Results are expressed as the mean of SI from 12 LVAD recipients and 15 NYHA Class IV heart failure controls ± SEM. B. Following TCR ligation with anti-CD3 monoclonal antibody, the mean SI of T cells from LVAD recipients was 83% lower than that of T cells from NYHA Class IV controls. Results are expressed as the mean of SI from 12 LVAD recipients and 15 NYHA Class IV heart failure controls ± SEM. C. Following T cell activation by non-TCR triggering, using PHA stimulation, T cell proliferation in both LVAD recipients and controls was similar. Results are expressed as the mean of SI from 12 LVAD recipients and 15 NYHA Class IV heart failure controls ± SEM.

induced cell death (AICD) following triggering via the TCR complex, we next investigated whether the observed defects in T cell proliferative responses in LVAD patients following TCR engagement might be related to AICD. A flow cytometric assay was used to detect the proportion of apoptotic T cells that underwent cell death (defined by propidium iodide staining) in a given individual after 24 hours of culture with either medium or anti-CD3 monoclonal antibodies (Fig. 3). The increase in T cell death following anti-CD3 activation was then compared in both experimental groups (LVAD patients and controls). Following activation of resting T cells with anti-CD3, the proportion of CD4-positive cells undergoing cell death increased by a mean of 3.2-fold among LVAD patients compared with only 1.2-fold in heart failure controls ($P<0.05$). These results clearly demonstrate that circulating CD4 T cells from LVAD recipients are more susceptible to AICD compared with those from heart failure controls.

LVAD Implantation as a Model for Diseases of Immune Deficiency

The development of defects in T cell immunity in LVAD patients shares some similarities with that in the human immunodeficiency virus type 1 (HIV-1) infection.

Stimulation with αCD3 mAbs Increases Annexin V and Pi Positivity preferentially in CD4 T Cell Subset

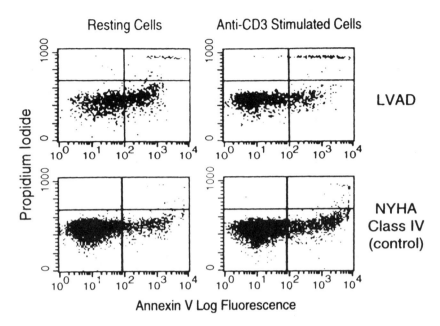

FIGURE 3. Circulating CD4 T cells from left ventricular assist device (LVAD) recipients demonstrate increased susceptibility to activation-induced cell death following T cell receptor engagement. Shown is an example of the flow cytometric assay used to detect the proportion of T cells in a given individual (LVAD recipient or Class IV control) that have undergone apoptosis (annexin V binding) and cell death (propidium iodide positive) after 24 hours of culture with either medium or anti-CD3 monoclonal antibody. Following 24 hours of culture with the latter, death of annexin-V–positive CD4 T cells in the LVAD recipient increased by threefold compared to medium, whereas no differences are observed in the death of CD4 T cells from the control patient under the two experimental conditions.

Progressive depletion of CD4 cells and immune dysfunction in HIV infection accompanies increases in viral burden within cells of various lineages, including T cells, macrophages, and dendritic cells.[25–27] One proposed mechanism is inappropriate induction of T cell apoptosis resulting from HIV-mediated interactions between CD95 and CD95L.[28–31] HIV-infected dendritic cells, a lineage highly specialized for cellular activation through the TCR complex, appear to be particularly effective at inducing T cell expression of CD95 and delivering apoptosis-inducing signals to uninfected T cells.[32,33] Since activation via the TCR complex increases CD95L expression,[34] T cells that express high surface levels of CD95 are particularly susceptible to AICD following TCR engagement by antigen-presenting cells.

It is reasonable to postulate that some aspects of the pathogenesis of AICD in LVAD recipients resemble those in HIV infected individuals. Cells of monocyte or dendritic origin are present on the LVAD surface at the time of explantation,[21] and are functionally activated as defined by NFkB expression and augmented production of cytokines and coagulation factors.[22] In addition, preactivated T cells expressing IL-2 receptors are interspersed among the macrophages and dendritic cells that are isolated at the time of LVAD explantation.[23] These results suggest that antigen-presenting cells that are aberrantly activated by the implanted LVAD deliver excessive costimulatory signals to T cells, inducing surface expression of CD95 and other markers of cellular activation. Rather than proliferate appropriately in response to subsequent antigenic stimulation, these cells presumably undergo AICD as a result of interactions between CD95 and newly expressed CD95L.

Alteration in T Cell Cytokine Profile in LVAD Recipients

Since T cells that are producing Th1-type cytokines (ie, IL-2 and IFN-gamma) have been reported to be selectively susceptible to CD95-mediated apoptosis,[34–38] we next used the reverse transcriptase-polymerase chain reaction to compare the pattern of Th cytokine gene expression in LVAD recipients and heart failure controls. Freshly obtained circulating peripheral blood mononuclear cells (PBMCs) from each of 12 NYHA Class IV controls expressed mRNA for both Th1-type cytokines and Th2-type cytokines (ie, IL-10 and transforming growth factor-β). In contrast, similarly obtained PBMCs from each of 12 LVAD recipients expressed mRNA for the Th2-type cytokines but not for the Th1 cytokines. Expression of IL-4 or IL-5 mRNA was not detected in any of the LVAD patients or control patients. These results suggest that the augmented levels of T cell apoptosis in LVAD recipients leads to a selective loss of T cells that produce Th1-type cytokines and to an unopposed T cell production of Th2-type cytokines.

B Cell Hyper-reactivity in LVAD Recipients

Since induction of autoimmunity, polyclonal B cell activation, and production of autoantibodies have been postulated to result from both excessive circulating apoptotic waste[39–41] and from a predominance of circulating Th2-type cytokines,[42,43] we investigated to determine whether LVAD recipients demonstrate prominent B cell hyper-reactivity. LVAD recipients had significantly higher frequencies of circulating antiphospholipid and anti-HLA antibodies in comparison to NYHA Class IV controls awaiting transplantation. Circulating antiphospholipid antibodies were detected in 9 of 20 (45%) LVAD recipients and in none of 20 controls ($P<0.0001$). Similarly, the frequencies of IgG antibodies against major histocompatibility complex (MHC) class I and II antigens were significantly higher in LVAD recipients than in controls awaiting transplantation (43% versus 3% and 33% versus 3%, respectively; both $P<0.0001$).

We next sought to determine whether production of these anti-MHC antibodies in LVAD recipients were a result of perioperative transfusion of blood products or related to host genetic factors. Sixty-three percent of patients who received more than 6 units of platelets were found to develop IgG antibodies against MHC class I antigens by 4 months post-LVAD implantation, compared with 8% of those receiving less than 6 units ($P<0.01$). Perioperative red blood cell (RBC) transfusions did not influence the production of these antibodies, presumably because donor RBCs contain less contaminating MHC class-I–expressing T cells than donor platelets. In contrast to anti-MHC class I antibodies, development of IgG antibodies against MHC class II antigens was not influenced by the number of perioperative platelet transfusions or by the number of RBC transfusions, presumably because contaminating T cells in the absence of activating signals do not express MHC class II antigens.

We next determined the influence of genetic factors on the development of anti-MHC antibodies. The median time to the appearance of anti-MHC class II IgG antibodies was significantly shorter for LVAD recipients with HLA-DR3 than for those without this particular haplotype (33 versus 103 days; $P = 0.03$). By 50 days post-LVAD implantation, 80% of HLA-DR3 individuals developed anti-MHC class II IgG antibodies compared with only 30% of DR3-negative patients. HLA-DR3 type was also associated with shorter time to developing anti-MHC class I IgG antibodies, although this finding did not reach statistical significance. No other HLA-DR type influenced the onset of anti-MHC antibody production. In additional studies, circulating antiphospholipid antibodies were detected in 7 of 9 (78%) HLA-DR3 LVAD recipients compared with only 5 of 15 (33%) LVAD recipients who were not HLA-DR3 ($P < 0.05$). Together, these results indicate that the inheritance of HLA-DR3 increases susceptibility of LVAD recipients to the development of B cell hyper-reactivity.

LVAD Implantation as a Model of Autoimmunity

A similar discordance between defects in T cell immunity and B cell hyper-reactivity characterizes two other immunologic disorders: systemic lupus erythematosus (SLE)[44–46] and HIV-1 infection.[47,48] A proposed mechanism to account for the coexistence of T cell defects and autoimmunity in these disorders is the inappropriate induction of apoptotic T cell death[28,29,40,41] due to heightened interactions between CD95 and CD95L.[32,33,49,50] Since these interactions appear to result in a selective loss of Th1 cytokine-producing CD4 T cells in both SLE[43,44] and HIV-1 infection,[35,51] the residual populations of CD4 T cells may induce B cell hyper-reactivity and dysregulated immunoglobulin syntheses by unopposed production of Th2 cytokines. Our results support the concept that excessive T cell apoptosis is a general mechanism underlying B cell hyper-reactivity, and suggest that this process is amplified in individuals with inheritance of immunogenetic haplotypes that encode high-level production of additional proapoptotic factors.

Maintenance of T cell homeostasis and peripheral tolerance to self-antigens following repeated lymphocyte stimulation is regulated by a form of apoptosis termed apoptosis-induced cell death. Activated CD4 T cells undergo apoptosis-induced cell death as a result of interactions between CD95 and CD95L molecules coexpressed after TCR engagement.[34–36] Following cross-linkage of CD95, the cytoplasmic domain of this receptor binds the adaptor molecule Fas-associated death domain protein (FADD),[52,53] enabling interactions with the protein-binding domain of another protein termed FLICE (caspase 8). Activation of the latter leads to catalytic activation of a cascade of caspases, with the ultimate result being cellular apoptosis.[54,55] The binding of FLICE to FADD can be competitively inhibited by another recently identified protein, FADD-like interleukin Iβ-converting enzyme inhibitory protein (FLIP), which negatively regulates apoptosis.[56,57] Cellular levels of FLIP are high in naive T cells that are resistant to CD95-mediated apoptosis, but are inhibited in activated T cells by IL-2.[58] Since IL-2 also enhances transcription of CD95L, these observations provide an explanation for the selective sensitivity of IL-2–producing Th1 cells, as well as resistance of Th2 cells, to apoptosis-induced cell death following CD95 engagement.[34–36] The absence of Th1-type cytokine mRNA expression in circulating mononuclear cells from LVAD recipients could therefore be consistent with a selective loss of IL-2–producing Th1 cells in these persons, consequent to induction of CD95-mediated apoptosis. Selective loss of Th1 cells through apoptosis would explain the high prevalence of disseminated fungal infections in vivo[59–61] as well as the observed defects in cell-mediated immunity in vitro in LVAD recipients. Since SLE patients also demonstrate a predominantly Th2-type cytokine profile with loss of IL-2–producing capability, a similar process may underlie the defects in cellular immunity that exist in this disorder.

In addition to the classic DNA fragmentation that accompanies apoptosis, a consequence of FLICE activation following CD95 ligation is the export of phosphatidylserine from the inner to the outer leaflet of the plasma membrane by a process that involves inhibition of mitochondrial phosphatidylserine decarboxylation.[62] Outer leaflet phosphatidylserine serves as a signal for engulfment of apoptotic cells by macrophages,[63] and may be shed from the cell surface within plasma membrane vesicles.[62]

Since high levels of T cell CD95 expression and apoptosis occur in SLE patients,[49,50] it has been postulated that B cell hyper-reactivity and autoantibody production in these patients is a consequence of heightened macrophage presentation of autoantigens, which have been altered by the apoptotic process, to Th2-type CD4 T cells. Indirect support of this hypothesis is the recent observation that intravenous injection of syngeneic apoptotic thymocytes in mice induces the production of antinuclear and antiphospholipid antibodies as well as glomerular IgG deposition.[64] In this context, LVAD implantation serves as an iatrogenic example of another human disorder of B cell hyper-reactivity accompanying excessive T cell apoptosis.

The association between HLA-DR3 and antibody production in LVAD recipients provides a striking parallel to patients with SLE, in whom elevated frequencies of HLA-DR3[65,66] or of HLA-DR3–associated extended haplotypes[67,68] have been well documented. In particular, cumulative observations have shown that inheritance of HLA-DR3 is associated with an extended haplotype that contains both C4 null alleles[65–68] and a particular TNF-α promoter polymorphism[69–71] that is associated with high levels of TNF-α gene transcription[72] and cytokine production,[73] particularly after monocyte stimulation with lipopolysaccharide.[74] The lipopolysaccharide receptor CD14 is used by monocytes to recognize and phagocytose apoptotic cells,[75] suggesting that HLA-DR3 individuals may produce higher levels of TNF-α following CD95-mediated T cell apoptosis than HLA-DR3-negative individuals. Since binding of TNF-α to TNF receptor-1 molecules is accompanied by further augmentation of the FADD/FLICE-dependent cell death pathway,[76] particularly in chronically activated T cells where IL-2 expression inhibits FLIP transcription,[58] this process is likely to lead to a vicious cycle of progressively increasing apoptosis of CD4 Th1 cells, unopposed Th2 cytokine production, and B cell hyper-reactivity in HLA-DR3 individuals.

Clinical Relevance of T Cell Defects and B Cell Hyper-reactivity in LVAD Recipients

We next investigated whether the in vitro defects in cellular immunity identified in LVAD recipients were related to infectious complications in vivo. In a Candidal infection prevalence study among 78 NYHA Class IV heart failure patients who were listed as United Network of Organ Sharing status I and were awaiting cardiac transplantation, the presence of LVAD implantation was associated with a significantly increased risk of developing disseminated Candida infection (defined as positive blood cultures either alone or in combination with positive cultures at extravascular sites).[24]

By 3 months post LVAD implantation, 28% of patients had developed disseminated Candida infection compared with only 3% of those without devices ($P = 0.0029$). Since the risk of developing disseminated Candida infection persisted throughout the duration of LVAD implantation, with 34% of patients developing an infection by 6 months and 45% by 9 months, this is a strong argument that the increased risk was associated with the implanted device rather than with any effects related to the surgery itself. Moreover, no cases of disseminated fungal infection were observed in an additional consecutive 425 patients who underwent cardiac bypass surgery at our institution over the past 12 months, with the same surgical team involved in LVAD implantation.

The clinical consequences of LVAD-related immune dysfunction, particularly disseminated fungal infections, are very serious. In order to prevent induction of defects in host immunity and to limit such infectious complications, novel strategies must be developed. In contrast to HIV-1 disease, in which the etiology of the immune dysfunction is multifactorial, the immune defects that accompany LVAD implantation appear to be far more limited and may therefore be amenable to reversal by therapeutic intervention. One potential approach to prevent apoptosis-induced cell death is the use of cyclosporine A (Sandimmune, Sandoz Pharmaceutical Corp., East Hanover, NJ) or FK506 (Fujizawa, Japan), two drugs that inhibit mRNA transcription of CD95L following T cell activation via the TCR complex.[77] We are currently evaluating these and other strategies to reduce abnormal immune activation that is present in LVAD recipients.

Antibodies in the serum of a cardiac allograft recipient that are directed against donor HLA class I MHC antigens constitutively expressed by allograft endothelium portend a significant risk for early graft failure (ie, within the first 24 to 48 hours, and poorer patient survival as a result of complement-mediated humoral rejection).[78–80] Since T cells constitutively express MHC class I antigens, the presence of preformed lymphocytotoxic antibodies, particularly of IgG isotype, detected in a routine T cell cross-match is considered a contraindication to solid organ transplantation.[78] In order to identify patients at high risk of having a positive donor-specific cross-match, cardiac transplantation candidates are screened for anti-MHC class I antibodies that are reactive with lymphocytes from a panel of volunteers representative of the major HLA allotypes, collectively referred to as panel reactive antibodies (PRA). Since patients with high PRA levels are considered to be sensitized to various alloantigens and require donor-specific cross-matches prior to transplantation at our institution, we investigated the effects of IgG anti-MHC class I antibodies on waiting time to cardiac transplantation. As expected, LVAD patients with IgG anti-MHC class I antibodies had a significantly longer waiting time than those without these antibodies (175 versus 90 days; $P = 0.009$).[81,82] In contrast, the presence of IgG anti-MHC class II antibodies did not affect the waiting time to transplantation (139 versus 144 days; $P = 0.5$).

The presence of IgG anti-MHC class II antibodies detected at the time of transplantation was highly predictive of early high-grade cellular rejection in the post-transplant period.[81] The median time for a high-grade rejection was 70 days for patients with IgG anti-MHC class II antibodies. In contrast, the actuarial freedom from rejection never fell below 50% in more than 1700 days of follow-up for patients without such antibodies (odds ratio 24.3; $P = 0.006$). The presence of IgG directed at class I antigens was also a moderate risk factor for a high-grade rejection; however this was not statistically significant ($P = 0.08$). Additionally, neither the presence of immunoglobulin M (IgM) anti-MHC class I nor that of IgM anti-MHC class II antibodies at the time of transplant influenced the time to high-grade cellular rejection ($P = 0.94$ and $P = 0.79$, respectively). By Cox proportional Hazard modeling for multivariable analysis, the only risk factors identified to predict an early high-grade cellular rejection were the presence of pre-transplant IgG anti-MHC class II antibodies ($P = 0.018$) and, to a lesser extent, IgG anti-MHC class I antibodies ($P = 0.086$). None of the other variables tested in this analysis were predictive of rejection in LVAD recipients, including T cell PRA, matching at the HLA-DR, -B, or -A loci, ischemic time, or donor age. Additionally, those patients with IgG anti-MHC class II antibodies at the time of transplantation had higher cumulative annual rejection frequencies than did those without these antibodies (0.846 versus 0.169 high-grade rejections per patient-year of follow-up). Among the demographic and immunologic variables examined, including the other antibody types, only the presence of pre-transplant IgG anti-MHC class II antibodies was predictive of a higher cumulative annual rejection frequency ($P = 0.002$).

The mechanism by which the presence of pre-transplant IgG anti-MHC class II antibodies relates to the post-transplant development of earlier and more frequent high-grade rejections remains conjectural. Recent cumulative evidence suggests that the indirect pathway of CD4 T cell activation plays a major role in acute and chronic cardiac allograft rejection, due to continuous shedding of donor alloantigenic HLA peptides and their processing by host antigen presenting cells (APC) such as macrophages and B cells. Acute cellular rejection is accompanied by the appearance, in the circulation and in the allograft, of recipient T cells that are reactive with donor HLA-DR peptides presented by self-APC.[83] Primary rejections appear to be invariably accompanied by indirect recognition of a dominant HLA-DR allopeptide,[83,84] whereas recurrent rejections appear to be accompanied by intermolecular spreading and T cell recognition of multiple donor HLA-DR alloantigenic determinants.[84] Similar patterns of progressive intramolecular and intermolecular HLA-DR epitope spreading can be detected in cardiac transplant recipients who are developing accelerated transplant-related coronary artery disease.[85] This diversification of the immune response has been postulated to be a result of activation of antigen-specific B cells by soluble HLA-DR molecules, and the subsequent efficient presentation of multiple HLA-DR allopeptides by self B cells to CD4 T cells.[86–88] Therefore, the relationship between recurrent high-grade cellular rejections and preexisting IgG anti-MHC class II antibodies documented in this study may in fact indirectly reflect the presence in sensitized cardiac transplantation candidates of circulating memory B cells with reactivity to allogeneic HLA-DR molecules.

Therapeutic Interventions

Recent studies have suggested that pooled human intravenous immunoglobulin (IVIg, Baxter Healthcare Corp.) is an effective modality to reduce allosensitization.[89–91] Postulated mechanisms include the presence in IVIg of anti-idiotypic antibodies,[92–94] antibodies against membrane-associated immunologic molecules such as CD4 or CD5,[95,96] or soluble forms of HLA molecules.[97,98] We investigated the effects of IVIg on serum reactivity to HLA class I molecules in LVAD recipients, and compared these effects to plasmapheresis, an alternative modality for the reduction of alloreactive antibodies.[99]

We first evaluated the efficacy of monthly IVIg courses (2 g/kg) combined with monthly infusions of cyclophosphamide (Cytoxan, Bristol-Myers Squibb, Princeton, NJ) (0.5 to 1.0 g/m^2) on reduction of reactivity of circulating IgG antibodies for allogeneic HLA class I molecules. Data were obtained from 16 patients who received one to three monthly courses of IVIg (total 28 courses). Each course of IVIg was evaluated as an independent event, and the effects of each course on IgG anti-HLA class I antibodies during the ensuing 4 weeks were analyzed. Within 1 week following infusion of IVIg in four divided daily doses, the reactivity of circulating IgG antibodies for allogeneic HLA class I molecules was reduced by a mean of 33% ($P = 0.01$). This was the maximal level of reduction in alloreactivity achieved during the 4 weeks post IVIg infusion, with the efficacy progressively decreasing by the end of the fourth week to a mean reduction in alloreactivity of 8 ± 7%. Sequential courses of IVIg did not cause an additive effect. Each course resulted in a similar level of reduction in alloreactivity compared to baseline, with mean decreases of 38%, 36%, and 35% accompanying first, second, and third courses of IVIg, respectively. Six of the 16 highly sensitized patients were found to be resistant to treatment with IVIg, with a mean reduction of only 4% in reactivity of circulating IgG antibodies with allogeneic HLA class II molecules per treatment course in this group. These patients were subsequently treated with one to two courses of high-dose (3 g/kg) IVIg therapy. In each patient treated, high-dose IVIg reduced reactivity with a mean reduction of 20% (range 16% to 24%) per treatment course ($P < 0.05$).

We next compared the effects of IVIg (2 g/kg) with plasmapheresis on reduction of reactivity of circulating IgG antibodies with allogeneic HLA class I molecules in LVAD recipients. Four sensitized patients received one to two monthly courses of plasmapheresis, administered two to three times per week (total six courses). Reactivity of circulating IgG antibodies with allogeneic HLA class I molecules was not significantly reduced within the first 2 weeks of initiation of therapy. Maximal reduction in alloreactivity occurred by the fourth week of plasmapheresis (38 ± 11%). These results show that IVIg has earlier onset of action and greater efficacy in reducing IgG anti-HLA alloreactivity compared with plasmapheresis.

The effect of IVIg (2 g/kg) plus Cytoxan (0.5 to 1.0 g/m^2) therapy on waiting time to transplantation was studied. The first three highly sensitized LVAD recipients to receive desensitization therapy had unsuccessfully been waiting for cardiac transplantation for a mean of 303 ± 25 days prior to the onset of therapy. This was a result of repeated positive donor-specific cross-matches (mean 33, range 24 to 43). Following initiation of combined IVIg and Cytoxan therapy, with or without additional plasmapheresis, all patients obtained negative donor-specific cross-matches and were successfully transplanted in a mean duration of 99 ± 8 days. On the basis of these results, a formal protocol was established to initiate monthly courses of combined therapy with IVIg and Cytoxan following initial detection of allosensitization. The duration from listing to cardiac transplantation was then compared between 28 sensitized patients who did not receive IVIg treatment and 16 sensitized patients who received treatment following detection of anti-HLA class I IgG antibodies. None of these patients received additional plasmapheresis. Whereas the mean duration to transplantation was 7.1 months (range 0.2 to 17.9 months) in patients with IgG antibodies against HLA class I molecules, this was significantly reduced to 3.3 months (range 0.3 to 6.2 months) in sensitized recipients receiving therapy ($P<0.05$). No patient in either group was transplanted across a positive donor-specific IgG T cell cross-match. This duration was similar to the waiting time to transplantation in 27 unsensitized patients (3.1 months, range 0.3 to 10.7).

We next evaluated the efficacy of immunosuppression using Cytoxan on post-transplant outcome in individuals with preexisting IgG anti-MHC class II antibodies. Standard immunosuppression with Sandimmune, prednisone, azathioprine (Imuran, Glaxo Wellcome Inc., Research Triangle Park, NC) or mycophenolate mofetil (CellCept, Roche Laboratories, Nutley, NJ) was used in 35 patients (group 1). In 10 patients, intravenous Cytoxan was administered monthly peri-transplant and for two to six doses post-transplantation together with Sandimmune and prednisone (group 2). In group 1, IgG anti-MHC class II antibodies increased post-transplantation in 52% of patients, whereas in group 2, IgG anti-MHC class II antibodies increased in only 10% ($P=0.02$). By Kaplan-Meier analysis, group 2 patients had a significantly longer time to a high-grade rejection than those in group 1 ($P = 0.03$). During the first post-transplant year, 58% of patients in group 1 had at least one high-grade rejection compared with only 1 patient in group 2. Moreover, the cumulative annual high-grade rejection frequency was significantly lower in group 2 than in group 1 (0.21 versus 0.53 high-grade rejection/year, $P<0.05$). Our results indicate that the use of Cytoxan in highly sensitized cardiac transplant recipients significantly improves clinical outcome, possibly involving mechanisms that reduce alloreactivity against HLA class II antigens.

Use of these therapies was not without morbidity (Table 1). IVIg therapy was

Table 1

Side Effects of Immunoglobulin Depletion Therapy

	IVIg	Plasmapheresis
Infectious	1/27 Staph aureus sepsis	3/6 Staph aureus and Acinetobacter sepsis
Immunologic	4/27 Immune complex disease (fever, rash, arthralgia)	2/6 Anaphylactic reactions
Renal	Reversable renal insufficiency (>50% increase in serum creatinine) 0/21 low-dose IVIg (2 g/kg) 4/6 high-dose IVIg (3 g/kg)	—

IVIg = immunoglobulin g.

associated with clinical manifestations of immune complex disease in 4 of 27 (15%) monthly courses, as evidenced by fevers, arthralgias, and maculopapular rashes. Only 1 in 27 courses was associated with systemic infection (*Staphylococcus sepsis*). High-dose IVIg therapy resulted in reversible renal insufficiency (defined as >50% rise in serum creatinine) in 4 of 6 courses. All cases resolved spontaneously over the ensuing 3 weeks post infusion. Renal insufficiency was not observed in any courses of low-dose IVIg. Systemic infection accompanied 3 of 6 (50%) courses of plasmapheresis. In addition, 2 of 6 courses (33%) of plasmapheresis were associated with systemic anaphylaxis, as defined by hypotension requiring pressor support. Together, these results suggest that low-dose IVIg has a better safety profile than does plasmapheresis in this group of patients. Intravenous Cytoxan was not associated with any infections, bleeding, or neoplastic complications.

Conclusions

The development of novel materials used for implant surgery and the increasing use of implanted devices had made it evident that improved biocompatibility of such materials will require a better understanding of the events occurring at the host–implant interface and in the host circulation. It has become evident that biomaterials in direct contact with the blood circulation elicit significant immunologic and thrombostatic alterations. LVAD implantation results in an aberrant state of monocyte and T cell activation, increased production of pro-inflammatory cytokines by these cells, heightened susceptibility of circulating CD4 T cells to AICD, progressive defects in cellular immunity, and increased risk for serious infection. A second consequence of the progressive loss of immunoregulatory CD4 T cells is unbridled Th2 helper cell activity resulting in polyclonal B cell hyper-reactivity manifested by excessive production of various antibodies, including those directed against HLA and phospholipid-related antigens. At a clinical level, the increased production of anti-HLA antibodies prolongs the waiting time of LVAD recipients for a suitable cardiac transplant donor, since these portend an increased risk of antibody-mediated allograft rejection. Protocols incorporating the use of intravenous γ-globulin and Cytoxan have proven to be effective at reducing anti-HLA alloreactivity, shortening cardiac transplant waiting time, and improving post-transplant outcome by reducing episodes of cellular rejection.

Since the number of patients with end-stage heart failure continues to grow, and cardiac transplantation remains a limited option due to donor organ shortage, permanent LVAD implantation has emerged as a potential therapeutic modality for these patients. However, the immune dysfunction identified in LVAD recipients will need to be addressed in order to achieve successful long-term LVAD implantation. Although the T cell defects identified in these patients resemble those found in individuals afflicted with the HIV infection, these appear to be relatively limited in scope in comparison to the broad multifactorial immune dysfunction accompanying HIV disease. Nevertheless, LVAD implantation serves as an iatrogenic model of immune deficiency due to excessive T cell activation and apoptosis, confirming this as one mechanism for the development of progressive CD4 T cell dysfunction and depletion in vivo. Since the immune dysfunction appears to be related to the effects of excessive biomaterial-related monocyte and T cell activation, future efforts will be directed toward either altering the physical properties of the materials interfacing with the host circulation or developing pharmacologic interventions to inhibit pathways of cellular activation. Together, these approaches to improving biocompatibility should have a positive impact on the long-term success of LVAD implantation.

References

1. Hakim RM. Clinical implications of hemodialysis membrane biocompatibility. *Kidney Int* 1993;44:484–494.
2. Radovich JM. Composition of polymer membranes for therapies of end-stage renal disease. *Contrib Nephrol* 1995;113:11–24.
3. Parnes EI, Shapiro WB. Anaphylactoid reactions in hemodialysis patients treated with AN69 dialyzers. *Kidney Int* 1991;40:1148–1152.
4. Lo SK, Detmers PA, Levin SM, Wright SD. Transient adhesion of neutrophils to endothelium. *J Exp Med* 1989;169:1779–1793.
5. Whele B, Bergstrom J, Kishimoto T, et al. β2-microglobulin and granulocyte release. *Nephrol Dial Transplant* 1993;8:20–24.
6. Brubacker L, Nolph K. Mechanisms of recovery from neutropenia induced by hemodialysis. *Blood* 1971;38:623–631.
7. Grooteman MPC, Nube MJ, Daha MR, et al. Cytokine profiles during clinical high-flux dialysis: No evidence for cytokine generation by circulating monocytes. *J Am Soc Nephrol* 1997;8:1745–1754.
8. Tielemans CL, Delville JPC, Husson CP, et al. Adhesion molecules and leukocyte common antigen on monocytes and granulocytes during hemodialysis. *Clin Nephrol* 1993;39:158–163.
9. Thylen P, Lundahl J, Fernivik E, et al. Mobilization of an intracellular glycoprotein (Mac-1) on monocytes and granulocytes during hemodialysis. *Am J Nephrol* 1992;12:393–400.
10. Schiller B, Ziegler-Heitbrock HWL, Meyer N, et al. Monocyte phenotype and interleukin-1 production in patients undergoing hemodialysis. *Nephron* 1991;59:573–579.
11. Ueki Y, Nagata M, Miyake S, Tominaga Y. Lymphocyte subsets in hemodialysis patients treated with recombinant erythropoietin. *J Clin Immunol* 1993;4:279–287.
12. Descamps-Latscha B, Herbelin A. Long-term dialysis and cellular immunity: A critical survey. *Kidney Int* 1993;43:S135-S142.
13. Paczek L, Schaefer M, Heidland A. Dialysis membranes decrease immunoglobulin and interleukin-6 production by peripheral blood mononuclear cells in vitro. *Nephrol Dial Transplant* 1991;(suppl 3):41–44.
14. Himmelfarb J, Hakim RM. Biocompatibility and risk of infection in hemodialysis patients. *Nephrol Dial Transplant* 1994;9:138–144.
15. Mailloux LU, Belluci AG, Wilkes BM. Mortality in dialysis patients: Analysis of the causes of death. *Am J Kidney Dis* 1991;3:326–335.
16. Didisheim P. Current concepts of thrombosis and infection in artificial organs. *ASAIO J* 1994;40:230–237.
17. Wagner WR, Johnson PC, Kormos RL, Griffith BP. Evaluation of bioprosthetic valve-associated thrombus in ventricular assist device patients. *Circulation* 1993;88:2023–2029.
18. Rose EA, Levin HR, Oz MC, et al. Artificial circulatory support with textures interior surfaces: A counterintuitive approach to minimizing thromboembolism. *Circulation* 1994;50:1187–1191.
19. Menconi MJ, Owen T, Dasse KA, et al. Molecular approaches to the characterization of cell and blood/biomaterial interactions. *J Card Surg* 1992;7:177–187.
20. Dasse KA, Chipman SD, Sherman CN, et al. Clinical experience with textured blood contacting surfaces in ventricular assist devices. *ASAIO Trans* 1987;33:418–425.
21. Spanier TB, Oz MC, Rose EA, et al. Activation of NFKb is central to the proinflammatory/procoagulant response in textured surface left ventricular assist device recipients and may be influenced by anti-inflammatory intervention with aspirin. *J Heart Lung Transplant* 1997;17:80.

22. Spanier TB, Oz MC, Levin HR, et al. Activation of coagulation and fibrinolytic pathways in patients with left ventricular assist devices. *J Thorac Cardiovasc Surg* 1996;112;1090–1097.

23. Spanier TB, Rose E, Schmidt AM, Itescu S. Interactions between dendritic cells and T cells on the surface of left ventricular assist devices leads to a Th2 pattern of cytokine production and B cell hyper-reactivity in vivo. *Circulation* 1996;94:1704.

24. Ankersmit J, Tugulea S, Spanier T, et al. Activation-induced T cell death and immune dysfunction after implantation of left ventricular assist device. *Lancet* 1999;354:550–555.

25. Pantaleo G, Graziosi C, Demarest JF, et al. HIV infection is active and progressive in lymphoid tissue during the clinical latent stage of disease. *Nature* 1993;362:355–358.

26. Perelson AS, Neumann AU, Markowitz M, et al. HIV-1 dynamics in vivo: Virion clearance rate, infected cell life-span, and viral generation time. *Science* 1996;271:1582–1586.

27. Safrit JT, Koup RA. The immunology of primary HIV infection: Which immune responses control HIV replication. *Curr Opin Immunol* 1995;7:456–461.

28. Ameisen JC, Capron A. Cell dysfunction and depletion in AIDS: The programmed cell death hypothesis. *Immunol Today* 1991;12:102–105.

29. Groux H, Torpier G, Monte D, et al. Activation-induced death by apoptosis in CD4 + T cells from human immunodeficiency virus infected asymptomatic individuals. *J Exp Med* 1992;175:331–340.

30. Katsikis PD, Wunderlich ES, Smith CA, Herzenberg LA. Fas antigen stimulation induces marked apoptosis of T lymphocytes in human immunodeficiency virus infected individuals. *J Exp Med* 1995;181:2029–2036.

31. Orlikowski T, Wang ZQ, Dudhane A, et al. Cytotoxic monocytes in the blood of HIV type-1 infected subjects destroy targeted cells in a CD95-dependent fashion. *AIDS Res Hum Retroviruses* 1997;13:953–960.

32. Cameron PU, Pope M, Gezelter S, Steinman RM. Infection and apoptotic cell death of CD4 + T cells during an immune response to HIV-1 pulsed dendritic cells. *AIDS Res Hum Retrovirus* 1994;10:61–71.

33. Finkel TH, Monks C, Casella C, et al. Apoptosis and HIV disease. *Nat Med* 1995;1:386–387.

34. Ju ST, Panka DJ, Cui H, et al. Fas(CD95)/FasL interactions required for programmed cell death after T-cell activation. *Nature* 1995;373:444–448.

35. Ledru E, Lecoeur H, Garcia S, et al. Differential susceptibility to activation-induced apoptosis among peripheral Th1 subsets: Correlation with bcl-2 expression and consequences for AIDS pathogenesis. *J Immunol* 1998;160:3194–3206.

36. Brunner T, Mogil RJ, LaFace D, et al. Cell-autonomous Fas (CD95)/Las-ligand interaction mediates activation-induced apoptosis in T-cell hybridomas. *Nature* 1995;373:441–444.

37. Dhein J, Walczak H, Baumler C, et al. Autocrine T-cell suicide mediated by APO-1 (Fas/CD95). *Nature* 1995;373:438–441.

38. Lenardo MJ. Interleukin-2 programs mouse alpha beta T-lymphocytes for apoptosis. *Nature* 1991;353:858–861.

39. Casiano CA, Martin SJ, Green DR, Tan EM. Selective cleavage of nuclear antigens during CD95 (Fa/Apo-1) mediated T-cell apoptosis. *J Exp Med* 1996;184:765–778.

40. Casciola-Rosen L, Rosen A, Petri M, Schlissel M. Surface blebs on apoptotic cells are sites of enhanced procoagulant activity: Implications for coagulation events and antigenic spread in systemic lupus erythematosus. *Proc Natl Acad Sci U S A* 1996;93:1624–1629.

41. Bach JF. Immunology: New clues to systemic lupus. *Lancet* 1997;350:SIII11.

42. Funauchi M, Ikopma S, Enomoto H, Horiuchi A. Decreased Th1-like and increased Th2-like cells in systemic lupus erythematosus. *Scand J Rheumatol* 1998;27:219–224.

43. Horwitz DA, Grgay JD, Behrendsen SC, et al. Decreased production of interleukin12 and other Th1-type cytokines in patients with recent onset systemic lupus erythematosus. *Arthritis Rheum* 1998;41:838–844.

44. Alcocer-Verela J, Alarcon-Segovia D. Decreased production of and response to Il-2 cultured lymphocytes from patients with systemic lupus erythematosus. *J Clin Invest* 1982;69:1388–1392.

45. Huang YP, Miescher PA, Zubler RH. The interleukin 2 secretion defect in vitro in patients with systemic lupus erythematosus is reversible in rested cultured T cells. *J Immunol* 1986;137:3515–3520.

46. Klinman DM, Shirai A, Ishigatsubo Y, et al. Quantitation of IgM and IgG secreting B cells in the peripheral blood of patients with SLE. *Arthritis Rheum* 1991;34:11–15.

47. Bernard C, Exquis B, Reber A, et al. Determination of anticardiolipin and other antibodies in HIV-1 infected patients. *J Acquir Immune Defic Syndr Hum Retrovirol* 1990;3:536–539.
48. Sollinger AM, Hess EV. Induction of autoantibodies by HIV infection and their significance. *Rheum Dis Clin North Am* 1991;17:157–176.
49. Mysler E, Bini P, Drappa J, et al. The APO-1/Fas protein in human systemic lupus erythematosus. *J Clin Invest* 1994;93:1029–1034.
50. Perniok A, Wedekind F, Herrmann M, et al. High levels of circulating early apoptotic peripheral blood mononuclear cells in systemic lupus erythematosus. *Lupus* 1998;7: 113–118.
51. Clerici M, Shearer GM. The Th1-Th2 hypothesis of HIV infection: New insights. *Immunol Today* 1994;15:575–581.
52. Boldin MP, Varfolomeev EE, Pancer Z, et al. A novel protein that interacts with the death domain of Fas/APO-1 contains a sequence motif related to the death domain. *J Biol Chem* 1995;270:7795–7798.
53. Chinnaiyan AM, O'Rourke K, Tewari M, Dixit VM. FADD, a novel death domain containing protein, interacts with the death domain of Fas and initiates apoptosis. *Cell* 1995;81: 505–512.
54. Boldin MP, Goncharov TM, Golstev YV, Wallach D. Involvement of MACH, a novel MORT1/FADD-interacting protease, in Fas/APO-1 and TNF receptor-induced cell death. *Cell* 1996;85:803–815.
55. Muzio M, Chinnaiyan AM, Kischel FC, et al. FLICE, a novel FADDD-homologous ICE/ CED-3-like protease, is recruited to the CD95 (fas/Apo-1) death-inducing signalling complex. *Cell* 1996;85:817–827.
56. Hu S, Vicenz C, Ni J, et al. I-FLICE, a novel inhibitor of tumor necrosis factor receptor-1 and CD95-induced apoptosis. *J Biol Chem* 1997;272:17255–17257.
57. Irmler M, Thorne M, Hahne M, et al. Inhibition of death receptor signals by cellular FLIP. *Nature* 1997;388:190–195.
58. Reafeli Y, Van Parijs L, London CA, et al. Biochemical mechanisms of IL-2 regulated Fas-mediated T cell apoptosis. *Immunity* 1998;8:615–623.
59. Goldstein DJ, El-Amir NG, Ashton RC, et al. Fungal infections in left ventricular assist device recipients: Incidence, prophylaxis and treatment. *ASAIO J* 1995;41:873–875.
60. Holmann WL, Murrah CP, Ferguson ER, et al. Infections during extended circulatory support: University of Alabama at Birmingham experience 1989 to 1994. *Ann Thorac Surg* 1996;61:366–371.
61. McCarthy PM, Schmitt SK, Vargo RL, et al. Implantable LVAD infections: Implications for permanent use of the device. *Ann Thorac Surg* 1996;61:359–365.
62. Aussel C, Pelassy C, Breittmayer JP. CD95 (Fas/APO-1) induces and increased phosphatidylserine synthesis that precedes its externalization during programmed cell death. *FEBS Lett* 1998;431:195–199.
63. Fadok VA, Voelker DR, Campbell PA, et al. Exposure of phosphatidylserine on the surface of apoptotic lymphocytes triggers recognition and removal by macrophages. *J Immunol* 1992;148:2207–2216.
64. Mevorach D, Zhou JL, Song X, Elkon KB. Systemic exposure to irradiated apoptotic cells induces autoantibody production. *J Exp Med* 1998;188:387–392.
65. Arnett FC, Reveille JD. Genetics of systemic lupus erythematosus. *Rheum Dis Clin North Am* 1992;18:865–892.
66. Davies EJ, Hillarby MC, Cooper RG, et al. HLA-DQ, DR and complement C4 variants in systemic lupus erythematosus. *Br J Rheumatol* 1993;32:870–875.
67. Kemp ME, Atkinson JP, Skanes VM, et al. Deletion of C4A genes in patients with systemic lupus erythematosus. *Arthritis Rheum* 1987;30:1015–1022.
68. Schur PH, Marcus-Bagley D, Awdwh ZL, et al. The effect of ethnicity on major histocompatibility complex complement allotypes and extended haplotypes in patients with systemic lupus erythematosus. *Arthritis Rheum* 1990;33:985–992.
69. Jacob CO, Fronek Z, Lewis GD, et al. Heritable major histocompatibility complex class II-associated differences in production of tumor necrosis factor-alpha: Relevance to genetic predisposition to systemic lupus erythematosus. *Proc Natl Acad Sci U S A* 1990;87: 1233–1237.
70. Wilson AG, de Vries V, Pociot F, di Giovane FS, et al. An allelic polymorphism within

the tumor necrosis factor alpha promoter region is strongly associated with LLA A1, B8, and DR3 alleles. *J Exp Med* 1993;177:557–560.

71. Wilson AG, Gordon C, di Giovane FS, et al. A genetic association between systemic lupus erythematosus and tumor necrosis factor alpha. *Eur J Immunol* 1994;24:191–195.

72. Wilson AG, Symons JA, McDowell TL, et al. Effects of a polymorphism in the human tumor necrosis factor alpha promoter on transcriptional activation. *Proc Natl Acad Sci U S A* 1997;94:3195–3199.

73. Bouma G, Crusius JB, Oudkerk-Pool M, et al. Secretion of tumor necrosis factor alpha and lymphotoxin in relation to polymorphisms in the TNF genes and HLA-DR alleles: Relevance for inflammatory bowel disease. *Scand J Immunol* 1996;43:456–463.

74. Louis E, Franchimont D, Prion A, et al. TNF gene polymorphism influences TNF-alpha production in LPS-stimulated whole blood cell culture in healthy humans. *Clin Exp Immunol* 1998;113:401–406.

75. Devitt A, Moffatt OD, Raykundalia C, et al. Human CD14 mediates recognition and phagocytosis of apoptotic cells. *Nature* 1998;392:505–509.

76. Chinnaiyan AM, Tepper CG, Seldin MF, et al. FADD/MORT1 is a common mediator of CD95 (Faas/APO-1) and tumor necrosis factor receptor-induced apoptosis. *J Biol Chem* 1996;271:4961–4965.

77. Brunner T, Yoo NJ, LaFace D, et al. Activation-induced cell death in murine T cell hybridomas. Differential regulation of Fas (CD95) versus Fas ligand expression by Cyclosporin A and FK 506. *Int Immunol* 1996;8:11017–11019.

78. Smith JD, Danskine AJ, Laylor RM, et al. The effect of panel reactive antibodies and the donor specific crossmatch on graft survival after heart and heart-lung transplantation. *Transplant Immunol* 1993;1:60–65.

79. Joysey VC. Tissue typing, heart and heart-lung transplantation. *Br J Biomed Sci* 1993;50:272–276.

80. Ratkovec RM, Hammond EH, O'Connell JB, et al. Outcome of cardiac transplant recipients with a positive donor-specific crossmatch—preliminary results with plasmapheresis. *Transplantation* 1992;54:651–655.

81. Itescu S, Tung T, Burke E, et al. Preformed IgG antibodies against major histocompatibility class II antigens are major risk factors for high-grade cellular rejection in recipients of heart transplantation. *Circulation* 1998;98:786–793.

82. Moazami N, Itescu S, Williams M, et al. Platelet transfusions are associated with the development of anti-major histocompatibility complex class I antibodies in patients with left ventricular assist support. *J Heart Lung Transplant* 1998;17:876–880.

83. Liu Z, Colovai AI, Tugulea S, et al. Indirect recognition of donor HLA-DR peptides in organ allograft rejection. *J Clin Invest* 1996;98:1150–1157.

84. Tugulea S, Ciubotariu R, Colovai Ai, et al. New strategies for early diagnosis of heart allograft rejection. *Transplantation* 1997;64:842–847.

85. Ciubotariu R, Liu Z, Itescu S, et al. Persistent allopeptide reactivity and epitope spreading in chronic rejection of organ allografts. *J Clin Invest* 1997;101:398–405.

86. Vanderlugt CJ, Miller SD. Epitope spreading. *Curr Opin Immunol* 1996;8:831–836.

87. Mamula MJ, Janeway CA Jr. Do B cells drive the diversification of immune responses? *Immunol Today* 1993;14:151–154.

88. Reed EF, Hong B, Ho E, et al. Monitoring of soluble HLA alloantigens and anti-HLA antibodies identifies heart allograft recipients at risk of transplant associated coronary artery disease. *Transplantation* 1996;61:556–572.

89. Glotz D, Haymann J, Sansonetti N, et al. Suppression of HLA-specific alloantibodies by high-dose intravenous immunoglobulins (IVIg). *Transplantation* 1993;56:335–337.

90. Tyan DB, Li VA, Czer L, et al. Intravenous immunoglobulin suppression of HLA alloantibody in highly sensitized transplant candidates and transplantation with a histoincompatible organ. *Transplantation* 1994;57:553–562.

91. Peraldi M, Akposso K, Hayman J, et al. Long-term benefit of intravenous immunoglobulins in cadaveric kidney retransplantation. *Transplantation* 1996;62:1670–1673.

92. Dwyer JM. Manipulating the immune system with immune globulin. *N Engl J Med* 1992;326:107–116.

93. Dietrich G, Algiman M, Sultan Y, et al. Origin of anti-idiotypic activity against anti-factor VIII autoantibodies in pools of normal human immunoglobulin G. *Blood* 1992;79:2946–2951.

94. Rossi F, Kazzzatchkine MD. Anti-idiotypes against autoantibodies in pooled normal polys-pecific Ig. *J Immunol* 1989;143:4104–4109.
95. Hurez V, Kaveri SV, Mouhoub A, et al. Anti-CD4 activity of normal human immunoglobu-lins for therapeutic use (IVIg). *Ther Immunol* 1993;1:269–278.
96. Vassilev T, Gelin C, Kaveri SV, et al. Antibodies to the CD5 molecule in normal immuno-globulins for therapeutic use. *Clin Exp Immunol* 1993;92:369–372.
97. Blasczyk R, Westhoff U, Grossewilde H. Soluble CD4, CD8, and HLA molecules in com-mercial immunoglobulin preparation. *Lancet* 1993;341:789–790.
98. Lam L, Whitsett CF, McNicholl JM, et al. Immunologically active proteins in intravenous immunoglobulin. *Lancet* 1993;342:678.
99. John R, Lietz K, Burke E, et al. Use of intravenous immunoglobulin to reduce allosensitiza-tion in LVAD recipients awaiting transplantation. *Circulation* 1999. In press.

Part II

Available Devices:
A. Extracorporeal Devices

Extracorporeal Support:

Centrifugal Pumps

Jack J. Curtis MD and Colette Wagner-Mann DVM, PhD

Introduction

Of the various cardiac assist devices presently available, centrifugal pumps are the most commonly used.[1] This is not surprising because these devices are available to all surgeons, they are relatively simple to operate, and they are inexpensive compared with other devices. Importantly, in the large group of patients receiving mechanical cardiac assist for postcardiotomy ventricular failure, survival seems more dependent on reversibility of myocardial pathology than on the type of mechanical assist device employed.[1–3]

Saxton and Andrews first suggested the attractiveness of a centrifugal design for a blood pump because of its autoregulatory pressure-flow performance.[4] The absence of occluding surfaces and multiple moving parts, as well as the absence of valves were traits that purported to reduce hemolysis and component wear.

A centrifugal blood pump that was capable of left heart bypass was described and tested in animals by Bernstein,[5] and first used clinically by Golding[6] and Pennington.[7] Although some patients were salvaged, the device caused excessive hemolysis and was abandoned. Worldwide, numerous centrifugal pumps with improved technology are presently available or in development for clinical use.[8–17]

Description of Centrifugal Pumps

Centrifugal pumps, also known as rotodynamic or radial-flow pumps, impart momentum to fluid by means of fast-moving blades, impellers, or concentric cones. Fluid enters the pump axially from an inlet pipe or tubing, and is caught up between vanes or stages and whirled outward. Rotation (rotary action) of the impellers or

From Goldstein DJ and Oz MC (eds). *Cardiac Assist Devices*. Armonk, NY: Futura Publishing Co., Inc.; ©2000.

stages causes the velocity of the fluid to change while it moves toward the periphery of the pump. As the fluid exits through the outlet port, pressure is increased. Centrifugal pumps can provide high flow rates with low pressure rises. Flow with centrifugal pumps is particularly sensitive to afterload. These pumps are ineffective in handling high-viscosity fluids (ie, efficiency drops sharply with increasing viscosity). Interested readers should refer to the comprehensive book on the engineering science of rotary pumps by Herbert Addison.[18]

Most centrifugal pumps have only one moving part. Consequently, disposable blood pumps can be manufactured inexpensively. Centrifugal pumps require priming and are susceptible to "air lock" depriming if air enters the system, a trait that

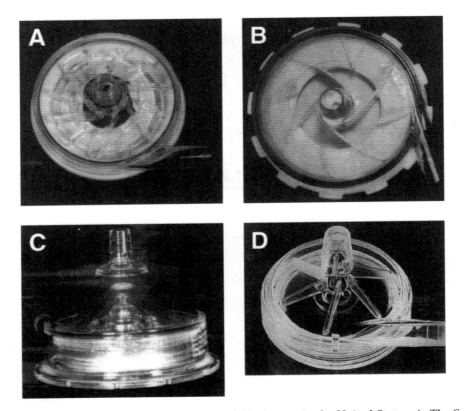

FIGURE 1. Centrifugal pumps currently available for use in the United States. A. The Sarns centrifugal pump is composed of a spinning impeller system to impart a rotary motion to incoming perfusate. B. The St. Jude Medical Lifestream centrifugal pump (Bard Cardiopulmonary Division, Haverhill, MA) uses a curved vane design and angled egress blood flow path, which purports to minimize turbulence, decrease hemolysis, and reduce periods of flow stasis. C. The Bio-Medicus BIO-PUMP centrifugal pump head (Medtronic Bio-Medicus, Inc., Eden Prairie, MN) consists of valveless rotator cones made to impart a circular motion to incoming blood by viscous drag and constrained vortex principles generating pressure and flow. The Carmeda-coated BIO-PUMP has the same appearance but has heparin covalently bonded to the blood contacting surfaces. D. The Nikkiso centrifugal pump (Nikkiso Co., Ltd., Shizuoka, Japan) consists of a semiopen-holed impeller with six straight vanes mounted to the magnet shaft. A through C reproduced from Reference 37, with permission from *Seminars in Thoracic and Cardiovascular Surgery*; D reproduced from Reference 16, with permission from *Artificial Organs*.

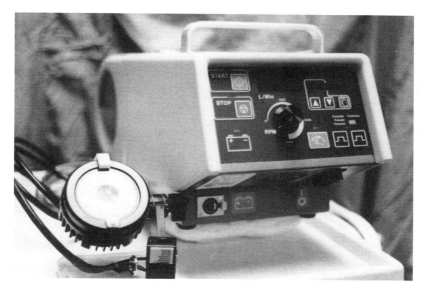

FIGURE 2. The Sarns perfusion system has four principal components: a sterile disposable centrifugal pump (see Fig. 1A) that is magnetically coupled to a motorized pump drive unit, an ultrasonic Doppler flow sensor that is placed around the outflow tubing of the centrifugal pump, and a microcomputer-based control console that regulates flow.

is desirable in human use because large air boluses are less likely to be propagated to patients with use of centrifugal pumps compared with roller pumps.

Figure 1 shows several centrifugal blood pumps that are available in the United States. Each of these systems consists of a disposable pump coupled to a motorized pump drive unit. Each has some system for monitoring and controlling blood flow. Figure 2 shows the Sarns centrifugal perfusion system (3M Health Care, Ann Arbor, MI) used at the University of Missouri Health Sciences Center. Table 1 lists the priming volume and propulsion mechanism of commonly available centrifugal pumps.

In Vitro Comparison of Centrifugal Pumps

Because early centrifugal pumps caused significant hemolysis, subsequent models have been designed to eliminate this problem. Marketing strategies of these

Table 1		
Characteristics of Centrifugal Pumps Currently Available for Clinical Use in the US		
	Prime (mL)	# Impellers
Sarns 3M	52	12
St. Jude	67	8
Nikkiso	25	6
Medtronic BioPump	87	2 concentric cones

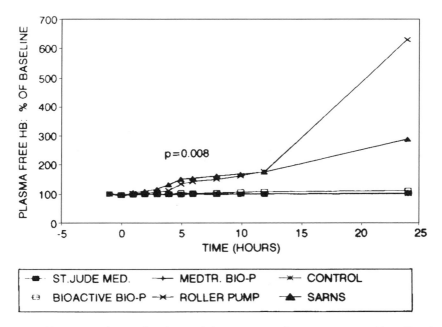

FIGURE 3. Change in plasma-free hemoglobin, expressed as percentage of baseline for each of the pump systems tested, including control, over the 24-hour in vitro experimental protocol. Reproduced from Reference 19, with permission from *International Journal of Angiology.*

pumps are often based on reliability, priming volume, and blood cellular destruction over time when compared with roller pumps.

We have compared four centrifugal pump systems (Sarns, St. Jude [Bard Cardiopulmonary Division, Haverhill, MA], BIO-PUMP [Medtronic Bio-Medicus, Eden Prairie, MN], and Carmeda BIO-PUMP [Medtronic Bio-Medicus]) with a standard roller pump in an in vitro trial designed to assess blood cell element destruction.[19] Identical circuits (n=7) primed with fresh, unpooled, citrated bovine blood were used to test each of the five systems for 24 hours at a flow of 4.5 L per minute. No mechanical mishaps were observed during the 24 hours of pumping with any of the five systems. Platelet counts decreased similarly among the groups. Of the monitored blood parameters, no significant differences were observed during the first 4 hours of pumping. By 5 hours, however, plasma-free hemoglobin and lactic dehydrogenase levels rose significantly with the roller pump and the Sarns centrifugal pump. With additional pumping, evidence of continued red blood cell destruction was observed with the roller pump (Fig. 3). Other comparisons of centrifugal pumps with roller pumps have shown that centrifugal pumps are less destructive to red blood cells.[20,21] Well designed in vitro comparisons of centrifugal pumps have been reported.[13,22,23] In general, all clinically available centrifugal pumps have superior blood handling characteristics when compared with roller pumps. Engineering efforts continue to improve geometric design, with the aim of further improving centrifugal pumps.[24,25]

In Vivo Comparison of Centrifugal Pumps

We compared four centrifugal pumping systems in a 96-hour left heart assist calf model, and evaluated mechanical function, hematologic effects, and incidence of thromboembolism.[26] Left atrial to thoracic aorta bypass was accomplished with the Sarns, St. Jude, BIO-PUMP, and Carmeda BIO-PUMP (n = 5 in each group) with use of techniques that have been previously described.[27] Left heart bypass was maintained for 96 hours at 3.5 L/min with continuous hemodynamic monitoring and frequent blood sampling. Heparin was used in the initial prime only. Compared with sham-operated controls, platelet counts dropped and complement (C3a) rose significantly but similarly with each pump. No significant differences were noted among the centrifugal pump groups with regard to changes in plasma-free hemoglobin or lactic dehydrogenase. All pumps functioned for 96 hours. Inspection of the pump heads at the end of 96 hours revealed detectable pump thrombus in 4 of 5 pump heads in each group. Gross and histopathologic findings at post mortem examination of the animals revealed frequent thromboembolism, confirming the need for strict anticoagulation strategies, as has been observed in other experimental and clinical experience with centrifugal mechanical assist.[28–36]

In summary, observations from in vitro and in vivo testing reveal no compelling features that would dictate clear superiority of one clinically available centrifugal pump over another.[37]

Implantation Techniques

Implantation techniques for centrifugal mechanical assist are simple but require great attention to detail. Our techniques have evolved based on potential and observed complications.[38–42]

Cannula Selection

A variety of cannulae have been used for centrifugal mechanical assist at the University of Missouri, and some of these are shown in Figure 4. To avoid kinking, we prefer wire-reinforced cannulae. The choice of cannula seems less important than the insertion technique, the route of exit from the mediastinum, and the fixation technique.

Insertion Technique

Table 2 lists reported sites, as well as our preferred sites, for left and right heart cannulation. Postoperative bleeding is common after centrifugal mechanical assist (CMA),[31,42,43] and the most common source of bleeding is at the cannulation sites. Meticulous cannulation technique is the most important factor in the avoidance of postoperative bleeding.

Concentric purse-string sutures are employed at all cannulation sites, with the innermost tied to prevent bleeding and the outermost left to be secured at the time of cannula removal. Bleeding at the cannulation sites is unacceptable. If bleeding is present after this technique has been accomplished, the second (outermost) purse-string is tied and others are added as needed.

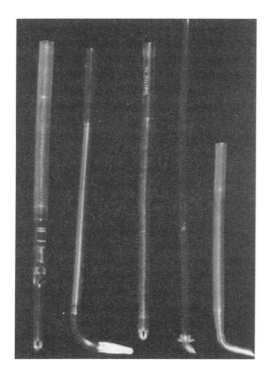

FIGURE 4. Cannulae that are frequently employed for centrifugal mechanical assist for postcardiotomy ventricular failure (from left to right): 36F wire-reinforced venoatrial (two-stage) cannula (Sarns) used for right atrial cannulation; DLP VAD 36F venous cannula (DLP, Inc., Grand Rapids, MI) used for cannulation of the left atrium at the entrance of the right superior pulmonary vein; 32F or 36F wire-reinforced straight venous return cannula (Sarns) used for cannulation of the left atrium, right atrium, or the pulmonary artery; 8-mm aortic arch cannula (Sarns) used for aortic cannulation and, less frequently, for pulmonary artery cannulation; and William Harvey wire-reinforced aortic perfusion cannula (CR Bard, Inc, Tewsbury, MA), which is less commonly used for aortic or pulmonary cannulation. Reproduced from Reference 40, with permission from *Annals of Thoracic Surgery*.

Table 2

Reported Sites for Left and Right Heart Cannulation for Centrifugal Mechanical Assistance

---

Left Heart Cannulation
 Egress
  *Junction of superior pulmonary vein with left atrium
  Left atrial appendage
  Left atrium between superior and inferior pulmonary veins
  Dome of left atrium
  Left ventricular apex
  Left ventricle via ascending aorta
 Return
  *Ascending aorta
  Aortic arch
  Subclavian artery
  Femoral artery
Right Heart Cannulation
 Egress
  *Low right atrium with tip pointed cephalad
  Right atrial free wall with ventricular cannulation across tricuspid valve
  Bicaval cannulation
  Right atrial appendage
 Return
  *Pulmonary artery
  Pulmonary artery via right ventricular outflow tract

---

* Indicates preferred cannulation site at the University of Missouri-Columbia.

Left Heart Bypass

Cannulation of the aortic arch distal to the left common carotid artery is theoretically attractive as a technique to reduce cerebrovascular thromboembolism. However, when the patient cannot be weaned from cardiopulmonary bypass, we usually accomplish left heart CMA using the existing aortic cannula.[40] Our preferred site for the left atrial cannulation is at the junction of the right superior pulmonary vein and the left atrium. This site may have been used intraoperatively for left ventricular venting. No attempt is made to cross the mitral valve with the venous cannula. A right-angled 36F cannula (Fig. 4) is a little bit more difficult to insert and remove, but provides excellent drainage. A 32F or 36F straight wire-reinforced venous catheter also functions satisfactorily.

Right Heart Bypass

For right ventricular CMA, the surgeon may use the existing 36F two-staged wire-reinforced venous return catheter that is employed during routine cardiopulmonary bypass. However, we prefer recannulation through concentric sutures placed low at the junction of the inferior vena cava and the right atrium, orienting the tip of the cannula superiorly. This allows the cannula direct exit from the mediastinum inferiorly through the abdominal wall, without kinking.

Our choice of blood return to the pulmonary circulation is by direct cannulation of the pulmonary artery just distal to the pulmonic valve. Although arterial cannulae can be used, we commonly use a 32F wire-reinforced "venous return" catheter at this site.

Cannula Fixation

It is important to avoid movement at the cannulation sites postoperatively in order to prevent bleeding. Exiting cannulae through the intercostal spaces should be avoided if possible, because chest wall excursion with ventilation or use of a sternal retractor can cause motion of the cannulae. We generally exit the aortic cannula from the median sternotomy incision superior to the sternum. The right and left atrial cannulae exit inferior to the right costal margin, and the pulmonary artery cannula inferior to the left costal margin. Indeed, it is easier to place the cannulae through the abdominal wall before cannulating the left and right atria and the pulmonary artery. Once adequate placement and function are confirmed, the cannulae are secured to the skin with heavy silk sutures. A schematic of biventricular CMA is depicted in Figure 5.

Postinsertion Considerations

Unless intraoperative physiology dictates otherwise, left heart CMA is always started first and slowly as right ventricular function is assessed. Rapid delivery of blood to the right heart can precipitate right ventricular dilation.

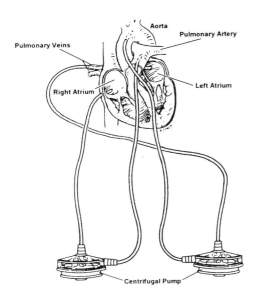

FIGURE 5. Schematic of biventricular centrifugal assist and preferred cannulation sites.

Although not preferred, the sternum is left open in most cases, because the cannulae and expanding lungs crowd the heart and interfere with venous drainage. The unopposed sternal edges can be a major source of bleeding in the patient with coagulopathy. Sternal edge bleeding is controlled in this situation by applying warmed bone wax. Skin closure is preferred. If the skin cannot be closed, transparent silicone sheeting is sutured to the edges, with use of continuous suture. An iodophor adhesive drape is placed over the silicone sheeting to make an airtight seal.

Mediastinal exploration to relieve tamponade or to control bleeding is performed in the intensive care unit, avoiding the difficult return trip to the operating room. This is accomplished by incision of the silicone sheath in midline, evacuation of the mediastinum, control of hemorrhage, irrigation with warm saline solution, closure of the silicone sheet, and application of an additional iodophor adhesive drape.

We routinely interpose a disposable plastic T-connector with Leur-Lok™ between the cardiac cannulae and the bypass tubing. This facilitates priming and air removal when elective or urgent device exchange is necessary.

Renal insufficiency and pulmonary edema are common after CMA. Incorporation of a hemofiltration filter in the centrifugal tubing circuit is a convenient and expedient technique for removal of excess intravascular volume. The ultrafiltration rate can be controlled by passing the effluent through an infusion pump, which controls the egress and avoids large intravascular volume shifts. We usually connect the hemofiltration filter to the right ventricular assist circuitry as shown in Figure 6.[44] This circuitry is also applicable when left ventricular assist only is employed.

Management of Anticoagulation

Anticoagulation strategies continue to evolve. In the setting of postcardiotomy CMA, coagulopathy is ubiquitous and bleeding is common. Our initial anticoagula-

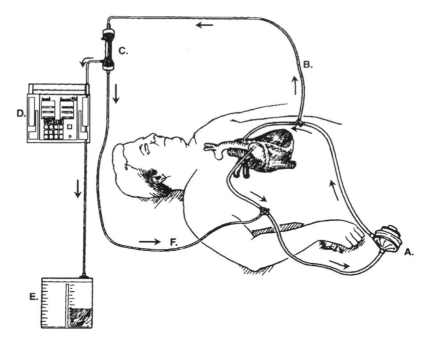

FIGURE 6. A centrifugal pump is used for postcardiotomy ventricular assist. A. The outflow limb of the ventricular assist device provides the driving pressure for ultrafiltration. B. A hollow-fiber filter removes excess intravascular volume. C. An intravenous infusion pump allows one to precisely control (D) the volume of effluent (E) taken from the ultrafiltration device. The inflow limb of the ventricular assist circuit receives outflow (F) from the filter. Reproduced from Reference 44, with permission from *Artificial Organs*.

tion strategy was to allow the coagulation profile to normalize and bleeding to subside before instituting heparin anticoagulation. This rarely occurred during the first 24 hours. It has become clear that this anticoagulation strategy will result in a significant incidence of thromboembolism.

We have reviewed the clinical course of 43 patients who failed to survive centrifugal mechanical assist, to compare the thromboembolism rate diagnosed clinically with that determined at autopsy. In the 35 patients who had no autopsy, there was one clinically apparent thromboembolic event (2.3%). In eight similar patients who had autopsy, there was no clinically apparent thromboembolism. At autopsy, however, 5 of these 8 patients (63%) had evidence of acute thromboembolic infarcts. There were 3 pulmonary thromboembolisms, 2 cerebral vascular infarctions, 2 liver infarcts, 2 splenic infarcts, 2 renal infarcts, and 1 each gastric, pancreatic, prostatic, adrenal, cervical, and ileal infarcts documented in this study.[28] Based on this evidence and on our animal research experience, it is clear that thromboembolism is much more common than is clinically apparent. It is also clear that any meaningful data on thromboembolism rates with any device must include autopsy data.

Our present anticoagulation strategy for postcardiotomy CMA is to completely reverse heparin with protamine in the operating room. Postoperatively, a heparin drip is begun when the partial thromboplastin time (PTT) drops below 60 seconds, a phenomenon that rarely occurs during the first 24 hours in this setting. The PTT is then maintained in the range between 40 and 60 seconds, ensuring that the PTT is in the higher range during weaning trials. This is coupled with an aggressive mediastinal reexploration policy, since most massive bleeding will be from surgical causes and not from coagulopathy. It remains to be seen if this more aggressive anticoagulation strategy translates into reduced thromboembolism.

Monitoring of Centrifugal Mechanical Assistance

Patients are monitored primarily in our Thoracic Intensive Care Unit by our nurses, staffed two nurses per patient. Nurses are comfortable with this responsibility having had minimal training, because of the few and simple controls on the devices. The centrifugal pump speed is set at the lowest revolutions per minute (rpm) that will accomplish the flow prescribed by the physician. Central venous pressure is maintained in the physiologic range by addition of fluids or blood as necessary. Flow at a given centrifugal pump speed is preload- and afterload-dependent. In the absence of adequate preload, the atrium will collapse about the inlet cannula, causing cessation of blood ingress. This is followed by release of the atrial wall as the atrium fills. With inadequate atrial volume, this process repeats rapidly, causing a "chunking" or "chattering" of the pump inlet tubing. This is managed by decreasing the rpm or administering fluid to the patient.

At a given pump speed, flow is dependent on vascular resistance. A sudden fall in flow may suggest a kinked outflow tubing rarely, or, more often, a pump failure. Line pressure is not monitored. As there is no reservoir to empty, the risk of air embolization is quite small, particularly if preload is maintained.

Oversight of CMA is provided by our cardiopulmonary perfusionists through periodic checks with overall control by the attending surgeon. Coagulation studies, hemoglobin, electrolytes, and arterial blood gases are monitored at intervals consistent with the patient's course. Plasma-free hemoglobin is not measured as long as the urine is clear. Nitric oxide is increasingly employed in cases of right heart failure or pulmonary hypertension.

Weaning of Centrifugal Mechanical Assistance

Because it is frequently difficult to discern why CMA was required, it is difficult to be dogmatic in dictating the minimal duration CMA should be maintained. Our goal is to remove the device(s) as soon as hemodynamic competence and stability return. This rarely occurs before 24 hours.

Weaning of left ventricular CMA is reasonably straightforward[37] Initially, the systemic arterial pressure trace without intra-aortic balloon pumping may show no contribution from the left ventricle. However, because left ventricular bypass is incomplete, as left ventricular function recovers, a pulse pressure will be observed at full flows and magnified as CMA flows are decreased. Thermodilution cardiac output measurements allow one to determine right ventricular output. By subtracting CMA flow, the portion of cardiac output contributed by the recovering left ventricle is easily determined. When a right ventricular index of 2.0 to 2.2 L/min/m^2 is accomplished with minimal inotropic drugs and left CMA at low flow, CMA on/off trials are performed and are repeated every 8 hours until recovery is ascertained.

Timing of weaning of biventricular CMA is more difficult. Because mixing does not occur in the right ventricle, cardiac output by thermodilution is inaccurate, and the relative contributions of the right and left ventricles to forward flow cannot be determined without CMA on/off trials. Pulmonary artery SVO_2, while helpful, may be misleading because of selective CMA pumping of more saturated inferior vena caval blood. However, an SVO_2 of less than 50% reflects inadequate tissue perfusion, provided both by CMA and the heart, assuming other causes of low SVO_2 have been ruled out. We observe for left ventricular recovery as described for left CMA. Then, with both devices temporarily decreased to the lowest rpm that will prevent flow reversal, CMA on/off trials are observed.

A finite window of opportunity for device removal, between myocardial recovery and device-induced complications, is possible and should not be missed.

Indications

Centrifugal pumps have been used for extracorporeal membrane oxygenation (ECMO), left heart bypass during surgery on the thoracic aorta, post cardiotomy ventricular failure, bridge to transplantation, right heart assist following cardiac transplantation, and as a bridge to more sophisticated, pulsatile assist devices. Some of these indications deserve comment.

Extracorporeal Membrane Oxygenation

Centrifugal pumps are less destructive to blood cellular elements than are roller pumps.[19–21] Consequently, for any clinical application that would require longer than 4 hours of mechanical assist, a centrifugal pump is preferable to roller pumps. ECMO is described in detail in Chapters 4 and 20.

Centrifugal Mechanical Assist for Surgery on the Thoracic Aorta

Centrifugal pumps are ideally suited for facilitation of surgery on the aortic arch or thoracic aorta, even though the need for assist is usually less than 1 hour.[9,45,46] Transsected aortas due to trauma or elective thoracic aortic aneurysm resection can be managed by cannulating the left atrial appendage using a 36F wire-reinforced cannula, gaining exposure through a small pericardiotomy. With use of short sections of tubing, the centrifugal pump can be placed near the operating field, returning

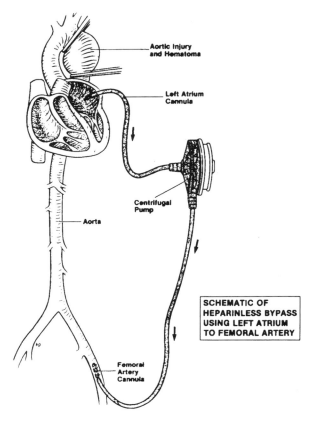

Aortic Injury
and Hematoma

Left Atrium
Cannula

Centrifugal
Pump

Aorta

SCHEMATIC OF
HEPARINLESS BYPASS
USING LEFT ATRIUM
TO FEMORAL ARTERY

Femoral
Artery
Cannula

FIGURE 7. Perfusion of the distal thoracic aorta by proximal cannulation of the left atrium with distal cannulation of the femoral artery using the Sarns centrifugal pump. This setup allows well controlled afterload reduction and permits good visualization of the operative site while maintaining distal perfusion pressure. Reproduced from Reference 45, with permission from *Journal of Trauma.*

blood either to the femoral artery or to the distal thoracic aorta (Fig. 7).[46] The right radial and right femoral arteries are used to monitor proximal aortic perfusion pressure provided by the heart, and distal thoracic aortic perfusion pressure provided by the centrifugal pump during aortic cross-clamping. By unloading the heart, clamp injuries to the proximal aorta should be lessened while adequate perfusion to abdominal viscera and the spinal cord can be maintained. A perfusion cannula can be constructed from the pump egress limb of tubing to allow selective perfusion of the left carotid artery or of the large intercostal arteries, if necessary.[9] In the case of traumatic thoracic aorta disruption associated with multisystem organ trauma, systemic heparinization is not employed.[47]

Postcardiotomy Ventricular Failure

The major indication for centrifugal mechanical assistance is the inability to wean from cardiopulmonary bypass secondary to left, right, or biventricular failure.[1,31] After the initial unsuccessful effort at weaning, the heart is allowed to rest on cardiopulmonary bypass while it is determined that the operative procedure cannot be improved. Low-dose inotropic agents are then initiated based on apparent physiology. If a repeat effort at separation from cardiopulmonary bypass is unsuccessful, intra-aortic balloon pumping is instituted. If the subsequent weaning effort is unsuccessful, high-dose multiple inotropes are instituted. If this effort fails and if the patient is faced with certain demise in the operating room, CMA is applied for salvage.

A less common indication for CMA following cardiac surgery is hemodynamic criteria that place the patient in jeopardy for survival, as described by Norman et al.[48] These criteria include a cardiac index less than 1.8 L/min/m^2, a blood pressure less than 90 mm Hg, atrial pressures greater than 20 mm Hg, systemic vascular resistance greater than 2100 dynes/sec/cm^{-5}, and low urinary output.

Bridge to Transplantation

Centrifugal pumps have been used successfully as a bridge to cardiac transplantation.[49–51] In the volunteer registry for the clinical use of mechanical ventricular assist pumps, sponsored by the American Society for Artificial Internal Organs-International Society for Heart Lung Transplants, 23 patients received left ventricular centrifugal pumps and 18 patients received biventricular centrifugal pumps with the intention to bridge to transplantation.[51] Overall, 32 patients (78%) were transplanted and 19 (46.3%) survived hospitalization. This represents a hospital discharge rate of 59.4% of those successfully bridged to transplantation. Total support time with centrifugal pumps averaged 8 days with a range of 1 to 29 days. Because donors are scarce and waiting times are long, centrifugal pumps are rarely chosen for bridge to transplantation if other mechanical assist devices are available.

"CMA Bridge to Bridge"

Presently, it is not possible to predict which patients who develop postcardiotomy shock are suffering from "stunned" myocardium and will recover after short-term mechanical cardiac assist.[52] Application of centrifugal pumps in this setting may allow for time to assess the patient's neurologic status and the function of other organ systems to determine if the patient is a candidate for cardiac transplantation. If so, switching to a pulsatile electric or air-driven mechanical assist device may allow for ambulation, rehabilitation, and successful bridge to cardiac transplantation.[53] In our experience, patients with postcardiotomy shock who show no evidence of myocardial recovery by 96 hours will not improve.[39]

Limitations

The presently available centrifugal pumps were not designed for long-term mechanical support. If they are used for this purpose, device mechanical failure should be anticipated. Seal disruption within the pump head occurs, allowing fluid to accumulate in the magnet chamber, and can interfere with pumping. Of our first 60 patients assisted for postcardiotomy failure, 9 (15%) encountered this problem.[54] The time to seal disruption was 10 to 144 hours with a median of 48 hours with the left ventricular assist, and 48 to 149 hours with a median of 83 hours with right ventricular assist ($P = 0.02$). Consequently, we recommend inspection of centrifugal pumps every 12 hours with left ventricular assist and every 24 hours with right ventricular assist. We have used a pump for 18 days without malfunction. Thus, prophylactic pump change is not recommended unless there is evidence of malfunction or thrombus formation.[31,43]

In general, patients require continued mechanical ventilation and sedation until the devices are removed. Therefore, the chief limitation of CMA is the inability to ambulate and rehabilitate patients.

Institutional Experience with Centrifugal Mechanical Assist for Postcardiotomy Ventricular Failure

Since 1986, we have had experience with 201 centrifugal pumps in 151 patients for a variety of indications including surgery of the thoracic aorta, support of cardiac

Table 3
Characteristics of 91 Patients Having Centrifugal Mechanical Assistance for Postcardiotomy Ventricular Failure

Demographics	
Age	58.5 (2–83)
Sex	75% male
Surgical Procedures	
CABG	68 (74.7%)
Valve	9 (10%)
CABG + Valve	8 (9%)
CABG + LVA	4 (4.4%)
Other	2 (2.2%)
Operative Urgency	
Elective	24 (26.4%)
Urgent	45 (49.5%)
Emergent	22 (24.1%)
Type of Assist	
RVAD	9 (10%)
Duration	
Mean	45.7 hrs
Range	12–84 hrs
LVAD	33 (36%)
Duration	
Mean	54.7 hrs
Range	1–342 hrs
biVAD	49 (54%)
Duration	
Mean	53.9 hrs
Range	1–434 hrs

CABG = coronary artery bypass grafting; LVA = left ventricular aneurysmectomy; RVAD = right ventricular assist device; LVAD = left ventricular assist device; biVAD = biventricular assist device.

allograft, ECMO for various indications, and for postcardiotomy ventricular failure. The latter is reviewed in detail below.

Between October of 1986 and April of 1998, 8019 patients had open heart surgery at the University of Missouri Hospital and Clinics in Columbia, Missouri. We used 140 Sarns centrifugal pumps as ventricular assist devices in 91 of these patients who developed severe hemodynamic compromise in the postcardiotomy setting. This represents an incidence of application of centrifugal assist of 1.13%. Ninety of these patients could not be separated from cardiopulmonary bypass despite extended attempts, multiple combinations of inotropes, and intra-aortic balloon pumping in all instances. Application of centrifugal mechanical assist was considered truly a salvage effort. Patients' ages ranged from 2 to 83 years, with a mean of 58 years. Sixty-eight males and 23 females underwent a variety of common operative procedures as listed in Table 3. The majority of these operative procedures were urgent or emergent. Forty-two patients (46%) recovered sufficient myocardial function that they could be weaned from the device(s). Nineteen patients (21%) survived hospitalization. The type and duration of assist, complications, and survival by type of assist are shown in Tables 3 and 4.

A meaningful comparison of clinical outcomes from different institutions and with different centrifugal pumps for postcardiotomy CMA is imperfect, if not impossible. This is because the indication for instituting ventricular mechanical assist varies from the truly salvage situation of inability to wean from cardiopulmonary bypass,

Table 4

Morbidity and Outcome of 91 Patients Undergoing Centrifugal Mechanical Assist for Postcardiotomy Failure

	n
Complications	
Bleeding	41 (45%)
Renal Failure	32 (35%)
Thromboembolism	4 (4.4%)
Infection	19 (21%)
Outcome by type of assist	
Weaned from CPB	90 (99%)
Weaned from device(s)	42 (46%)
Hospital survival	19 (21%)
RVAD (n = 9)	
Weaned	9 (100%)
Survived	2 (22%)
LVAD (n = 33)	
Weaned	16 (48.5%)
Survived	8 (24.3%)
biVAD (n = 49)	
Weaned	22 (44.9%)
Survived	9 (18.4%)

biVAD = biventricular assist device; CPB = cardiopulmonary bypass; LVAD = left ventricular assist device; RVAD = right ventricular assist device.

Table 5

Review of Large Series in the Literature Reporting Outcomes of Centrifugal
Mechanical Assistance in the Setting of Postcardiotomy Cardiac Failure

Author/Reference	Device	Patients	% Biventricular	Mean Duration of Support (range)	Weaned	Survived
Noon [57]	Biomedicus	129	17	3.8 (1–22)	56%	21%
Magovern [30]	Biomedicus	77	46.8	2.2 (<1–7.7)	56%	35%
Joyce[1] [56]	Sarns	34	NR	NR	62%	41%
Univ. of MO[2]	Sarns	91	54	2.2 (<1–18)	46%	21%
Combined registry[3]	All	559	NR	NR	45%	26%

[1] Results of this series includes transplanted patients; [2] University of Missouri-Columbia; [3] Volunteer Registry established by the American Society for Artificial Organs-ISHLT.

to support for postcardiotomy in patients with marginal hemodynamics, to placement of mechanical support with the intention to bridge to transplantation.[30,43,51,55,56] With this qualification, several published reports of outcomes with postcardiotomy centrifugal assist are listed in Table 5.

In summary, 20% to 25% of patients who would have been perioperative fatalities can be salvaged with CMA. Patients who survive postcardiotomy mechanical assist ultimately do reasonably well regardless of the type of assist device used.[57,58] From the combined registry experience, 82% of hospital survivors were alive at 2 years and 86% were in New York Heart Association functional Class I or II.[1] Figure 8 shows the actuarial survival of hospital survivors in the University of Missouri experience.

Conclusions

Centrifugal pumps are relatively inexpensive, simple to use, and available to all surgeons. All currently available centrifugal pumps have superior blood-handling

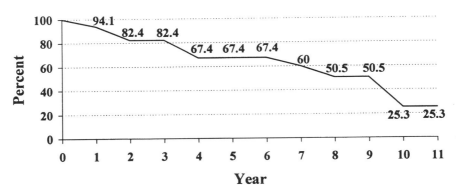

FIGURE 8. Eleven-year actuarial survival graph of hospital survivors who underwent postcardiotomy centrifugal assist as a salvage procedure.

characteristics compared with extended use of roller pumps. Presently, there are no compelling clinical data to support a claim of superiority of any of the centrifugal pumps in clinical use. In the setting of postcardiotomy ventricular failure, centrifugal mechanical assist in anticipation of myocardial recovery is equally efficacious as more sophisticated and costlier devices. The high morbidity associated with the use of centrifugal pumps can be decreased through improvements in insertion, anticoagulation, and weaning strategies. While presently available disposable models are not suitable for long-term use, centrifugal pumps should be a part of the armamentarium of all thoracic surgeons.

References

1. Pae WE Jr, Miller CA, Matthews Y, et al. Ventricular assist devices for postcardiotomy cardiogenic shock. *J Thorac Cardiovasc Surg* 1992;104:541–553.
2. Adamson RM, Dembitsky WP, Reichman RT, et al. Mechanical support: Assist or nemesis? *J Thorac Cardiovasc Surg* 1989;98(5 Pt .2):915–921.
3. Curtis JJ, Walls JT, Schmaltz R, Boley TM, et al. Experience with the Sarns centrifugal pump in postcardiotomy ventricular failure. *J Thorac Cardiovasc Surg* 1992;104(3):554–560.
4. Saxton GA Jr, Andrews CB. An ideal heart pump with hydrodynamic characteristics analogous to the mammalian heart. *Trans Am Soc Artif Intern Organs* 1960;6:288–290.
5. Bernstein EF, Dorman FD, Blackshear PL, Scott DR. An efficient compact pump for assisted circulation. *Surgery* 1970;68:105–115.
6. Golding LR, Groves LK, Peter M, et al. Initial clinical experience with a new temporary left ventricular assist device. *Ann Thorac Surg* 1980;29:66–69.
7. Pennington DG, Merjavy JP, Swartz MT, et al. Clinical experience with a centrifugal pump ventricular assist device. *ASAIO Trans* 1982;28;93–99.
8. Bianchi JJ, Swartz MT, Raithel SC, et al. Initial clinical experience with centrifugal pumps coated with the Carmeda process. *ASAIO J* 1992;38(3):M143-M146.
9. Coselli JS, LeMaire SA, Ledesma DF, et al. Initial experience with the Nikkiso centrifugal pump during thoracoabdominal aortic aneurysm repair. *J Vasc Surg* 1998;27(2):378–383.
10. Curtis J, Wagner-Mann C, Mann F, et al. Subchronic use of the St. Jude centrifugal pump as a mechanical assist device in calves. *Artif Organs* 1996;20(6):662–665.
11. Magovern GJ Jr. Use of the BioMedicus pump in postoperative circulatory support. In Ott RA, Gutfinger DE, Gazzaniga AB (eds): *Cardiac Surgery: State of the Art Review*. Volume 7. Philadelphia: Hanley & Belfus α·93:249–264.
12. Magovern GJ, Christlieb IY, Kao RL, et al. Recovery of the failing canine heart with biventricular support in a previously fatal experimental model. *J Thorac Cardiovasc Surg* 1987;94:656–663.
13. Mendler N, Podechtl F, Bernhard A, et al. Zentrifugalpumpen im Vergleich: Hydraulische Leistung und Blutschadingung. *Kardiotechnik* 1998;2:31–36.
14. Naganuma S, Yambe T, Sonobe T, et al. Development of a novel centrifugal pump: Magnetic rotary pump. *Artif Organs* 1997;21(7):746–750.
15. Ohtsubo S, Naito K, Matsuura M, et al. Initial clinical experience with the Baylor-Nikkiso centrifugal pump. *Artif Organs* 1995;19(7):769–773.
16. Taguchi S, Yozu R, Mori A, et al. A miniaturized centrifugal pump for assist circulation. *Artif Organs* 1994;18(9):664–668.
17. Takami Y, Ohara Y, Otsuka G, et al. Pre-clinical evaluation of the Kyocera Byro centrifugal blood pump for cardiopulmonary bypass. *Perfusion* 1997;12(5):335–341.
18. Addison H. *Centrifugal and Other Rotodynamic Pumps*. 3rd Ed. London: Chapman & Hall Ltd.; 1966.
19. Curtis JJ, Wagner-Mann CC, Turpin TA, et al. In vitro evaluation of five commercially available perfusion systems. *Int J Angiol* 1994;3:128–133.
20. Hoerr HR Jr, Kraemer MF, Williams JL, et al. In vitro comparison of the blood handling by the constrained vortex and twin roller blood pumps. *J Extracorpor Technol* 1987;19:316–321.

21. Iatridis E, Chan T. An evaluation of vortex, centrifugal and roller pump systems. *Proceedings: International Workshop on Rotary Blood Pumps*. Vienna, Austria: September 1991.
22. Naito K, Suenaga E. Cao Z-L, et al. Comparative hemolysis study of clinically available centrifugal pumps. *Artif Organs* 1996;20(6):560–563.
23. Kawahito K, Nose Y. Hemolysis in different centrifugal pumps. *Artif Organs* 1997;21(4):323–326.
24. Schima H, Muller MR, Papantonis D, et al. Minimization of hemolysis in centrifugal blood pumps: Influence of different geometries. *Int J Artif Organs* 1993;16(7):521–529.
25. Mulder MM, Hansen AC, Mohammad SF, et al. Thoughts and progress: In vitro investigation of the St. Jude Medical Isoflow centrifugal pump: Flow visualization and hemolysis studies. *Artif Organs* 1997;21(8):947–960.
26. Curtis JJ, Wagner-Mann CC, Mann FA, et al. A 96 hour comparative study of centrifugal pumps used for left ventricular assist. *Proceedings of the Fifth Congress of the International Society for Rotary Blood Pumps*. 1997;11. Abstract.
27. Mann FA, Wagner-Mann CC, Curtis JJ, et al. A calf model for left ventricular mechanical assist. *Artif Organs* 1996;20:670–677.
28. Curtis JJ, Walls JT, Boley TM, et al. Autopsy findings in patients on postcardiotomy centrifugal ventricular assist. *ASAIO J* 1992;38(3):M688-M690.
29. Killen DA, Poichler JM, Borkon AM, et al. BioMedicus ventricular assist device for salvage of cardiac surgical patients. *Ann Thorac Surg* 1991;52:230–235.
30. Magovern GJ Jr. The BioPump and postoperative circulatory support. *Ann Thorac Surg* 1993;55:245–249.
31. Noon GP, Ball JW Jr, Papaconstantinou HT. Clinical experience with BioMedicus centrifugal ventricular support in 172 patients. *Artif Organs* 1995;19(7):756–760.
32. Orime Y, Takatani S, Sasaki T, et al. Cardiopulmonary bypass with Nikkiso and BioMedicus centrifugal pumps. *Artif Organs* 1994;18(1):11–16.
33. Takarabe K, Yoshikai M, Murayama J, et al. Clinical evaluation of the centrifugal pump in open heart surgery: A comparative study of different pumps. *Artif Organs* 1997;21(7):760–762.
34. Tayama E, Ohtsubo S, Nakazawa T, et al. Thoughts and progress: In vitro thrombogenic evaluation of centrifugal pumps. *Artif Organs* 1997;21(5):418–420.
35. Tominga R, Harasaki H, Golding LAR. Blood coagulability and hematological changes in calves with chronic centrifugal biventricular bypass pumps. *J Surg Res* 1994;56:13–19.
36. Wagner-Mann C, Curtis J, Mann F, et al. Subchronic centrifugal mechanical assist in an unheparinized calf model. *Artif Organs* 1996;20(6):666–669.
37. Curtis JJ. Centrifugal mechanical assist for postcardiotomy ventricular failure. *Semin Thorac Cardiovasc Surg* 1994;6(3):140–146.
38. Curtis JJ, Walls JT, Demmy TL, et al. Clinical experience with the Sarns centrifugal pump. *Artif Organs* 1993;17(7):630–633.
39. Curtis JJ, Walls JT, Schmaltz RA, et al. Improving clinical outcome with centrifugal mechanical assist for postcardiotomy ventricular failure. *Artif Organs* 1995;19(7):761–765.
40. Curtis JJ, Walls JT, Schmaltz RA, et al. Use of centrifugal pumps for postcardiotomy ventricular failure: Technique and anticoagulation. *Ann Thorac Surg* 1996;61:296–300.
41. Curtis JJ, Walls JT, Wagner-Mann CC, et al. Centrifugal pumps: Description of devices and surgical techniques. *Ann Thorac Surg* 1999;68:666–671.
42. Curtis JJ, Wagner-Mann CC, Mann FA, et al. In vivo left ventricular assist induced coagulation derangements: Comparison of Sarns-3M and St. Jude medical circuits. *ASAIO J* 1997;43(5):M414-M417.
43. Golding LAR, Crouch RD, Stewart RW, et al. Postcardiotomy centrifugal mechanical ventricular support. *Ann Thorac Surg* 1992;54:1059–1064.
44. Curtis JJ, Deese LR, Walls JT, Boley TM. The use of a rate limited ultrafiltration circuit with centrifugal ventricular assist. *Artif Organs* 1994;18(6):465–466.
45. Walls JT, Curtis JJ, Boley T. Sarns centrifugal pump for repair of thoracic aortic injury: Case reports. *J Trauma* 1989;29:1283–1285.
46. Walls JT, Boley TM, Curtis JJ, et al. Experience with four surgical techniques to repair traumatic aortic pseudoaneurysm. *J Thorac Cardiovasc Surg* 1993;106:283–287.
47. Walls JT, Boley T, Curtis J, et al. Centrifugal pump support for repair of thoracic aortic injury. *Missouri Med* 1991;811–813.

48. Norman JC, Cooley DA, Igo SR, et al. Prognostic indices for survival during postcardiotomy intra-aortic balloon pumping. *J Thorac Cardiovasc Surg* 1977;74:709–720.
49. Bolman RM III, Cox JL, Marshall W, et al. Circulatory support with a centrifugal pump as a bridge to cardiac transplantation. *Ann Thorac Surg* 1989;47(1):108–112.
50. Golding LAR, Stewart RW, Sinkewich M, et al. Nonpulsatile ventricular assist bridging to transplantation. *ASAIO Trans* 1988;34:476–479.
51. Mehta SM, Aufiero TX, Pae WE Jr, et al. Combined registry for the clinical use of mechanical ventricular assist pumps and the total artificial heart in conjunction with heart transplantation: Sixth official report—1994. *J Heart Lung Transplant* 1995;14:585–593.
52. Braunwald E, Kloner RA. The stunned myocardium: Prolonged, postischemic ventricular dysfunction. *Circulation* 1982;66:1146–1149.
53. Derose JJ Jr, Umana JP, Argenziano M, et al. Improved results for postcardiotomy cardiogenic shock with the use of implantable left ventricular assist devices. *Ann Thorac Surg* 1997;64(6):1757–1763.
54. Curtis JJ, Boley TM, Walls JT, et al. Frequency of seal disruption with the Sarns centrifugal pump in postcardiotomy assist. *Artif Organs* 1994;18(3):235–237.
55. Joyce LD, Kiser JC, Eales F, et al. Experience with generally accepted centrifugal pumps: Personal and collective experience. *Ann Thorac Surg* 1996;61:287–290.
56. Noon GP, Ball JW Jr, Short HD. BioMedicus centrifugal ventricular support for postcardiotomy cardiac failure: A review of 129 cases. *Ann Thorac Surg* 1996;61:291–295.
57. Pennington DG, Bernhard WF, Golding LR, et al. Long-term follow-up of postcardiotomy patients with profound cardiogenic shock treated with ventricular assist devices. *Circulation* 1985;72(suppl 2):216–226.
58. Curtis JJ, Walls JT, Schmaltz RA, et al. Prognosis of hospital survivors after salvage from cardiopulmonary bypass with centrifugal cardiac assist. *ASAIO Trans* 1990;36(3):552–554.

Chapter 18

Extracorporeal Support:

The ABIOMED BVS 5000

G. Kimble Jett, MD and Robert R. Lazzara, MD

Introduction

The ABIOMED BVS 5000, an extracorporeal cardiac assist device manufactured by ABIOMED Cardiovascular Inc. (Danvers, MA), was the first cardiac assist device approved by the Food and Drug Administration (FDA) for support of postcardiotomy patients. Since its approval in 1992, it has been used in more than 3000 patients and it has rapidly become the second (after the intra-aortic balloon pump) most popular mechanical support for patients with postcardiotomy ventricular dysfunction.

Device Description

The BVS 5000 biventricular support system is an external pulsatile ventricular assist device that is capable of providing short-term left, right, or biventricular support. The system is composed of three components: 1) transthoracic cannulae; 2) disposable external pumps; and 3) a microprocessor-controlled pneumatic drive console (Fig. 1).

Transthoracic Cannulae

The cannulae have evolved since early trials to be more user-friendly; their size has been reduced without compromising flow. This evolution was made possible by the advent of thin wall cannula technology. Transthoracic cannulae provide drainage

From Goldstein DJ and Oz MC (eds). *Cardiac Assist Devices*. Armonk, NY: Futura Publishing Co., Inc.; ©2000.

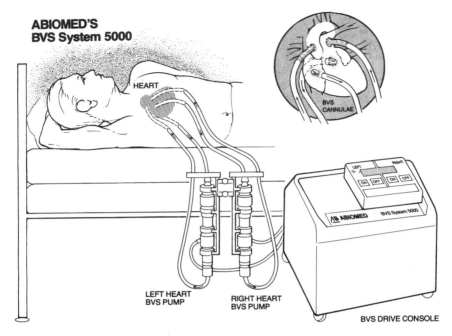

FIGURE 1. ABIOMED BVS 5000 system. With permission from ABIOMED Inc., Danvers, MA.

from the right atrium, left atrium, or left ventricle for inflow to the pump. Outflow from the pump to the patient is then provided by cannulae attached to the right ventricular outflow tract, the pulmonary artery, or the aorta.

Inflow cannulae are made of wire-reinforced polyvinyl chloride, and are 40 cm long. A variety of sizes are available: a 32F right-angle light-house tip, a 36F malleable open tip, and a 42F or 46F right-angle light-house tip (Fig. 2). The 32F and 36F cannulae have the same internal diameter as do the 42F and 46F cannulae, the difference related to thin wall technology. Outflow cannulae only differ from inflow cannulae by the presence of a precoated Dacron™ graft that is attached to the end, allowing anastomosis to the great vessel (pulmonary artery or aorta). The graft is precoated with a polymer that renders it somewhat stiff but impermeable, with zero porosity. Outflow cannulae are either 12 mm graft/42F cannulae or 14 mm graft/46F cannulae (Fig. 2). Each cannula has the same internal diameter, again the difference being thin wall technology. External surfaces of the inflow and outflow cannulae incorporate a Dacron velour sleeve at the skin interface. This promotes tissue ingrowth, and adherence fixes the cannulae to the integument and prevents ascending infection.

The Pump

The device is a dual-chamber pump contained in a hard polycarbonate housing. The upper (atrial) chamber is a passive, gravity-filled reservoir and the lower chamber is the pumping chamber. Blood drains from the atria by gravity into the blood

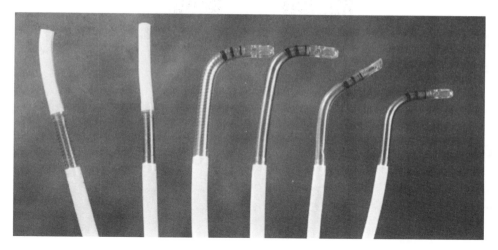

FIGURE 2. Inflow and outflow cannulae. With permission from ABIOMED Inc., Danvers, MA.

pump, which is externally located by the bedside. This passive filling avoids native atrial collapse, inflow cannula suction of air, and hemolysis. Each chamber contains a smooth surface polyurethane bladder (volume 100 mL), and the ventricular or pumping chamber is isolated by two polyurethane trileaflet valves, which ensure unidirectional blood flow. A compressed air drive line connects the console with the blood pump's ventricular chamber. Compressed air enters the blood pump's ventricular chamber during pump systole, causing bladder collapse and thus returning its blood volume to the patient. During diastole, air is vented through the console to the atmosphere, allowing ventricular bladder filling. A single blood pump supports one side of the heart (Fig. 3).

Atrial bladders operate in a fill-to-empty mode. Adequate intravascular volume is mandatory for optimal flows. Inadequate atrial filling occurs if the external blood pump position is too high; on the other hand, prolonged filling may occur if the blood pump position is too low or if the patient is volume overloaded. Atrial filling is inspected visually at the bedside, and the pump height is adjusted as needed. Typical height is approximately 25 cm below the patient's atria. In some biventricular cases, it is necessary to adjust right and left pump heights independently. The system takes 2 minutes to equilibrate after each height change. It is important to balance the flows to prevent excessive right-sided flow and pulmonary overload.

The Console

The BVS console is an automated, self-regulating, pulsatile support device controlled by a microprocessor. It operates asynchronously relative to the native cardiac rhythm. The console automatically adjusts external pump beat rate as well as the duration of the pump diastole and systole to compensate for changes in preload and afterload, respectively. The BVS maintains a constant stroke volume (approximately 80 mL) and can provide a maximal output of 6 L/min if patient hydration is adequate.

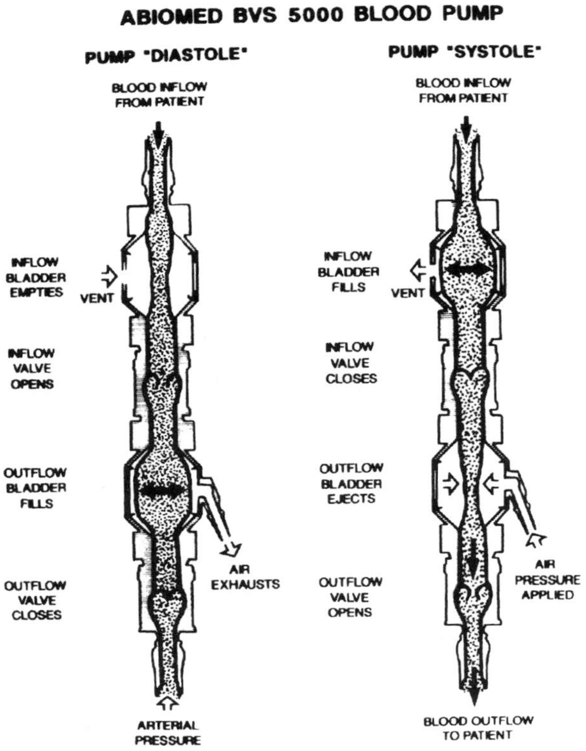

ABIOMED BVS 5000 BLOOD PUMP

FIGURE 3. Schematic illustration of the BVS 5000 blood pump during pump systole and diastole. Ventricular bladder collapses during pump systole and fills during diastole. Atrial bladder fills continuously. With permission from ABIOMED Inc., Danvers, MA.

The console reports pump rate, stroke volume, and flow to the operator. The microprocessor makes adjustments based on external system compressed air flow. The console senses bladder filling and returns blood to the patient whenever the ventricular chamber is full. The pumps are sensitive to both preload and afterload conditions.

The BVS 5000 pumps independently of the heart, simplifying its operation and minimizing the need for operator intervention. System operation is fully automated and therefore does not require operator input during normal operations. Several controls are provided for flow reduction during weaning attempts. The drive console operates on alternating current or internal battery and contains a safety back-up system for the microprocessor and a foot pump for completely manual operation. A single BVS console can operate and adjust one or two blood pumps. In the biventricular support mode, the console controls right and left pumps independently.

There were some design goals for the BVS 5000. These goals were to be safe, simple, and effective. The safety of the pump is due to its design: a dual-chamber pump with a built-in reservoir. There is no vacuum, as blood drains merely by gravity. Experience with the device has demonstrated no significant hemolysis.

The BVS 5000's automated control system with on and off operation automatically adjusts for changes in the patient preload and afterload, and it requires minimal operator intervention. This simplicity renders the device easier for nurses to manage than an intra-aortic balloon pump and, unlike other external devices, it requires no added personnel for device management.

The dual-chamber, two-valve design mimics a natural heart and fully decompresses the ventricle while providing pulsatile flow to the major organs. The pulse pressures exhibited are physiologic. During support, the device will allow withdrawal of inotropes to rest the heart.

Implantation Techniques

Careful cannula insertion is important for successful intraoperative and postoperative results with the ABIOMED BVS 5000. The newer, smaller cannulae have made insertion easier. Each cannula must be inserted in a fashion that allows unimpeded device filling and does not obstruct venous drainage. In addition, since the device is afterload sensitive, the outflow graft must not be kinked or impaired. Implantation is usually done while the patient is supported on cardiopulmonary bypass. Standard biventricular cannulation is demonstrated in Figure 4.

Outflow Cannulation

Outflow cannulation is usually performed first while the patient is supported on cardiopulmonary bypass. The anastomoses are constructed prior to externalizing

BIVENTRICULAR SUPPORT CANNULATION

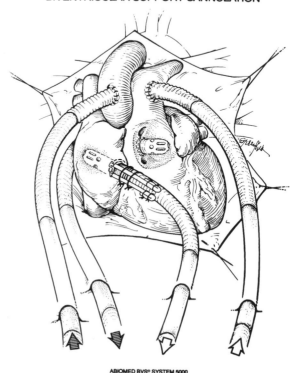

ABIOMED BVS® SYSTEM 5000

FIGURE 4. Standard inflow and outflow cannulation. With permission from ABIOMED Inc., Danvers, MA.

the cannulae, which aids in performing the anastomosis. Bleeding around the aortic cannula frequently occurs and can be prevented by incorporating Teflon pledgets or a pericardial strip into the anastomosis around the aortic aspect. Usually, a 4–0 monofilament suture is used. Once the cannula is anastomosed, it is vigorously de-aired, as air tends to hide in the interstices of the graft. The cannula is then externalized, allowing enough slack on the graft to avoid tension on the anastomosis but not enough to permit kinking of the graft. The cannulae are usually externalized to the far left and right of the midline.

Right-Sided Outflow

The right-sided outflow cannula is usually anastomosed to the main pulmonary artery. This is performed while the patient is on cardiopulmonary bypass, and thus no vascular clamp is needed. Once an arteriotomy is made in the main pulmonary artery, care is taken to avoid incorporating a leaflet of the pulmonary valve or the pulmonary artery catheter in the anastomosis. The graft can be trimmed with an acute angle to make it lie flat and close to the right ventricle in order to avoid impinging overlying bypass grafts.

If the pulmonary artery is inaccessible, a 36F malleable cannula can be inserted through the right ventricular outflow tract and advanced through the pulmonary valve.[1] In this case, the cannula should be externalized before it is inserted. A double purse-string pledgetted suture is used. A right-sided outflow cannula is usually externalized to the far left of the patient's midline.

Left-Sided Outflow

The left-sided outflow cannula is usually anastomosed to the anterolateral aspect of the aorta. A side-biting clamp is used for this purpose. A pericardial strip is commonly used on the aortic aspect to buttress the anastomoses. If a patient is operated on with compromised left ventricular function, an area of the anterolateral aspect of the aorta should be left available should the BVS be needed. The anterior aspect of the aorta near the aortic valve may be used if transplantation is an expected outcome (cardiomyopathy, myocarditis). The left-sided outflow cannula is then externalized subcostal and to the far right of the patient's midline.

Inflow Cannulation

Once the outflow cannulae are inserted, the inflow cannulae are placed. Each inflow cannula must be secured to the atrium or the ventricle to prevent inadvertent removal and subsequent air emboli. A double-pledgetted purse-string suture with tourniquets applied over the suture (3–0 or 4–0 polypropylene) has been effective for cannula securing and for allowing easy removal once a patient is weaned from mechanical support. Cannula removal usually does not require cardiopulmonary bypass. Volume loading of the atrium or ventricle that is being cannulated is important for preventing intracardiac introduction of air. The inflow cannula should be under fluid during initiation of support to prevent introduction of air into the inflow cannula. In addition, the external blood pump should be positioned level with the patient during initiation of support to prevent generation of negative atrial pressure.

The inflow cannula is usually externalized prior to its insertion in order to avoid placing tension on the purse-string suture during insertion. These cannulae are usually externalized subcostal just off the midline and medial to the outflow cannulae.

Right-Sided Inflow

Right-sided inflow cannulation is usually through the mid right atrial wall. The tip of the cannula is directed toward the inferior vena cava and not through the tricuspid valve. If the atrial appendage is used for inflow cannulation, it may become sucked up in the cannula, leading to poor drainage; this is therefore not advised. If the patient is on cardiopulmonary bypass with a two-stage single venous cannula inserted through the atrial appendage, insertion of the inflow cannula through the midatrial wall may be aided by repositioning the tip of the two-stage cannula through the tricuspid valve. This will open up the body of the atrium. If the free wall of the atrium has been used for cardiopulmonary bypass, then the cannula may be traded out with the pump's inflow cannula once cardiopulmonary bypass is discontinued. Alternatively, the right ventricular free wall can be cannulated.

Left-Sided Inflow

Left-sided inflow cannulation may be achieved through either the left atrium or the left ventricular apex. The choice depends on ease of insertion and the presence of a mitral prosthesis. Left ventricular cannulation is preferred if the left atrium is not accessible due to small size or scarring from prior operations, or in the presence of an atriotomy in the case of a mitral valve operation.[2] In addition, if there is a mechanical mitral prosthesis, left ventricular cannulation is preferred to maintain flow across the prosthesis and preserve leaflet motion in order to reduce the chance of thromboembolism.

Three sites are available for left-sided atrial inflow cannulation: 1) below the interatrial groove between the right superior and inferior pulmonary veins; 2) the left atrial appendage; and 3) the dome of the left atrium. The left atrial appendage in a normal heart is usually thin-walled and is not acceptable for inflow drainage. It may be used, however, in patients with cardiomyopathy. The standard approach has been to cannulate the left atrium below the interatrial groove. In our experience, however, the dome approach is preferred because it is technically easier in a normal or small-sized left atrium and it also provides better drainage than the standard approach below the interatrial groove.[3] Moreover, the latter approach provides good

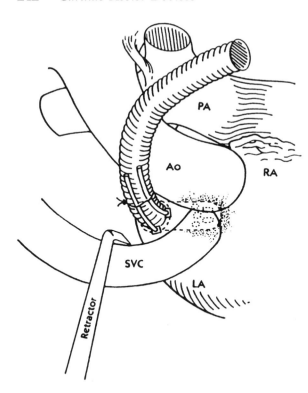

FIGURE 5. Completed cannulation of the dome of the left atrium with a 46F wire-reinforced right-angle cannula. Ao = aorta; LA = left atrium; PA = pulmonary artery; RA = right atrium; SVC = superior vena cava. Reprinted, with permission, from Jett GK. Atrial cannulation for left ventricular assistance: Superiority of the dome approach. *Ann Thorac Surg* 1996;61:1014–1015.

visualization should bleeding occur after decannulation, and it requires less manipulation of the heart, thereby preventing further circulatory instability (Fig. 5).

In the setting of previous coronary bypass grafting to right coronary artery branches, care must be taken during atrial cannulation for left ventricular support. If the saphenous vein graft comes off the aorta anteriorly, then a cannula placed in the dome of the left atrium may compress the graft as it crosses the heart. Cannulation below the interatrial groove would avoid the saphenous graft and would be preferable in this case. However, if the saphenous vein graft comes off the right side of the aorta, then the graft may well be away from the cannula placed in the dome of the left atrium. Use of the 36F malleable cannula may also avoid compression of bypass grafts because it can be carefully shaped.

Left ventricular apical cannulation is usually performed on the anterior aspect of the left ventricular apex (Fig. 6). The apex is elevated by placing a laparotomy pad underneath the heart. Double-pledgetted purse-string sutures are then placed in the anterior aspect of the apex, using a monofilament suture. If the inflow cannula is to be externalized subcostally, this should be done before its insertion to prevent inadvertent decannulation or tearing of the purse-string sutures. The cannula is usually externalized just to the left of the midline. If a right-sided device has been inserted, then the pulmonary artery outflow cannula is externalized to the far left of the midline and the left ventricular cannula crosses over the pulmonary artery cannula as it enters the left ventricular apex.

The heart is volume loaded and a Valsalva maneuver is performed while a cruciate stab wound is made in the center of the purse-string suture. The cannula is

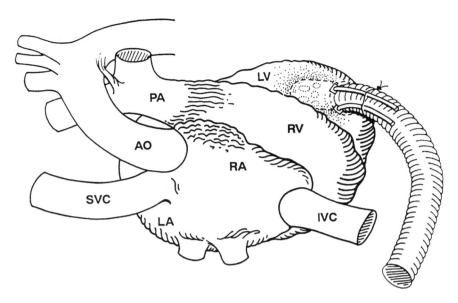

FIGURE 6. Completed cannulation of the left ventricular apex with a 46F wire-reinforced right-angle cannula. AO = aorta; IVC = inferior vena cava; LA = left atrium; LV = left ventricle; PA = pulmonary artery; RA = right atrium; RV = right ventricle; SVC = superior vena cava. Reprinted, with permission, from Jett GK. Left ventricular apical cannulation for circulatory support. *J Card Surg* 1998;13:51–55.

inserted and the tourniquets are tightened and secured to the cannula. If a malleable 36F cannula has been used, the bevel should be directed away from the interventricular septum. Position of the cannula can be confirmed by transesophageal echocardiography. The cannula is then evacuated of air and connected to the device.

The left atrium is chosen most frequently as a site for cannulation, in order to prevent damage to the left ventricle. However, when the left ventricular apex is cannulated, as previously described,[2] it does not appear to impair apical contraction. A core of myocardium is not excised as is done with other ventricular assist devices.[4]

Apical cannulation may offer advantages over left atrial cannulation. Apical cannulation has been shown to more completely decompress the left ventricle, thus enhancing ventricular recovery.[5] In addition, there appear to be fewer thromboemboli with apical cannulation, due to less stagnation of blood in the ventricle.[6] To assess myocardial recovery with transesophageal echocardiography, the ventricle must to be volume loaded. This requires reducing or transiently discontinuing circulatory support with atrial cannulation. With apical cannulation, the volume passes freely through the ventricle and the ejection fraction is the same on full or partial support.

As the cannulae are being inserted, the blood pumps are primed by the perfusionist and the scrub nurse. This is done with either lactated Ringer's solution for univentricular support or blood for biventricular pumps. The fluid should be warmed to prevent a sudden drop in the patient's temperature once support is initiated. Inspection for air in the pump should be diligently performed, especially around the sinuses of the valves. All air bubbles should be removed.

Once the cannulae are inserted and connected to the blood pumps, they are tested. The heart is volume loaded, the patient is placed in the Trendelenburg position, and the chest is filled with fluid. Several ejections are performed by foot compression, and the inflow cannula is carefully inspected for air. If air is visualized, the cannula is immediately clamped and de-aired and the procedure is repeated. Each pump is tested separately. The foot pedal is then replaced in the console and support is initiated as cardiopulmonary bypass is discontinued.

Once the patient is off cardiopulmonary bypass and BVS support has been initiated, the heparin is completely reversed in order to achieve a normal activated clotting time. All cannulation sites are inspected for bleeding. Chest closure is always possible with biventricular assist devices; however, when only one ventricle is supported, chest closure may compromise the unsupported ventricle. We prefer chest closure because we believe there are advantages: 1) it helps to obtain hemostasis; 2) it maintains body temperature; 3) it prevents infection; and 4) it allows for extubation while the patient is on mechanical support.

Explantation Techniques

Once cardiac recovery has been confirmed by clinical and echocardiographic criteria, the patient is taken back to the operating room. The explantation procedure usually does not require cardiopulmonary bypass. The patient is volume loaded and the chest is opened. Care is taken to avoid inadvertent decannulation as the tourniquets are separated. Ten thousand units of heparin are then administered and dobutamine (Dobutrex, Eli Lilly & Company, Indianapolis, IN) is started at 5 μg/kg/min for inotropic support.

The pump supporting the recovered side of the heart is removed first. Usually, this is the right ventricular assist device. The inflow cannula is clamped to allow as much blood as possible to return to the patient. Hemodynamics, including central venous pressure, blood pressure, and left-sided pump flow, are carefully watched. If stable, the inflow cannula is removed as the purse-string sutures are secured. Approximately 100 mL should be expelled from the atrium prior to securing the sutures in order to allow removal of any panus that may have formed during mechanical support. The anesthesiologist is instructed to advance a pulmonary artery catheter. The outflow graft is then divided close to the anastomosis with a vascular stapler, thereby leaving a small nub of graft. Clamping of the great vessel and complete removal of the Dacron graft is not necessary and may compromise ventricular function. If, however, transplantation is the outcome, then all the of graft material should be removed.

Once the first device is removed and the patient is hemodynamically stable, the other device can be removed in a similar fashion. Once both devices are removed, the heparin is reversed and the sternum debrided. The chest is then closed along with its cannulation sites. Only once in our experience has an intra-aortic balloon pump been needed to support a patient when the ventricular assist devices were removed. Also, we have been able to close the chest in all cases except one, but we were able to close the latter several days later. Vigorous diuresis to the preoperative weight prior to device removal helps to ensure that chest closure is possible.

Indications for BVS Support

The ABIOMED BVS 5000 was initially approved by the FDA in 1992 for postcardiotomy support.[7] Since that time, the indications have been expanded to include support of all forms of recoverable heart failure (Table 1). This includes acute myocardial infarction, myocarditis, cardiac trauma, and right ventricular support with an implantable left ventricular assist device as and as a bridge to recovery or bridge to transplantation in failed transplant.

The BVS 5000 is best used as a bridge to recovery when short-term support is needed. Postcardiotomy support is the most common indication, comprising approximately 63% in the Worldwide Registry. We have previously described the selection of recipients for postcardiotomy support,[8] and it is briefly summarized below.

The classic hemodynamic criteria for mechanical support were established 20 years ago by Norman et al,[9] who suggested that the only alternative to support was death. These criteria probably account for the low survival rate with ventricular assist devices used in FDA-approved studies.[7] These rigid hemodynamic criteria should be more flexible. We believe that mechanical support should be considered if the cardiac index is less than 2.2 $L/min/m^2$, the systolic blood pressure is less then 90 mm Hg, the pulmonary capillary wedge pressure or central venous pressure is greater than 20 mm Hg, and if the patient requires two or more high-dose inotropic drugs. Frequently, we will not use an intra-aortic balloon pump first; we will proceed directly with the implantation of the BVS system. The mortality when the patient is taking two or more high-dose inotropes[10] or when an intra-aortic balloon pump is needed to separate from cardiopulmonary bypass is in excess of 50%,[11] and improved results may be obtained with the insertion of a ventricular assist device.

Several risk factors have been associated with poor outcome in patients receiving ventricular assist devices. These include a technically unsuccessful operation, preoperative myocardial infarction, biventricular failure, and advanced age. In addition, relative contraindications to the insertion of the ventricular assist devices have been advanced (Table 2). The timing of the insertion of the device is the most critical determinant of survival.[12]

In addition to postcardiotomy support, other forms of heart failure may be supported to recovery. Acute myocardial infarction with cardiogenic shock has recently been supported with the Abiomed BVS 5000, and the early experience with heart rest is impressive, with greater than 70% survival.[13] Since our initial case report of

---

Table 1

Indications for Placement of the ABIOMED BVS 5000

Postcardiotomy low cardiac output
Acute myocardial infarction
Acute myocarditis
Donor heart dysfunction/failure
Right heart failure after placement of implantable LVAD
Cardiac Trauma
Cardiomyopathy

LVAD = left ventricular assist device

Table 2

Relative Contraindications to the Institution
of Mechanical Circulatory Support

Anuria on cardiopulmonary bypass
Persistent acidosis on cardiopulmonary bypass
Symptomatic cerebrovascular disease
Cancer with extensive metastasis
Advanced liver failure
Known hypercoagulable state
Severe infection resistant to therapy

BVS support for myocarditis,[14] many patients worldwide have been supported and bridged to recovery for acute myocarditis.

If recovery has not occurred, then the ABIOMED BVS 5000 may be used to bridge to another device for long-term support or bridge to transplantation. The BVS 5000 may be used for pulsatile right-sided support when an implantable left ventricular assist device has been inserted. Also, in cases donor heart failure the BVS has been used to either bridge to recovery or to bridge to retransplantation.

The ABIOMED BVS 5000 is a valuable device for use in the community hospitals. It is easy to operate and will allow the operating team to continue with their busy schedule while a patient is on support, especially since additional personnel are not required for management or operation of the device. Transplant centers have developed transfer protocols for patients who do not exhibit myocardial recovery and may need to be bridged to transplantation or bridged to another device.[15]

Limitations

The ABIOMED BVS 5000 is best used for short-term support. Although patients have been supported for as long as 90 days, mobility is limited. Patients may dangle at the bedside, may be moved from bed to a chair, and occasionally may be walked with the BVS in place. Mobility with the BVS is much more limited than that achievable with current implantable devices (TCI HeartMate [Thermo Cardiosystems, Woburn, MA], Novacor [Baxter Healthcare Corp., Oakland, CA]) or even with extracorporeal pumps intended for bridge to transplantation (Thoratec [Thoratec Laboratories Corp., Berkeley, CA]).

The ABIOMED BVS 5000 has limited flow capability. It can achieve flows of 6 L/min, and in most cases this is adequate. However, in cases of increased oxygen consumption (ie, sepsis or large patient size) flow may be inadequate with the BVS 5000.

Insertion of the BVS 5000 does require an operation—either a sternotomy or a minimally invasive insertion via a right parasternal approach or left thoracotomy. Moreover, removal of the device requires a second operation. Unfortunately, all of the current devices that are capable of providing full cardiac support require an invasive approach for insertion and removal.

The BVS 5000 also requires full anticoagulation. Thrombus can form at the sinuses of the valves if the patient is suboptimally anticoagulated. Most of the thromboemboli that we have seen have originated from the native left ventricle. Left atrial cannulation does result in stasis in the native left ventricle. Perhaps left ventricular apical cannulation can prevent ventricular stasis and thrombus formation.[6]

Despite some limitations of the ABIOMED BVS 5000, there are many advantages.[12] Some of the advantages were covered in the device description. The BVS 5000 has been demonstrated to be a safe device. The majority of the complications seen with the device are patient-related, especially in postcardiotomy patients with prolonged cardiopulmonary bypass time before the insertion of the device. The device is very simple to operate, and requires minimal operator intervention. In addition, no added personnel are required for management of the device. It has also been shown to be quite effective for circulatory support. It has demonstrated support of the circulation, allowing the heart to rest and recover from its insult. Another advantage of the BVS lies in its physiologic pulsatile nature.

Outcome

Institutional Experience

We have used the ABIOMED BVS 5000 in approximately 55 patients. In 40 of these patients, the device was inserted and managed by our team.

The indications for insertion in our experience were postcardiotomy (28), failed transplant (8), acute myocardial infarction (2), myocarditis (1), and failed automatic implantable cardioverter defibrillator insertion (1). The average age of our patients was 52 and the average ejection fraction 30%. The mean duration of support was 7 days. Given our specific patient population, 83% of the patients were weaned from the BVS and 45% were discharged home.

The best determinant of survival was early insertion of the device with 86% wean rate and 57% discharged versus 25% wean rate and 0% survival with late insertion. Early insertion of the BVS limits myocardial and end organ damage and limits the complications associated with prolonged cardiopulmonary bypass. This is particularly true in the older patient population, in whom the heart may very well recover but other organs probably will not. Complications were seen in our patient population, as with other devices. Approximately 40% of patients required additional operations for bleeding. Fifty percent of BVS patients had respiratory complications consisting of pneumonia or prolonged intubation. However, 40% of our patients were extubated on support. There was no evidence of thrombus within the pump, although 25% of our patients had neurologic complications. These were due to preoperative cardiac arrest with diffused neurologic injury, cerebral emboli from native left ventricular thrombus, or a case of postoperative cerebral hemorrhage due to anticoagulation 1 week after the devices were removed.

Worldwide Registry Experience

ABIOMED maintains a voluntary Worldwide Registry with the BVS 5000. There are currently 1391 patients entered in the registry. The majority of patients (63%) are postcardiotomy patients. Other indications incude bridge to transplant patients with cardiomyopathy (15%). Most of that experience has been accrued from European centers. In addition, patients have been supported with acute myocardial infarction (7%), failed transplantation (9%), myocarditis (2%), and other indications (4%). Interestingly, since the FDA approval of the BVS, the percentage of postcardiotomy patients has increased. This is probably due to the experience in the United States. Before the approval, the majority of experience was in Europe with bridge to transplantation, as the BVS 5000 represents the most cost-effective device available.

The average age among postcardiotomy patients was 56 years and 43 years for cardiomyopathy patients. The mean duration of support was 5 days for postcardiotomy patients and slightly more than 8 days for cardiomyopathy patients. The short support time for cardiomyopathy patients relates to the European experience, where the wait time for donor organs is much less than it is in the United States. The majority of patients (52%) in the Worldwide Registry have been supported with biventricular assist devices, with 34% left ventricular assist devices and 14% right assist devices. The majority of cardiomyopathy patients have required biventricular assist devices, whereas postcardiotomy patients have been evenly divided between biventricular and left ventricular assist devices. Also of interest is that half of the patients supported for myocarditis have been supported with left ventricular assist devices alone. Despite the fact that myocarditis is a biventricular process, most of these patients have been young, have had normal pulmonary vasculature, and therefore have been able to be supported with a left ventricular assist device only.

Complications have been most common in postcardiotomy patients. This is due to the prolonged cardiopulmonary bypass time before the insertion of the device in these patients. Cardiomyopathy patients have experienced much less bleeding and other complications than have postcardiotomy patients. The majority of postcardiotomy patients have been weaned, although some have been bridged to transplantation. In contrast, most of the cardiomyopathy patients have been bridged to transplantation. The overall survival with the BVS 5000 is displayed in Figure 7.

Survival is related to the type of support. Recipients of univentricular support have generally fared better than patients requiring biventricular support. This observation likely relates more to the extent of damage to the heart before the insertion of the device than to the presence of a second device.

The Worldwide Registry has also demonstrated improved survival with early intervention. When the device was inserted within 3 hours of the decision to implant, the survival was 60%, versus 20% when device insertion was delayed. In addition, if the decision is made within 3 hours, the likelihood that a left ventricular assist device will be sufficient is greater than when the decision is delayed. As the decision is delayed, biventricular damage supervenes and the likelihood of the patient requiring biventricular support increases.

Worldwide experience has also demonstrated that better results can be expected from experienced centers. The center at Bad Oyenhausen, Germany has a 62% survival compared with 42% survival seen in less experienced centers.[8] This reflects a learning curve associated with this device as with any other technique or device. The ABIOMED BVS 5000 postmarket study has continued to demonstrate the safety and effectiveness of the device. Fifty percent of patients have been weaned and 7% have been transplanted. The overall survival is 34% (Fig. 7).

Postcardiotomy patients have a 31% discharge rate compared to 40% for cardio-

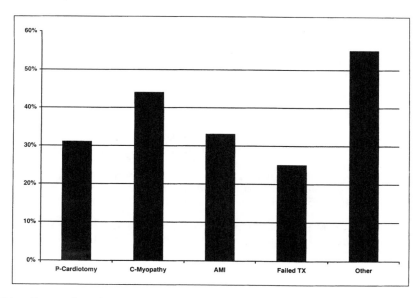

FIGURE 7. Survival to discharge from BVS (postmarket data). Demonstrated as discharge rate for each patient category. AMI = acute myocardial infarction; C-myopathy = cardiomyopathy; P-cardiotomy = postcardiotomy; TX = transplantation.

myopathy patients. Acute myocardial infarction discharge rate is close to 33%. The dismal results seen with donor heart failure mirror our own experience.

Conclusions

The ABIOMED BVS 5000 is a widely available extracorporeal cardiac assist device that has been approved by the FDA for all forms of recoverable heart failure. It is best used for short-term support as a bridge to recovery. Its effectiveness, safety, and simplicity have been demonstrated in the Worldwide Registry with more than 1000 implants. Its design makes it ideal for use in the community as an initial method of circulatory support. For patients who fail to recover, the device is well suited for easy transfer to specialized heart failure centers where long-term devices and transplantation can be offered.

References

1. Dewey TM, Chen JM, Spanier TB, Oz MC. Alternative techniques of right-sided outflow cannula insertion for right ventricular support. *Ann Thorac Surg* 1998;66:829–830.
2. Jett GK. Left ventricular apical cannulation for circulatory support. *J Card Surg* 1998;13:51–55.
3. Jett GK. Atrial cannulation for left ventricle assistance: Superiority of the dome approach. *Ann Thorac Surg* 1996; 61:1014–1015.
4. Arubia FA, Paramesh V, Toporoff B, et al. Biventricular cannulation for the Thoratec ventricular assist device. *Ann Thorac Surg* 1998;66:2119–2120.

5. Lohmann BP, Swartz RC, Pendelton DJ, et al. Left ventricular versus left atrial cannulation for the Thoratec ventricular assist device. *ASAIO J* 1990;36:M545-M548.
6. Holman WL, Bourge RC, Murrah CP, et al. Left atrial or ventricular cannulation beyond thirty days for a Thoratec ventricular assist device. *ASAIO J* 1995;41:M17-M22.
7. Guyton R, Schonberger J, Everts P, et al. Postcardiotomy shock: Clinical evaluation of the BVS 5000 biventricular support system. *Ann Thorac Surg* 1993;56:346–356.
8. Jett GK. Postcardiotomy support with ventricular assist devices: Selection of recipients. *Semin Thorac Cardiovasc Surg* 1994;6:136–139.
9. Norman JC, Cooley DA, Igo SR, et al. Prognostic indices for survival during postcardiotomy intra-aortic balloon pumping. *J Thorac Cardiovasc Surg* 1997;74:709–720.
10. Samuels L. Pharmacologic criteria for ventricular assist device insertion with the ABIOMED BVS 5000. *J Cardiac Med* In press.
11. Baldwin RT, Slogoff S, Noon GP, et al. A model to predict survival at time of postcardiotomy intraaortic balloon pump insertion. *Ann Thorac Surg* 1993;55:908–913
12. Jett GK. ABIOMED BVS 5000: Experience and potential advantages. *Ann Thorac Surg* 1996;61:301–304
13. Grossman DS, Levy N, Sears N. Temporary ventricular assist using the ABIOMED system as a new option for cardiogenic shock due to myocardial infarction. *Heart Failure Summit IV.*
14. Jett GK, Miller A, Savino D, Gonwa T. Reversal of acute fulminant lymphocytic myocarditis with combined technology of OKT3 monoclonal antibody and mechanical circulatory support. *J Heart Lung Transplant* 1992;11:733–738
15. Oz MC, Derose JJ, Chen JM, et al. Left ventricle assist device bridge-to-transplantation network improves survival following failed cardiotomy. *Ann Thorac Surg* 1999 In press.

Chapter 19

Extracorporeal Support:

The Thoratec Device

D. Glenn Pennington, MD, Timothy E. Oaks MD, and Douglas P. Lohmann, M.Eng.

Introduction

The Thoratec ventricular assist device (VAD) (Thoratec Laboratories Corp., Berkely, CA) is based on the original design by Drs. William Pierce and James Donachy at Penn State University,[1] and was first used clinically in 1982 for postcardiotomy support,[2] and in 1984 as a bridge to cardiac transplantation.[3] Twelve years later, in 1996, the Thoratec VAD system received premarketing approval by the Food and Drug Administration (FDA) for use as a bridge to cardiac transplantation and, more recently, for bridge to cardiac recovery; the Thoratec system is presently the only dually approved device on the market. To date, the Thoratec device has been implanted in more than 800 patients.

Device Description

The Thoratec VAD System consists of four main components: a drive console, inflow cannulae, outflow cannulae, and a pump. The pump is positioned in a paracorporeal position with cannulae piercing the skin below the costal margin, crossing the diaphragm, and going into the mediastinum, where they are connected to the heart and great vessels. The pump connects to a dual drive console to monitor and control pump operation. Alternating positive and negative air pressures actuate a flexible blood sac within the rigid outer casing of the Thoratec pump. Monostrut tilting delrin disc mechanical valves in the inflow and outflow ports ensure unidirec-

From Goldstein DJ and Oz MC (eds). *Cardiac Assist Devices*. Armonk, NY: Futura Publishing Co., Inc.; ©2000.

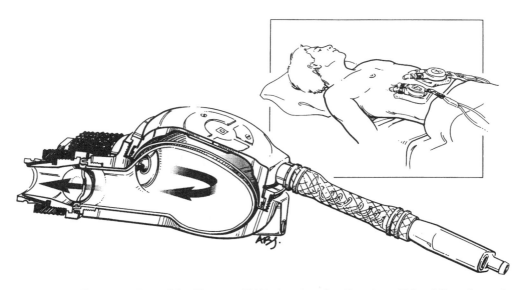

FIGURE 1. Cutaway view of the Thoratec VAD showing the direction of blood flow through the blood sac and tilting disc mechanical valves. The flexible diaphragm separates the blood sac from the compressed air used to drive the device. Also shown is the positioning of biventricular assist devices on a patient's abdomen with cannulae insertion sites just below the costal margins.

tional blood flow through the device (Fig. 1). Left and/or right heart support is possible with the Thoratec VAD. Blood is drained by the device from the left atrium or the left ventricle and is pumped to the ascending aorta. Clinically, higher pump flows are usually achieved with the ventricular cannula, but cannula selection is often influenced by myocardial recovery, left ventricular geometry, presence of left ventricular thrombus, and surgeon's preference (Table 1). With right-sided support, the Dacron™ graft is sewn to the pulmonary artery and blood is withdrawn from

Table 1

Factors that Determine Choice of Cannulation Site

Condition	Preferred Cannulation Site	Reason
Bridge to transplant	Left ventricle	Capture most of cardiac output, long-term support
Bridge to recovery	Left atrium	Ease of removal, short-term support
Recent myocardial infarction	Left atrium	Small and friable left ventricle
Presence of prosthetic mitral valve	Left atrium	Preserve flow across mitral valve, prevent thrombosis
Presence of prosthetic aortic valve	Left atrium	Not all cardiac output captured, preserving some flow across valve, reduce chance of thrombosis
Presence of left ventricular thrombus	Left ventricle	Can remove thrombus through cannulation site

the right atrium. Right ventricular cannulation is used in some cases. Cannulae are available in a limited number of shapes and sizes. All cannulae are wire-reinforced along the area where the cannula crosses the skin. The external surface of the same area is covered with velour to promote tissue in-growth and to reduce the incidence of infection. The cannulae are made from a proprietary polyurethane, with the exception of the distal end of the outflow cannula, which is a polyester Dacron graft for anastomosis to the aorta or pulmonary artery. This Dacron section of the outflow cannula must be preclotted prior to implantation.

The console provides the alternating positive and negative pressure to the pump via a pneumatic drive line. To maintain physiologic blood flow, the "volume" (or "fill-to-empty") mode of operation allows the pump to change speed as needed. Although asynchronous to the heart, this mode is recommended over the other two modes (fixed rate and electrocardiogram [ECG] synchronous) for most indications. The other two modes of operation are used mostly for de-airing procedures during implantation or weaning prior to explantation. In the volume mode, the pump operates on a fixed stroke volume with a variable pump rate, producing a variable pump output. Increased pump filling causes an increase in pump rate, which results in a higher pump output. The operator may change settings and drive pressures to increase operational efficiency or to compensate for changes in blood pressure, but after the first or second postoperative day, very few changes are necessary.

Although some physicians favor intracorporeal VADs, Thoratec's paracorporeal position has proven itself beneficial for many reasons. This position permits identification of clots within the pump, which if necessary, can be exchanged for a new pump without invasive surgery in most cases.[4] Because the cannulae are the only internal components, biventricular assistance is possible and the device can be implanted in much smaller patients. The favorable positioning characteristics of the Thoratec and the FDA approval for bridge to transplantation and bridge to recovery, as well as the option of left or right atrial or ventricular cannulation contribute to the great versatility of this device.

Implantation Technique

The most common method of implantation[5,6] uses cardiopulmonary bypass with standard venous and arterial cannulation. Bicaval cannulation for cardiopulmonary bypass is necessary in patients with a patent foramen ovale, especially if only a left VAD (LVAD) is inserted. Failure to close the patent foramen ovale in the face of left ventricular support and right ventricular failure often results in significant right-to-left shunting with resulting arterial hypoxemia. Intraoperative transesophageal echocardiography may be invaluable in detecting a patent foramen ovale.

It is important to carefully select the percutaneous exit sites for the cannulae. These sites should be chosen so that the pump or pumps rest on the anterior abdominal wall and not laterally, to avoid chronic tension on the cannula where it exits the skin site. The length of the cannula pair is dictated by the atrial cannula (if an atrial cannula is used). The outflow and ventricular cannulae may be trimmed in length, but the atrial cannula cannot be trimmed. The preclotted outflow cannula is trimmed to appropriate length by beveling the Dacron graft. The felt covering on the outflow cannula should extend 1 to 2 cm beyond the skin exit site.

The outflow cannula is attached first to the ascending aorta. The site selected on the aorta must be made with consideration to previously placed bypass grafts. If the device is used as a bridge to transplantation, the anastomosis should be placed as close to the aortic valve as possible in order to permit excision of all Dacron material at the subsequent transplant procedure. A partial occlusion clamp is placed on the aorta and the anastomosis is constructed with 4–0 polypropylene suture. Some investigators have reported that wrapping the dacron graft within a Hemashield® graft (Boston Scientific Corporation, Natick, MA) will decrease persistent oozing and bleeding through the wall of the dacron graft.[7] Inflow cannulation is performed next. Left atrial cannulation may be accomplished by placement in the left atrial appendage, the left atrial roof, or the interatrial groove. We prefer to cannulate the left atrium by placing a double pledgeted purse-string suture of 2–0 ethibond just behind the interatrial groove (Fig. 2) and with the cannula exiting below the right costal margin. The cannula is inserted through a small stab wound and the purse-string sutures are snared and tied over sterile buttons. This allows for expedient cannula removal at the time of device explantation. In patients who require a right VAD (RVAD), the right atrium provides inflow to the pump.

Left ventricular apical cannulation, when possible, is preferred in the bridge-to-transplant patients, as it provides high VAD flows at decreased preload.[8] Additionally, there is some evidence that neurologic events may be more common with left atrial cannulation in patients supported for prolonged periods.[9]

Left ventricular cannulation begins with placement of circumferential horizontal mattress sutures of 2–0 pledgeted polyester around the left ventricular apex. A small stab wound is made in the apex and a large Foley catheter is inserted. The Foley balloon is distended with saline and pulled snugly against the apex. A circular trocar

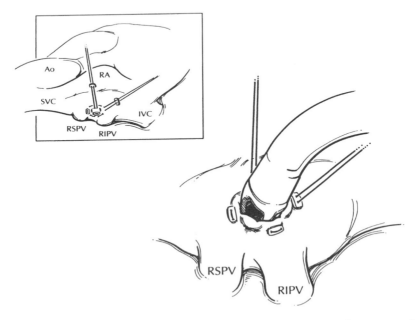

FIGURE 2. The left atrial cannula is inserted just behind the interatrial groove and secured with double pledgeted purse-string sutures placed at 90° apart.

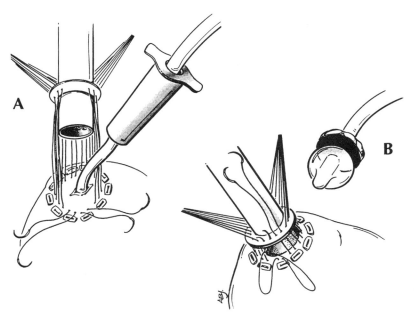

FIGURE 3. A. A Foley catheter is placed in the left ventricular apex. The trocar will cut a circular portion of myocardium, allowing insertion of the left ventricular cannula. B. The Foley catheter is removed along with the excised portion of myocardium. The pledgeted sutures placed through the felt cuff of the cannula can now be tied to secure the cannula to the apex of the left ventricle.

previously placed over the Foley is used for removal of a circular portion of myocardium. The interior of the left ventricle is visually and manually inspected and any thrombus is removed. The inflow cannula is inserted and the circumferential pledgeted 2–0 braided polyester sutures are placed through the felt washer of the inflow cannula and tied to secure the cannula to the myocardium (Fig. 3). The inflow cannulation site must be absolutely hemostatic, as it is very difficult to place additional sutures once the cannula has been brought out through the skin exit site.

After all cannulae have been brought out through the skin, the pumps are brought onto the operative field. The prosthetic ventricle is attached first to the inflow cannula. A small purse-string with a snare is placed in the outflow cannula graft, and a balloon-tipped vascular catheter with an aspiration port is placed through the graft, retrograde across the valve and into the prosthetic ventricle. It is important to pass the catheter through the larger valve orifice. The outflow cannula is then attached to the prosthetic ventricle. With release of the inflow cannula and aspiration of the catheter, air can be removed from the prosthetic ventricle. The vascular catheter is then removed and the purse-string suture on the graft material is snared. The prosthetic ventricle should now be free of any air and ready to begin ejection.

The pump or pumps are begun in the fixed rate mode while blood is being diverted from the cardiopulmonary bypass circuit into the heart. The pumping sacs are carefully observed for air bubbles and for the extent of filling and emptying. The VAD pumping rate is increased slowly as cardiopulmonary bypass is discontinued. Negative pumping pressure is used cautiously, because air may be in entrained around the cannula sites. Negative pressure, if necessary, is kept above -10 mm Hg. The pericardium is filled with saline in order to avoid air embolization.

After separation from cardiopulmonary bypass, careful management of the drive console is required. Diastolic vacuum, systolic duration, and drive line pressure may be manipulated to provide optimal cardiac output and complete emptying of the pump. Careful inspection of all cannulation sites is done to insure optimal hemostasis. Protamine is used to completely reverse the effects of heparin. A small left atrial pressure line may be inserted to give adequate preload readings of the LVAD. The chest is closed in standard fashion using stainless steel wires to approximate the sternum.

Postoperative care of these patients is similar to that of other cardiovascular patients. Careful attention to coagulation status, chest tube drainage, urine output, and hemodynamic parameters is imperative. With properly functioning VADs, the hemodynamics should be easy to control. An attempt is made to mobilize patients as soon as possible. Extubation is accomplished as soon as arterial blood gases demonstrate adequate gas exchange, and invasive catheters are removed as soon as feasible.

Anticoagulation protocols vary from institution to institution, but we begin low molecular weight dextran at 25 mL/h when the chest tube drainage has fallen to less than 100 mL/h for 3 consecutive hours. We begin warfarin on postoperative day 3 or 4 and attempt to maintain the international normalized ratio between 3.0 and 3.5. For patients who are unable to tolerate oral feedings, heparin may be administered with an attempt to maintain the partial thromboplastin time at twice normal.

It is important that patients who remain on VADs receive a minimal number of blood products. Many investigators have demonstrated that sensitization to human leukocyte antigens may occur with transfusion of blood products. We therefore use stringent criteria for blood product usage and utilize leuko-poor filters for all transfusions. We believe that this will decrease the rate and amount of sensitization in the patients who are bridged to cardiac transplantation and thereby make subsequent cross-matching of potential donor organs more feasible.

Indications

The Thoratec VAD is currently FDA-approved for temporary support for native cardiac recovery and as a bridge to cardiac transplantation. In recent years, reports of cardiac recovery in the bridge-to-transplantation population after a long duration of support has rekindled attempts to support patients until cardiac recovery occurs.[10,11] This is most likely a byproduct of the increasing waiting times for cardiac transplantation due the shortage of donor organs. Patients with diverse etiologies for advanced heart failure have benefited from temporary support with a Thoratec VAD. Ischemic cardiomyopathy is the most common, with idiopathic, viral, postpartum, congenital, and drug-induced cardiomyopathies also reported. Occasional cases of native cardiac recovery after moderately long duration of VAD support in patients with viral myocarditis as well as idiopathic and postpartum cardiomyopathies have been documented. Of course, there are many reports of post-coronary-bypass patients requiring VAD support for short duration to allow native recovery of the heart.[12,13]

Limitations

The major limitation of the Thoratec device lies in the restricted mobility and independence afforded to the patient. The main mobility-restricting factor is the large drive console, which must accompany the patient. At present, patients receiving the approved device as a bridge to transplantation must remain hospitalized until the time of transplantation. Efforts to address this issue are being actively pursued; indeed, a new smaller, portable driver is expected to be available shortly and should drastically improve this limitation.[14]

A limiting technical factor involves the preclotting of the Dacron outflow graft prior to implantation, which can delay placement of the device, thereby requiring additional time on cardiopulmonary bypass.

At present, all available VAD systems require a connection from the heart to a console or to the device itself. This transcutaneous connection represents a potential risk for infection. Electrical devices have an advantage over pneumatic systems in that they can potentially be completely implanted, hence greatly reducing the risk of infection. The recently developed transcutaneous energy transfer systems, which avert the need for transcutaneous power cables, will likely be present in the next generation of implantable circulatory support devices.

While the device has been used in adult patients with a wide range of body habitus, as well as in some adolescent patients (body surface area 0.73 to 2.5 m^2), it is too large for pediatric support. Finally, due to the need for chronic anticoagulation in patients maintained with the Thoratec device, patients with contraindications to systemic anticoagulation (ie, recent history of gastrointestinal or central nervous system bleeding) should not receive this device.

The Thoratec Device for Pulmonary Circulatory Support

There are few clinical indications for pulmonary mechanical circulatory support in the absence of significant left ventricular failure. However, isolated right ventricular failure may occur, and surgeons should be familiar with treatment options. Inotropic agents, pulmonary vasodilators, and volume loading are the first line of therapy. If these fail, intra-aortic balloon counterpulsation may be useful in the management of right ventricular failure because it unloads the left ventricle and, hence, reduces left atrial pressure (and thereby improves passive flow across the pulmonary bed) and improves coronary perfusion.[15] Direct balloon counterpulsation of the pulmonary artery has also been shown to increase pulmonary blood flow in several open-chest animal models of right ventricular failure,[16,17] and was first used clinically in 1980.[18] However, the improvement in pulmonary blood flow is modest at best, and more aggressive forms of mechanical circulatory support may be required. The recent availability of inhaled nitric oxide as a selective pulmonary vasodilator has reduced the incidence of right ventricular support after LVAD placement and presumably should benefit the rare patient with isolated right ventricular failure.

In an elegant animal model of profound right ventricular failure, four methods of providing pulmonary blood flow were compared quantitatively: 1) passive flow through the pulmonary artery due to a right atrial to left atrial pressure gradient; 2) pulmonary artery pulsation with an intra-aortic–type balloon within a graft anastomosed to the main pulmonary artery; 3) pulmonary artery pulsation with a single-port, valveless, sac-type pulsatile assist device; and 4) right atrial to pulmonary arterial bypass via a valved pneumatic pulsatile pump (Thoratec VAD).[19] Only the latter increased cardiac output to a satisfactory level and was the author's recommended method of pulmonary circulatory support for profound right ventricular failure.

Other forms of mechanical circulatory support may also be used in isolated profound right ventricular failure. Roller pumps or centrifugal pumps may be used for short-term support, but the Thoratec Device is particularly useful when the duration of right ventricular failure is expected to last more than a few days.

Bridging To Cardiac Transplant

Although sudden death may occur in patients awaiting cardiac transplantation, many patients present with acute exacerbation of their chronic congestive heart failure. Medical therapy for these decompensated patients includes elimination of any potentially reversible factors such as myocardial ischemia, infection, thyroid disease, and medical noncompliance. Pharmacologic therapy typically consists of inotropic drugs, vasodilators, and diuretics, but "tailored therapy" should be closely followed.[20] If these measures fail, an intra-aortic balloon pump may be beneficial. Unfortunately, the intra-aortic balloon pump provides only a modest increase in hemodynamic stability and cannot fully support the circulation. Patients who continue to deteriorate and become hemodynamically unstable while receiving maximum medical therapy and an intra-aortic balloon pump should be considered for advanced forms of mechanical circulatory support as a "bridge" to cardiac transplantation. At this juncture, consideration must be given to the patient's current medical condition as a transplant recipient before an assist device is implanted. Particular attention to the patient's pulmonary, renal, and hepatic functions is imperative. Although it may be very difficult to determine preoperatively, irreversible renal or hepatic dysfunction is a contraindication to implantation of a VAD. In an attempt to determine predictors of irreversible hepatic or renal dysfunction, a multi-institutional study of 193 patients receiving Thoratec VADs as bridges to transplantation was reviewed.[21] There were no factors that predicted the development of irreversible hepatic or renal dysfunction, although for patients ultimately undergoing transplantation, renal and hepatic function improved in most patients after 1 to 3 weeks of support. The most common cause of death in patients who died without transplantation was multiorgan failure, and these patients typically had higher levels of blood urea nitrogen, creatinine, and bilirubin during support when compared with patients who underwent transplantation. In a similar multi-institutional study of 186 patients supported with the Thoratec VAD as a bridge to cardiac transplantation, pre-implant blood urea nitrogen levels were found to be a sensitive predictor of survival to transplantation.[22] Elevations in serum creatinine and total bilirubin were also associated with decreased survival, although not statistically significant. Therefore, it would appear that there were no absolute predictors of irreversible end-organ dysfunction, although higher levels of blood urea nitrogen, creatinine, and bilirubin at the time of VAD implantation are likely to predict a decrease in survival to cardiac transplantation.

Once the decision has been made to proceed with VAD implantation, it is important to assess the need for univentricular or biventricular support. Most patients can be successfully bridged to transplantation with an LVAD and pharmacologic support of the right ventricle. Often it is not possible to predict preoperatively which patients will require biventricular assist device insertion. However, patients with clinically severe right heart failure, elevated pulmonary vascular resistance, and intractable ventricular arrhythmias should be strongly considered for biventricular support. The addition of an RVAD to an LVAD does not appear to increase operative mortality or morbidity and provides near complete control of the circulation. The final decision of whether to use biventricular support must be made intraoperatively only after insertion of the LVAD. The interaction of the right and left ventricles is complex and the response of the right ventricle after LVAD insertion cannot be fully predicted. If there is evidence of insufficient LVAD flow because of right heart failure, an RVAD should be inserted.

The Thoratec device can provide biventricular support, whereas the available implantable devices provide univentricular (left) support only. When mechanical right ventricular support is required after insertion of an implantable device, a hybrid system must be used; this increases the complexity of mechanical support and post-operative care.

Due to the fact that there are no reliable preoperative predictors of right heart failure with isolated LVAD support, and because there is no consensus on how to best select univentricular and biventricular devices for the total patient population requiring mechanical circulatory support, Farrar and colleagues[23] performed a retrospective study to determine whether there were any differences in populations of patients who require biventricular versus univentricular support.[23] The study consisted of 213 patients who received left ventricular or biventricular support with a Thoratec VAD System at 35 medical centers. Patients were divided into three groups: group 1 (n = 74) received isolated LVAD support; group 2 (n = 37) initially received an LVAD but subsequently had profound right heart failure and required an RVAD; group 3 (n = 102) received biventricular devices at the outset, based on the surgeon's judgment. Patients in the biventricular support groups (2 and 3) had a lower cardiac index and higher pulmonary capillary wedge pressure before the device was inserted; however, there was no difference in right heart hemodynamic values between the groups. Patients in the biventricular support groups also had higher creatinine and bilirubin levels preoperatively compared with those in the LVAD group. In addition, biventricular support recipients were more likely to require mechanical ventilatory and intra-aortic balloon pump support before VAD insertion, and were more likely to undergo implantation under emergency conditions. Univentricular support patients were more likely to survive to transplantation (74% versus 58% for biventricular support recipients); however, there was no difference between the groups regarding post-transplantation survival to hospital discharge. Results from this study indicate that patients who received isolated LVADs were less severely ill in the preoperative period and consequently had a lower mortality rate after the operation. This is consistent with the belief that the earlier the decision is made to proceed with VAD support, before major organ dysfunction occurs, the more likely that univentricular support will be all that is required. This study, however, failed to demonstrate preoperative hemodynamic parameters that would predict the need for univentricular versus biventricular support. These results are in agreement with a previous report, which concluded that the need for biventricular support is more dependent on the patient's clinical status than on hemodynamic parameters.[24]

The complications reported for the bridge-to-transplant patients are similar to those reported for the postcardiotomy patients. In a recent multicenter review, the most common complications were bleeding (42%), renal failure (36%), infection (36%), hepatic failure (24%), hemolysis (19%), respiratory failure (17%), multiorgan failure (16%), nonthromboembolic neurologic events (14%), and embolic neurologic events (8%).[25] Similar complications have been reported in single-center studies.[26,27]

The Thoratec device has been extremely beneficial in supporting patients to transplantation. In a large multicenter study, 74% of LVAD patients and 58% of biventricular patients survived to transplantation, with a hospital discharge rate of 89% and 81%, respectively.[23] Large single-center experiences have been even more encouraging, with hospital discharge rates approaching 100%[26,27] and long-term survival rates equivalent to those in patients transplanted without pre-transplant mechanical support.[27,28] Other investigators have found somewhat different results. In a series of 39 patients supported with either an intra-aortic balloon pump (n = 13), a VAD (n = 7), or a total artificial heart (n = 19), survival rates were significantly lower when compared with those of patients maintained on oral or intravenous medications prior to transplantation. Survival to discharge after transplantation decreased with increasing complexity of mechanical circulatory support,[29] although this finding did not reach statistical significance.

In summary, the Thoratec device is a versatile pump that is capable of providing biventricular support. Its timely use in appropriate candidates can result in short- and long-term survival after transplantation that is equivalent to that of conventional transplant recipients without major differences in post-transplant complications.

Future Directions

In the past several years, two problems have been identified with the Thoratec device when used to treat the entire spectrum of patients requiring mechanical circulatory support. First, the size of the cannulae and prosthetic pump preclude its use in small children. Second, the large, cumbersome device console has made it difficult for patients to be very mobile or even to be discharged to home. These two areas are the subjects of ongoing investigation.

A pediatric pneumatic, paracorporeal VAD similar to the Thoratec device has been developed. The "Berlin Heart" (see Chapter 21) has been successfully used in patients as small as 3.2 kg.[30] Unfortunately, this device is not available in the United States. Efforts to "scale down" the adult version of the Thoratec VAD have been hampered by the lack of sufficiently small commercially available valves and the tendency for thrombus to develop in small pumps. Studies are currently focusing on the complex flow patterns within the pediatric VAD as well as the relationship between blood contacting surfaces and thrombus formation.[31] More encouraging results have been obtained in the development of a portable pneumatic device console for the Thoratec VAD. Farrar and colleagues[14] have developed a briefcase-sized portable device unit called the Thoratec TLC-II Portable VAD Device. The TLC-II measures 33 cm × 34 cm × 13 cm, weighs 8 kg, and can be carried by hand, with a shoulder strap, or pushed on a wheeled mobility cart. The TLC-II consists of an electronic motor-driven air compressor for supplying positive and negative air pressure. Four power sources are provided: external direct current power, two rechargeable battery packs, and an emergency battery that drives an independent electronic back-up system. The TLC-II has been tested in animals[32] with excellent results and has been used successfully in the clinical setting.[33] The importance of patient mobility with VAD support has been well documented[34] and, hence, the availability of a smaller "wearable" device may enhance rehabilitation, improve the quality of life, and perhaps increase survival following transplantation. From an economic perspective, the prospect of being able to discharge patients to their homes with Thoratec VADs while they await cardiac transplantation is particularly attractive.

References

1. Pierce WS, Brighton JA, O'Bannon W, et al. Complete left ventricular bypass with paracorporeal pump: Design and evaluation. *Ann Surg* 1974;180:418–426.
2. Pennington DG, Bernhard WF, Golding LR, et al. Long-term follow-up of postcardiotomy patients with profound cardiogenic shock treated with ventricular assist devices. *Circulation* 1985;72(3 Pt. 2): II216-II226.
3. Hill JD, Farrar DJ, Hershon JJ, et al. Use of prosthetic ventricle as a bridge to cardiac transplantation for postinfarction cardiogenic shock. *N Engl J Med* 1986;314:626–628.
4. Lohmann DP, McBride LR, Pennington DG, Swartz MT. Replacement of paracorporeal ventricular assist devices. *Ann Thorac Surg* 1992;54(6):1226–1227.
5. Ganzel BL, Gray LA, Slater AD, Mavroudis C. Surgical techniques for the implantation of heterotopic prosthetic ventricles. *Ann Thorac Surg* 1989;47:113–120.
6. Holman WL, Bourge RC, McGiffin DC, Kirklin JK. Ventricular assist experience with a pulsatile heterotopic device. *Semin Thorac Cardiovasc Surg* 1994;6:147–153.
7. Minami K, Arusoglu L, Koyanagi T, et al. Successful implantation of Thoratec assist device: Wrapping of outflow conduit in Hemashield graft. *Ann Thorac Surg* 1997;64:861–862.
8. Lohmann DP, Swartz MT, Pennington DG, et al. Left ventricular versus left atrial cannulation for the Thoratec ventricular assist device. *ASAIO Trans* 1990;36:M545-M548.
9. Holman WL, Bourge RC, Murrah CP, et al. Left atrial or ventricular cannulation beyond 30 days for a Thoratec ventricular assist device. *ASAIO* 1995;41:M517-M522.
10. Holman WL, Bourge RC, Kirklin JK. Case report: Circulatory support for seventy days with resolution of acute heart failure [letter]. *J Thorac Cardiovasc Surg* 1991;102(6):932–934.
11. Loebe M, Hennig E, Muller J, et al. Long-term mechanical circulatory support as a bridge to transplantation, for recovery from cardiomyopathy, and for permanent replacement. *Eur J Cardiothorac Surg* 1997;11(suppl):S18-S24.
12. Korfer R, El-Banayosy A, Posival H, et al. Mechanical circulatory support with the Thoratec assist device in patients with postcardiotomy cardiogenic shock. *Ann Thorac Surg* 1996; 61(1):314–316.
13. Pennington DG, McBride LR, Swartz MT, et al. Use of the Pierce-Donachy ventricular assist device in patients with cardiogenic shock after cardiac operations. *Ann Thorac Surg* 1989;47(1):130–135.
14. Farrar DJ, Buck KE, Coulter JH, Kupa EJ. Portable pneumatic biventricular driver for the Thoratec ventricular assist device. *ASAIO J* 1997;43(5):M631-M634.
15. Kopman EA, Ramirez-Inawat RC. Intra-aortic balloon counterpulsation for right heart failure. *Anesth Analg* 1980;59:74–76.
16. Kralios AC, Zewart HHJ, Moulopoulos SD, et al. Intrapulmonary artery balloon pumping. *J Thorac Cardiovasc Surg* 1970;60:215–232.
17. Jett KG, Siwek MD, Picone AL, et al. Pulmonary artery balloon counterpulsation for right ventricular failure. *J Thorac Cardiovasc Surg* 1983;86:364–372.
18. Miller DC, Moreno-Cabral RJ, Stinson EB, et al. Pulmonary artery balloon counterpulsation for acute right ventricular failure. *J Thorac Cardiovasc Surg* 1980;80:760–763.
19. Gaines WE, Pierce WS, Prophet GA, Holtzman K. Pulmonary circulatory support: A quantitative comparison of four methods. *J Thorac Cardiovasc Surg* 1984;88:958–964.
20. Stevenson LS. Patient selection for mechanical bridging to transplantation. *Ann Thorac Surg* 1996;61:380–387.
21. Farrar DJ, Hill JD. Thoracic ventricular assist device principal investigators: Recovery of

major organ function in patients awaiting heart transplantation with Thoratec ventricular assist devices. *J Heart Lung Transplant* 1994;13:1125–1132.

22. Farrar DJ. Thoracic ventricular assist device principal investigators: Preoperative predictors of survival in patients with Thoratec ventricular assist devices as a bridge to heart transplantation. *J Heart Lung Transplant* 1994;13; 93–101.

23. Farrar DJ, Hill JD, Pennington DG, et al. Preoperative and postoperative comparison of patients with univentricular and biventricular support with the Thoratec ventricular assist device as a bridge to cardiac transplantation. *J Thorac Cardiovasc Surg* 1997;113:202–209.

24. Kormos RL, Gasior TA, Kawai A , et al. Transplant candidate's clinical status rather than right ventricular function defines need for univentricular versus biventricular support. *J Thorac Cardiovasc Surg* 1996;111:773–783.

25. Farrar DJ, Hill JD. Univentricular and biventricular Thoratec ventricular assist device support as a bridge to transplantation. *Ann Thorac Surg* 1993;55:276–282.

26. Korfer R, El-Banayosy A, Posival H, et al. Mechanical circulatory support: The Bad Oeynhausen experience. *Ann Thorac Surg* 1995;59: S56-S63.

27. Pennington DG, McBride LR, Peigh PS, et al. Eight years' experience with bridging to cardiac transplantation. *J Thorac Cardiovasc Surg* 1994;107:472–481.

28. Mehta SM, Boehmer JP, Pae WE Jr, et al. Bridging to transplant equals extended survival for patients undergoing LVAD support when compared with long-term medical management. *ASAIO J* 1996;42:M406-M410.

29. Masters RG, Hendry PJ, Davies RA, et al. Cardiac transplantation after mechanical circulatory support: a Canadian perspective. *Ann Thorac Surg* 1996;61:1734–1739.

30. Ishino K, Loebe M, Uhlemann F, et al. Circulatory support with paracorporeal pneumatic ventricular assist device (VAD) in infants and children. *Eur J Cardiothorac Surg* 1997:11: 965–972.

31. Daily BB, Pettitt TW, Sutera SP, Pierce WS. Pierce-Donachy pediatric VAD: Progress in development. *Ann Thorac Surg* 1996;61:437–443.

32. von Segesser LK, Tkebuchava T, Leskosek B, et al. Biventricular assist using a portable driver in combination with implanted devices: preliminary experience. *Artif Organs* 1997; 21:72–75.

33. Farrar DJ, Korfer R, El-Banayosy A, et al. First clinical use of the Thoratec TLC-II Portable VAD Driver in ambulatory and patient discharge settings. *ASAIO J* 1998;44:35A.

34. Reedy JE, Swartz T, Lohmann DP, et al. The importance of patient mobility with ventricular assist device support. *ASAIO J* 1992;38:M151-M153.

Chapter 20

Extracorporeal Membrane
Oxygenation in Adults

Richard J. Kaplon, MD and Nicholas G. Smedira, MD

First reported in 1965, extracorporeal membrane oxygenation (ECMO) is a system of mechanical assistance that may provide both cardiac and pulmonary support.[1] The concept of ECMO is to provide circulatory and/or pulmonary support for a short time, ie, days to weeks, while native heart or lung function recovers. The basic configuration of an ECMO circuit consists of a venous drainage cannula, reservoir, centrifugal or roller pump, oxygenator, and either an arterial or second venous return cannula.

While ECMO was initially used primarily for pulmonary support for patients with respiratory failure, its benefits—including versatility, portability, and ease of peripheral cannula insertion—have resulted in an expanded role for its use. This chapter reviews the use of adult ECMO, focusing on the indications for ECMO placement, techniques of cannulation, pump and patient management, risks and complications of mechanical assistance, and the results of long-term ECMO support.

Background

ECMO was first successfully used as mechanical support for a patient suffering "shock-lung" after traumatic aortic rupture.[2] Subsequently, from 1975 to 1979, a trial sponsored by the National Heart and Lung Institute randomized patients with refractory respiratory failure to ECMO versus medical therapy. The trial was abandoned prior to completion due to dismal results for both study cohorts, with survivals less than 10%.[3] Nonetheless, Dr. Bartlett and colleagues at the University of Michigan continued to investigate the efficacy of ECMO use in both neonates and adults.

Because of size constraints, ECMO is presently the only form of mechanical circulatory assist available to neonates. Further, neonatal pulmonary pathology such as meconium aspiration syndrome, hyaline membrane disease, and congenital diaphragmatic hernia makes these patients particularly well suited to this type of tempo-

From Goldstein DJ and Oz MC (eds). *Cardiac Assist Devices*. Armonk, NY: Futura Publishing Co., Inc.; ©2000.

rary, limited respiratory support. Zapol and colleagues[4] have reported their 20-year experience with ECMO for neonatal respiratory failure in 460 patients, reporting an impressive 87% overall survival.

As experience with neonatal ECMO progressed, so did the willingness to take the lessons learned with this population and apply them to the adult population. In 1994, Shanley et al[5] reported their experience with 65 adult patients over a 5-year period. In their institutional experience treating 51 patients with severe respiratory failure and 14 patients with cardiac failure, a 52% overall survival was documented. This and other similar reports demonstrated the feasibility of adult ECMO and heralded the current era of adult ECMO use.[6-8]

Indications for ECMO

In brief, the indications for ECMO include the need for mechanical assistance in the face of respiratory or cardiac failure refractory to medical management. Typical scenarios in which ECMO assistance would be required include postcardiotomy cardiac or pulmonary support, cardiac arrest, cardiogenic shock, primary respiratory failure, and during the period after heart or lung transplantation or left ventricular assist device (LVAD) placement.

Postcardiotomy Cardiac Support

Despite advances in surgical technique and myocardial preservation, postcardiotomy cardiogenic shock occurs in approximately 2% to 6% of patients undergoing either myocardial revascularization or valve operation.[9-12] With the concurrent use of inotropes, especially the phosphodiesterase inhibitors, intra-aortic balloon pumping allows 75% to 85% of these patients to be weaned from cardiopulmonary bypass.[13,14] The hospital survival for this population of patients is approximately 55%. Despite these interventions, there remains 1% of patients who will not respond to this therapy.[15,16] For this select population, various types of mechanical assistance have been used to allow time for recovery of "stunned" myocardium.[1,17-19]

Early experience with centrifugal pump ventricular assistance for this patient population at our institution was reported.[20] Of 91 patients requiring support from 1979 to 1991, 49 (62%) were successfully weaned from cardiopulmonary bypass; however, only 20 (25.3%) survived hospitalization.[20] The predominant morbidity associated with this type of support was bleeding (87.3%), and for this reason, we changed our mode of postcardiotomy support to ECMO, using a heparin-coated circuit to minimize the need for systemic anticoagulation.

From 1992 to 1997, we supported 72 patients in postcardiotomy cardiogenic shock with a heparin-coated ECMO circuit using minimal systemic heparinization. Thirty-two patients (45%) were weaned from support and 28 (40%) survived hospitalization.[21] Reports from other groups using heparin-coated ECMO circuits have described similar findings.[8]

Postcardiotomy Pulmonary Support

Pulmonary edema and acute lung injury are not uncommon sequelae after cardiopulmonary bypass, particularly in patients who are critically ill preoperatively. The need for ventilatory support with high levels of positive end-expiratory pressure (PEEP) often compromises right ventricular function and impairs systemic venous return to the heart with chest closure. Experience with venovenous (V-V) ECMO for primary respiratory failure has shown that ventilatory requirements may be markedly reduced, allowing time for recovery of pulmonary function.[22] From 1994 to 1997, we supported nine patients with V-V ECMO for postcardiotomy respiratory failure. Preoperatively, 5 (56%) of these patients were intubated, 3 (33%) were supported with an intra-aortic balloon pump, and 5 (56%) were on preoperative venoarterial (V-A) ECMO. Postoperatively, all patients were weaned from ECMO and six (67%) survived to hospital discharge.[23] ECMO placement allowed for reduced pressor support thus improving organ perfusion, and reduced ventilatory support thus minimizing barotrauma. Peripheral cannula insertion permitted chest closure in all patients, helping to minimize postoperative bleeding and allowing for device removal at the bedside without the need for an additional trip to the operating room.

Cardiac Arrest/Cardiogenic Shock

The portability of the small ECMO pumps and the ease and rapidity of peripheral cannulation have expanded the role of ECMO, making it ideal for use as temporary mechanical support in patients following cardiac arrest or in acute cardiogenic shock. Animal studies have suggested that ECMO may be more efficacious than open cardiac massage for resuscitation following protracted cardiac arrest and that ECMO, in conjunction with epinephrine, may be a highly effective intervention when conventional techniques of external compression and defibrillation fail to reverse cardiac arrest.[24,25]

Between 1986 and 1995, Willms and colleagues[26] used V-A ECMO to resuscitate 81 patients after cardiac arrest (n = 68) or in cardiogenic shock (n = 13). Thirty-five (43%) of these patients survived more than 24 hours after ECMO support was withdrawn and 20 (25%) survived long term.

In this study, Willms et al refer to ECMO use at "various locations in the hospital." In our experience, ECMO for cardiac resuscitation has proved particularly useful as temporary support for patients undergoing percutaneous cardiac interventions who become unstable and for in-hospital, inotrope-dependent patients awaiting heart transplantation who suffer a cardiac arrhythmia and arrest. In the former group of patients, ECMO placement offers excellent hemodynamic support while an operating room and surgical team are readied. In the latter group, ECMO support offers the chance to confirm adequate neurologic recovery prior to implantable LVAD placement.

From 1991 to 1996, we used ECMO to support 25 patients who were in cardiogenic shock prior to LVAD placement.[27] LVAD patients who did not require pre-LVAD ECMO during the same time period had an 81% survival to transplantation; comparatively, 17 patients (68%) bridged to LVAD with ECMO were transplanted.

Post LVAD implantation, 7 of these patients (28%) required ECMO for right ventricular support and 4 of these 7 (57%) survived to transplantation.

Primary Respiratory Failure

As discussed earlier, primary respiratory failure was the indication for which ECMO was first developed. Its success in the pediatric population has been clearly established. Zapol's group[4] reported their 20-year, 460-patient experience, with an 87% overall survival and 80% of children growing and developing normally.

In the adult setting, and despite improvement in ventilator design and management during the past 10 years, severe respiratory failure is still associated with a mortality in excess of 60%.[28] In this group of patients, ECMO has shown a steady improvement in outcome. Kolla et al[29] from the University of Michigan reported their experience with V-V ECMO in 100 adult patients with severe respiratory failure from 1991 to 1996. In this study, 94 patients required ECMO for hypoxemic respiratory failure (paO_2/FiO_2 ratio of 55.7 ± 15.9; transpulmonary shunt [Qs/Qt] of $55 \pm 22\%$) and six for severe hypercarbia ($paCO_2$ 84 ± 31.5 mm Hg), despite maximal ventilatory support. Primary diagnoses included pneumonia (49 cases; 26 survivors), adult respiratory distress syndrome (45 cases, 23 survivors), and airway support (6 cases, 5 survivors). Overall survival in this otherwise moribund group was 54%. In this study, advanced age, pre-ECMO days of mechanical ventilation, and pre-ECMO paO_2/FiO_2 ratio were identified as independent predictors of survival.

Post-Transplantation/LVAD

The need for ECMO placement after heart transplantation is unusual; however, post-lung-transplant or post-LVAD ECMO support is, unfortunately, not uncommon.

Glassman et al from the University of Pittsburgh[30] reported 17 cases of ECMO placement in 16 patients who underwent lung transplantation from 1991 to 1995. ECMO was placed within 7 days of transplant in 10 patients and after 1 week for late graft dysfunction in the remaining six patients. Of those patients requiring early ECMO support, eight (80%) survived long term. There were no survivors in the late graft dysfunction group.

The incidence of right ventricular failure necessitating right ventricular assist device (RVAD) placement after LVAD implantation ranges from 10% to 30%.[31] While hemodynamic indices have not been able to predict which subset of patients in this group will go on to require RVAD support, preoperative factors such as fever, pulmonary edema, high-dose inotropes, and rising serum creatinine have been shown to be reliable predictors of the need for post-LVAD RVAD.[32] Similarly, patients requiring intra-aortic balloon counterpulsation or ECMO pre-LVAD are more likely to require postoperative right ventricular support; however, interestingly, preoperative pulmonary hypertension has been shown not to correlate with postoperative RVAD use.[33]

From 1991 to 1996, we implanted 100 LVADs; 11 patients required RVAD support postoperatively.[34] As no specific preoperative indicators accurately predicted which patients would require RVAD placement, we found ECMO to be a versatile approach for these patients. Prior to surgery, 84 patients were on an intra-aortic balloon pump, 62 were intubated, and 25 were on ECMO. Eleven patients required V-A ECMO for right ventricular support post LVAD implant and three required V-V ECMO for respiratory failure. Eighty-one percent of patients supported with only an LVAD were successfully bridged to transplant; however, only 45% of patients requiring ECMO post LVAD were transplanted. While ECMO-RVAD use after transplantation or LVAD implant is associated with reduced survival, it helps to salvage these critically ill patients.

ECMO Circuit and Cannulation

Circuit

As discussed earlier, the basic ECMO circuit consists of a venous drainage cannula, reservoir, centrifugal or roller pump, oxygenator, and either an arterial or second venous return cannula. At our institution, as at most others, a roller pump is used for pediatric support while a centrifugal pump is used for adults. Our current adult circuit consists of a pump console (550 Bio-Console with TX50 Bio-Probe flow transducer, Medtronic Bio-Medicus Inc., Eden Prairie, MN); a heat exchanger (Bio-Cal 370 Blood Temperature Control Module, Medtronic Bio-Medicus), a pump cart (Bio-Medicus PBS Cabinets), a centrifugal pump (Bio-Pump BP-80, Medtronic Bio-Medicus Inc., Minneapolis, MN), a hollow-fiber oxygenator (Maxima Plus PRF, Medtronic Cardiac Surgery, Medtronic Inc., Cardiopulmonary Division, Anaheim, CA), and an oxygen blender (Sechrist Industries, Inc., Anaheim, CA). The pump tubing, pump head, and oxygenator are heparin-coated (Carmeda BioActive Surface, Medtronic Blood Systems Inc., Anaheim, CA) as are the cannulae and connectors (Duraflo, Baxter Bentley, Irvine, CA).

Cannulation

Cannulation for ECMO may be performed centrally using the right atrium for venous drainage and the great vessels for arterial return; however, the unique advantage of this system is its ability to cannulate peripherally. Peripheral cannulation may be performed either percutaneously or via open "cut-down" on the femoral artery and either the femoral or internal jugular vein.

V-A Mode

V-A ECMO is used primarily for cardiac or cardiorespiratory support. Cannulation is typically achieved via the common femoral artery using 16F to 20F arterial cannulae (Duraflo and Fem-flex II, Research Medical Inc., Midvale, UT) and 18F to 28F venous drainage cannulae (Duraflo and Fem-flex II) placed in the common femoral vein and advanced into the right atrium (Fig. 1, panel A). In order to avoid lower

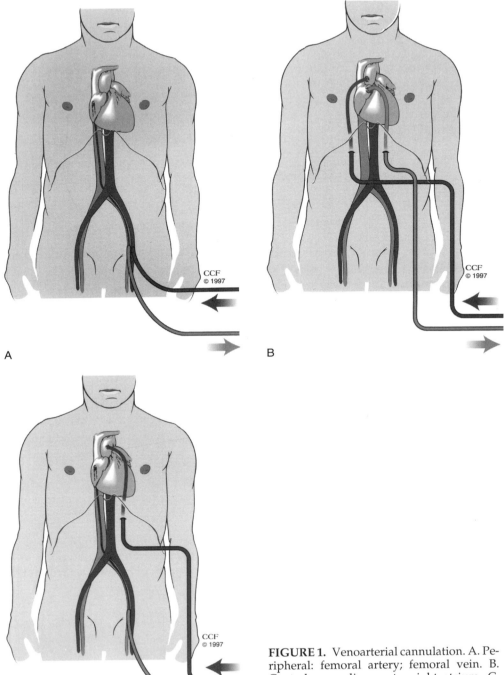

FIGURE 1. Venoarterial cannulation. A. Peripheral: femoral artery; femoral vein. B. Central: ascending aorta; right atrium. C. Hybrid: ascending aorta; femoral vein. Reproduced from Reference 21, with permission with permission.

limb ischemia, a 10F pediatric aortic cannula (Medtronic Bio-Medicus Inc.) is spliced into the arterial side of the circuit and advanced into the superficial femoral artery directed distally. Transthoracic cannulation is typically accomplished with an arterial cannula in the ascending aorta; venous drainage may be from either the right atrium or femoral vein (Fig. 1, panels B and C). With proper cannula placement, flows of 4 to 6 L/min are usually attained at 3000 to 3200 rpm.

V-V Mode

V-V ECMO is used solely for respiratory support. Cannulation for this mode of ECMO may be achieved in two ways: 1) with a 23F drainage cannula placed in the internal jugular vein (Medtronic Bio-Medicus Inc.) and return cannula (Duraflo, Fem-flex II) in the common femoral vein and advanced into the inferior vena cava (Fig. 2, panel A) or 2) with a drainage cannula (Duraflo, Fem-flex II) placed in common femoral vein and return cannula (Duraflo, Fem-flex II) in the contralateral common femoral vein and advanced into the right atrium (Fig. 2, panel B). V-V ECMO was

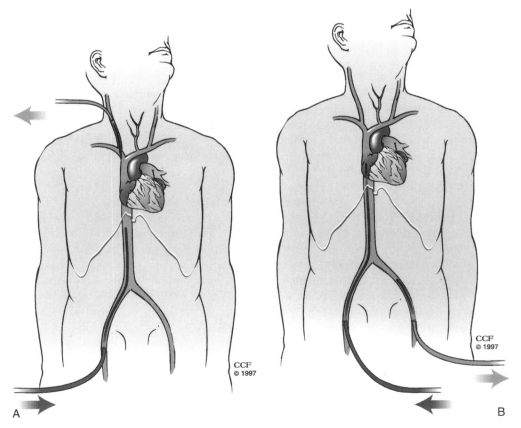

FIGURE 2. Venovenous cannulation. A. Internal jugular vein; femoral vein. B. Femoral vein; femoral vein. Reproduced from Reference 21, with permission.

traditionally performed with atrial drainage and femoral reinfusion (atriofemoral flow); however, Rich et al[35] have shown that flow reversal with femoral drainage and atrial reinfusion (femoroatrial flow) provides higher maximal extracorporeal flow and higher pulmonary arterial mixed venous oxygen saturation, and requires comparatively less flow to maintain an equivalent mixed venous oxygen saturation when compared to atriofemoral flow.

Patient Management

Prior to cannulation, patients placed on V-A ECMO are systemically anticoagulated with at least 5000 units of heparin. Heparin is repeatedly administered to maintain activated clotting times (ACTs) of 180 to 220 seconds. While not mandatory, some heparin is preferred for patients on V-V ECMO; however, these patients can be managed without any systemic anticoagulation.

Duration of ECMO typically ranges 2 to 3 days; however, we have successfully supported patients for as long as 13 days. While on support, end organ function is optimized. Ventilator tidal volumes and pressures are reduced to avoid barotrauma. Adjustment of ECMO and ventilator FiO_2, as well as ECMO gas sweep rates, ensures normal arterial blood gases. Patients are aggressively diuresed to remove third-space fluid. Patients who are unable to adequately diurese and those with renal dysfunction undergo ultrafiltration or dialysis via circuits that are easily spliced into the arterial and venous return lines.

Because V-A ECMO increases afterload to the left ventricle, patients on this mode of support for left ventricular compromise should have an intra-aortic balloon pump placed. Once on ECMO, inotropes are reduced, however, care is taken to maintain ventricular ejection by adjusting inotropes and ECMO flow while observing the arterial waveform. Maintaining ejection reduces the risk of thrombus formation and ventricular distension.

Thermodilution cardiac outputs from pulmonary artery catheters are unreliable while on ECMO because the injectate may be withdrawn into the venous return. Mixed venous oxygen saturation greater than 70%, however, is indicative of adequate systemic flow. Ideally, flows of 2 L/min/m^2 are maintained at the lowest necessary pump speeds; this will minimize trauma to the blood elements.

When ventricular recovery is suspected due to decreased inotropic dosage, improved ventricular ejection on the arterial waveform, and declining filling pressures, ECMO flows are reduced. Heparin dose is increased while flows are less than 1 L/min to avoid thrombus formation. If support is not easily weaned, transesophageal echocardiography is performed to assess ventricular function. If possible, ECMO is removed; otherwise conversion to an implantable VAD may be necessary.

Patients on V-V ECMO may be helped by adequate sedation and paralysis. Flows of approximately 4 L/min are usually necessary to achieve an arterial blood saturation of 90%. Improvement in pulmonary function is aided by reduction in mechanical ventilator FiO_2 less than 0.5, end-inspiratory pressure ≤35 mm Hg and PEEP less than 10 mm Hg at a rate of four to six breaths per minute. When native lung recovery is adequate to support approximately 75% of gas exchange, V-V ECMO is weaned.

Complications

Early in our experience using V-A ECMO for 30 patients with cardiogenic shock, we found that complications while on ECMO were common. In one series,[36] 24 patients were cannulated peripherally (femoral vein to femoral artery) and six were cannulated centrally (right atrium to ascending aorta, n = 5; femoral vein to ascending aorta, n = 1). All of the patients cannulated peripherally had percutaneously placed cannulae, whereas all of the patients cannulated centrally had their chests left open. None of the patients had distal leg perfusion catheters placed. Only five patients were systemically heparinized, and in these patients, ACTs greater than 200 seconds were maintained.

Limb ischemia was the most common complication and was found only in patients with femoral artery cannulation. Twenty-one patients (70%) had clinical signs of leg ischemia; however, only 10 (33%) required surgical intervention. Renal dysfunction was common; 17 patients (57%) required dialysis or ultrafiltration. Twelve of 23 patients (40% of total population) on ECMO for postcardiotomy cardiogenic shock required reexploration, including the six patients whose chests were left open. Seven patients (23%) suffered bacteremic episodes and one patient (3%) developed mediastinitis.

Oxygenator failure occurred in 13 patients (43%). The mean time to oxygenator failure was 42 hours; the mean number of oxygenator changes was 2.25. Two patients (6%) had pump heads changed because clot was detected within the pump head. Six patients (20%), none of whom were heparinized, developed intracardiac clot.

While complications during V-A ECMO remain problematic, several have been addressed. The placement of a distal leg perfusion catheter is now standard and has essentially eradicated the incidence of leg ischemia. Patients are routinely cannulated peripherally, even when ECMO is placed intraoperatively. This has dramatically reduced the incidence of infection and bleeding, and has removed the need for a return trip to the operating room at the time of ECMO removal. All patients on V-A ECMO are systemically heparinized to maintain ACTs 180 to 220 seconds; this, in conjunction with intra-aortic balloon counterpulsation, seems to have controlled the incidence of intracardiac clot formation. Despite these improvements, prolonged support remains a race between potential recovery and complications. Conversion to implantable LVAD is recommended if early recovery is not apparent.

Comparatively, patients on V-V ECMO have a lower incidence of significant complications. Kolla et al[29] reported that cannula site bleeding occurred in 39 patients (39%); this was associated with an increased incidence in mortality. However, in that series, other complications were not significant with regard to overall survival.

Summary

Between 1992 and 1998, we used ECMO in 200 patients. V-A ECMO was used in 177 patients and V-V ECMO in 23. Indications for ECMO included postcardiotomy (n = 87), cardiac arrest or cardiogenic shock (n = 63), primary respiratory failure (n = 24), post heart transplantation (n = 8), post lung transplantation (n = 5), and post-LVAD placement (n = 13). Duration of support ranged from 15 minutes to 13 days;

average time on ECMO was 3 days. Of the patients supported, 58 survived to hospital discharge.

Our results with ECMO, like results from other centers, demonstrate that ECMO is a flexible, effective means of providing cardiopulmonary support. Three distinct advantages to ECMO are that it may be used rapidly via peripheral insertion, it can provide either pulmonary, univentricular, or biventricular support, and, in patients unable to be weaned from V-A support, it has been shown to be an effective bridge to LVAD. We recognize that the use of ECMO introduces complications unique to itself; however, we believe that ECMO allows for salvage of patients who would otherwise not survive.

References

1. Spencer FC, Eisman B, Trinkle JK. Assisted circulation for cardiac failure following intracardiac surgery with cardiopulmonary bypass. *J Thorac Cardiovasc Surg* 1965;49:56–73.
2. Smedira NG, Hlozek C, McCarthy PM. Mechanical support after cardiac surgery. *Semin Cardiovasc Anesth* 1998;2:66–77.
3. Hill JD, O'Brien TG, Murray JJ, et al. Extracorporeal oxygenation for acute posttraumatic respiratory failure (shock-lung syndrome): Use of the Bramson Membrane Lung. *N Engl J Med* 1972;286:629–634.
4. Zapol WM, Snider MT, Hill JD, et al. Extracorporeal membrane oxygenation in severe respiratory failure. *JAMA* 1979;242:2193–2196.
5. Shanley CJ, Hirschl RB, Schumacher RE, et al. Extracorporeal life support for neonatal respiratory failure. A 20-year experience. *Ann Surg* 1994;220(3):269–280.
6. Pranikoff T, Hirschl RB, Steimle CN, et al. Efficacy of extracorporeal life support in the setting of adult cardiorespiratory failure. *ASAIO J* 1994;40(3):M339-M343.
7. Hill JG, Bruhn PS, Cohen SE, et al. Emergent applications of cardiopulmonary support: A multiinstitutional experience. *Ann Thorac Surg* 1992;54:699–704.
8. Stolar CJH, Delosh T, Bartlett RH. Extracorporeal Life Support Organization 1993. *ASAIO Trans* 1993;39:976–979.
9. Magovern GJ, Magovern JA, Benckart DH, et al. Extracorporeal membrane oxygenation: Preliminary results in patients with postcardiotomy cardiogenic shock. *Ann Thorac Surg* 1994;57(6):1462–1471.
10. Pennington DG, Swartz MT, Codd JE, et al. Intra-aortic balloon pumping in cardiac surgical patients: A nine year experience. *Ann Thorac Surg* 1983;36:125–131.
11. Bolooki H. Balloon pumping in cardiac surgery. In Bolooki H (ed): *Clinical Applications of Intra-Aortic Balloon Pump.* Mount Kisco, NY: Futura Publishing Co., Inc.; 1984:373–394.
12. Downing TP, Miller DC, Stofer R, Shumway NE. Use of intra-aortic balloon pump after valve replacement. *J Thorac Cardiovasc Surg* 1986;92:210–217.
13. Norman JC, Cooley DA, Igo SR, et al. Prognostic indices for survival during postcardiotomy intra-aortic balloon pumping. *J Thorac Cardiovasc Surg* 1977;74:709–720.
14. McEnany TM, Kay HR, Buckley MJ, et al. Clinical experience with intra-aortic balloon pump support in 782 patients. *Circulation* 1978;58(2):1124–1132.
15. Sanfelippo PM, Baker NH, Ewy HG, et al. Experience with intra-aortic balloon counterpulsation. *Ann Thorac Surg* 1986;41:36–41.
16. Rose DM, Colvin SB, Culliford AT, et al. Long-term survival with partial left heart bypass following peri-operative myocardial infarction and shock. *J Thorac Cardiovasc Surg* 1982; 83:483–492.
17. Pennington DG, Merjavy JP, Swartz MT, et al. The importance of biventricular failure in patients with post-operative cardiogenic shock. *Ann Thorac Surg* 1985;39:16–26.
18. Zumbro GL, Shearer G, Kitchens WR, Galloway RF. Mechanical assistance for biventricular failure following coronary bypass operations and heart transplantation. *J Heart Transplant* 1985;4:348–352.

19. Dennis C, Hall P, Morena JR, Senning A. Reduction of the oxygen utilization of the heart by left heart bypass. *Circ Res* 1962;10:298–305.
20. Pennock JL, Pierce WS, Wisman CB, et al. Survival and complications following ventricular assist pumping for cardiogenic shock. *Ann Surg* 1983;198:469–478.
21. Smedira NG, Hlozek CC, McCarthy PM. Mechanical support after cardiac surgery. *Semin Cardiothorac Vasc Anesth* 1998;2(1):66–77.
21. Golding LAR, Crouch RD, Stewart RW, et al. Postcardiotomy centrifugal mechanical ventricular support. *Ann Thorac Surg* 1992;54:1059–1064.
22. Delius R, Anderson H, Schumacher R, et al. Venovenous compares favorably with venoarterial access for extracorporeal membrane oxygenation in neonatal respiratory failure. *J Thorac Cardiovasc Surg* 1993;106:329–338.
23. Smedira NG, Wudel JH, Hlozek CC, et al. Venovenous extracorporeal life support for patients after cardiotomy. *ASAIO J* 1997;43:M444-M446.
24. Gazmuri RJ, Weil MH, Terwilliger K, et al. Extracorporeal circulation as an alternative to open-chest cardiac compression for cardiac resuscitation. *Chest* 1992;102(6):1846–1852.
25. Gazmuri RJ, Weil MH, von Planta M, et al. Cardiac resuscitation by extracorporeal circulation after failure of conventional CPR. *J Lab Clin Med* 1991;118(1):65–73.
26. Willms DC, Atkins PJ, Dembitsky WP, et al. Analysis of clinical trends in a program of emergent ECLS for cardiovascular collapse. *ASAIO J* 1997;43(1):65–68.
27. Smedira NG, Wudel JH, Hlozek CC, et al. Extracorporeal life support as a bridge to left ventricular assist device. *ASAIO J* 1997;43:33.
28. Bartlett RH. Extracorporeal life support for cardiopulmonary failure. *Curr Probl Surg* 1990; 27:621–705.
29. Kolla S, Awad SS, Rich PB, et al. Extracorporeal life support for 100 adult patients with severe respiratory failure. *Ann Surg* 1997;226(4):544–564.
30. Glassman LR, Keenan RJ, Fabrizio MC, et al. Extracorporeal membrane oxygenation as an adjunct treatment for primary graft failure in adult lung transplant recipients. *J Thorac Cardiovasc Surg* 1995;110(3):723–726.
31. Kanter KR, McBride LR, Pennington DG, et al. Bridging to cardiac transplantation with pulsatile ventricular assist devices. *Ann Thorac Surg* 1988;46:134–140.
32. Kormos RL, Gasior TA, Kawai A, et al. Transplant candidate's clinical status rather than right ventricular function defines need for univentricular versus biventricular support. *J Thorac Cardiovasc Surg* 1996;111:773–783.
33. Smedira NG, Massad MG, Navia JL, et al. Pulmonary hypertension is not a risk factor for RVAD use and death after left ventricular assist system. *ASAIO J* 1996;42:M733-M735.
34. McCarthy PM, Smedira NG, Vargo RL, et al. One hundred patients with the Heartmate left ventricular assist device: Evolving concepts and technology. *J Thorac Cardiovasc Surg* 1998;115:904–912.
35. Rich PB, Awad SS, Crotti S, et al. A prospective comparison of atrio-femoral and femoro-atrial flow in adult venovenous extracorporeal life support. *J Thorac Cardiovasc Surg* 1998; 116(4):628–632.
36. Muehrke DD, McCarthy PM, Stewart RW, et al. Complications of extracorporeal life support using heparin bound surfaces. *J Thorac Cardiovasc Surg* 1995;110:843–851.

Chapter 21

Extracorporeal Support:

The Berlin Heart

Matthias Loebe MD, PhD, Friedrich Kaufmann, and
Roland Hetzer MD, PhD

Introduction

The Berlin Heart assist device, produced by Mediport Kardiotechnik (Berlin, Germany), is a pneumatically driven paracorporeal support system that can be used to provide univentricular (left or right) or biventricular support. The system, which was developed at the Westend Hospital of the Free University Berlin under the guidance of E.S. Buecherl, has undergone extensive bench and animal testing. In 1988, the first clinical application of the Berlin Heart assist device as a bridge to heart transplantation took place.[1] Our discouraging early results with a total artificial heart (Buecherl) led us to concentrate our efforts on the development of paracorporeal assist devices, which offer two major advantages: first, the patient's natural heart could serve as a back-up system in the event of device failure; second, since major fitting problems were observed with the fully implantable devices, the paracorporeal assist systems enabled a broad variety of patients to be supported. In 1992, the Berlin Heart became the first commercially available pulsatile assist device for small children, when miniaturized pumps with stroke volumes of approximately 10 to 30 mL were introduced into clinical use.[2]

Today, the system can be implanted in patients with a broad variety of sizes and clinical characteristics. As with most other devices, the major indication is as a bridge to transplantation; however, a few patients have been supported with the perspective of subsequent myocardial recovery and weaning. Indeed, several patients with postcardiotomy heart failure and children with acute severe myocarditis, as well as a few patients with primary dilated cardiomyopathy (see Chapter 10) have demonstrated recovery of native cardiac function allowing for weaning from Berlin Heart support.

From Goldstein DJ and Oz MC (eds). *Cardiac Assist Devices.* Armonk, NY: Futura Publishing Co., Inc.; ©2000.

A number of patients have been on biventricular support for more than 1 year with the Berlin Heart assist device. Some have been able to leave the hospital and return to their homes. No major technical problems with the pumps or the driving units have been encountered during our extensive experience with the device. The incidence of thromboembolic events has been virtually zero in recent years, thanks to modified anticoagulation and aggressive pump cleaning. Infections at the skin exit sites of the cannulae have occasionally impaired patients' mobility and well-being. These infections, however, have never precluded subsequent heart transplantation.

Presently, a wearable driving unit is under clinical investigation. It is expected that availability of a portable system will greatly enhance the applicability of this very safe and reliable Berlin Heart assist system.

The Berlin Heart: System Description

The Berlin Heart ventricular assist device system consists of a paracorporeal air-driven blood pump, cannulae for the connection of the pump to the heart chambers and the great vessels, and the electropneumatic driving systems (Fig. 1). Within the semi-rigid polyurethane housing, the blood chamber and the air chamber are separated by a multilayer flexible polyurethane membrane. Both the blood chambers and the polyurethane ports are transparent to allow for transillumination detection of thrombotic deposits and for the control of the chamber filling and emptying. Since 1994, all blood contacting polyurethane surfaces have been heparin-coated (Carmeda, Stockholm, Sweden).

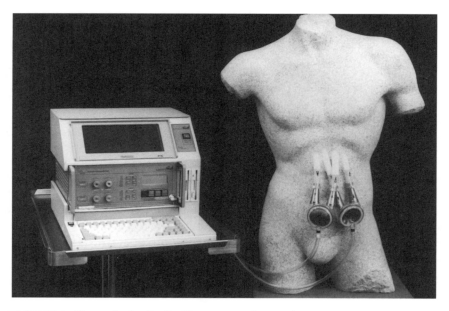

FIGURE 1. Biventricular Berlin Heart assist device the Heimes HD 7 drive unit.

Cannulae

A set of atrial and arterial silicone cannulae is now available with inner diameters ranging from 3.2 to 12.7 mm, enabling individual system assembly according to the patient's anatomy. The arterial cannulae are supplied with a basket tip at three different angles (45°, 60°, and 85°) and a sewing ring (Fig. 2). The arterial return cannulae have a sewing rim covered with Dacron® velour (C.R. Bard, Haverhill, PA) that permits end-to-side anastomosis to either the aorta or the pulmonary artery. The middle portion of the cannula is surrounded by a Dacron velour surface, which promotes tissue ingrowth and reduces the likelihood of ascending infection along the subcutaneous tunnel.

Atrial cannulae have small cages (22 to 26 mm long), which are inserted into the atrium. A matching mandrin enables the safe and quick insertion of the soft small atrial cage. Steel reinforcement prevents the soft silicone cannula from kinking, and can be used for ideal positioning of the cannula within the chest. Apical cannulae are also available for left ventricular drainage.

A transmitral cannula is also offered that corresponds in size to a normal atrial cannula, but which also has an extension from the small atrial cage with an anatomically correct angle of 110°. This extension, also made of silicone, is flexible enough to allow safe insertion through the mitral valve. This flexibility ensures that the mitral valve is not damaged or opened so wide that unwanted mitral valve insufficiency results. The length and inner diameter of the cannula have been designed so that

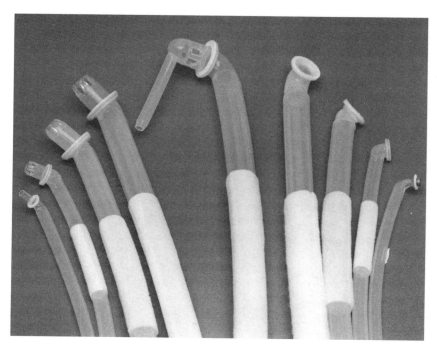

FIGURE 2. Berlin Heart cannulae. Flat metal tip "press-button" type pediatric arterial cannula with sewing ring (far right), small infant type atrial cannula (fare left), and transmitral atrial cannula (middle).

adequate pressure relief is achieved during pump operation with a quasi-constant flow from the ventricle into the left atrium. The majority of the pump volume is removed from the left atrium.

The Berlin Heart cannulae are made of silicon rubber and, due to the high flow rates, do not need heparin coating.

Blood Pumps

Membrane blood pumps for the Berlin Heart system are available in 80, 60, 50, 30, 25, and 12 mL sizes (Fig. 3); this permits a wide range of device applications. The membrane, which keeps the air and blood separated, has a three-layer construction, ensuring high durability. When compared with a single layer membrane of similar strength, it offers enhanced safety and greater flexibility. Two of the three membranes are drive membranes that absorb mechanical stress; the thinner membrane, which is in contact with the blood, remains free from stress because of its special size and because it is only moved by the drive membranes. The membranes are separated from one another with a graphite powder lubricant.

The membrane blood pumps are made of polyurethane with smooth blood contact surfaces. Recently, the pumps have been subjected to heparin coating, according to the Carmeda method, in order to further improve antithrombogenicity.[3] Heparin coating involves covalent bonding of partially degraded heparin with one end on an

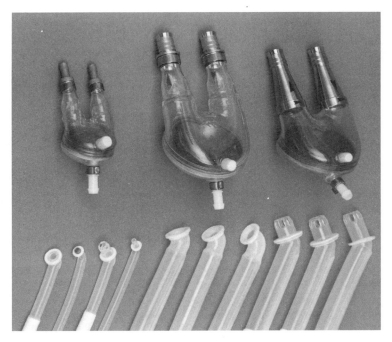

FIGURE 3. Adult size (80 mL) pump with tilting disk mechanical valves (right) and polyurethane ports, which include polyurethane trileaflet valves (middle), and 12 mL pump with polyurethane ports and valves (left). Spectrum of available atrial cannulae (right) and arterial cannulae (left) with different angles, and pediatric cannulae (left four cannulae).

amino group of the plastic surface. Thus, the chemically stable immobilized heparin molecules are free to move. The reactive sites on which antithrombin III is activated are not influenced,[3] and the long-term stability of the coating has been verified by measuring the residual coating activity after explantation of the Berlin Heart pumps. Although the ability to bind with antithrombin III had decreased to approximately 10% of the value before pump implantation, it remained within the same range regardless of whether the pump had been in operation for a few hours, several days, or 6 months.[3]

Valves are integrated in the inflow and outflow sides of the blood pump to ensure unidirectional blood flow. The three large pumps for cardiac support in adults and adolescents are available with mechanical valves (monoleaflet tilting disc valves, Sorin Biomedica, Turin, Italy), as well as with polyurethane trileaflet valves. The advantage of tilting disc valves lies in their proven operative safety and low thrombogenicity with long-term use. The newly developed polyurethane trileaflet valves are marked by their especially flat construction, which provides optimal washout behind the leaflets. Bulbs can be avoided, resulting in lowered dead volume, thus bringing about a reduced tendency toward thromboembolism. The valve profile is cylindrical, such that only two-dimensional folding occurs during opening. The bending stress and opening resistance are accordingly low. Another feature is that the valves are produced in one piece, thus absolutely uniform surface properties are attained. Since the valves are of the same polyurethane material as the pumps, an altogether homogenous blood contact surface is produced, which is advantageous particularly for heparin coating of the surface. Furthermore, the valve is cut in a closed condition, ie, the sectional planes match one another exactly. When closed, the valve is almost completely leak proof, enhancing the system's efficacy. In the miniaturized pediatric pumps, this feature is of even greater importance. The 30, 25, and 12 mL pumps for use in children and newborns are manufactured exclusively with polyurethane trileaflet valves. Mechanical tilting disk valves with the small diameters required would have too much leakage, resulting in suboptimal pump efficiency.[4]

Titanium used for the cone that supports the respective tilting disc valves allows a more even course at a smaller angle because of its high stability, as opposed to the polyvinyl chloride connectors normally used in cardiovascular settings, such that almost junction-free connections can be made to the cannula. Experience has taught us that these connection sites are a major source of thrombus formation. Therefore, we aggressively clear and correct pump-to-cannula connections whenever clots become visible.

Berlin Heart blood pumps have a de-airing nipple at the blood chamber through which air can be easily removed with a special de-airing cannula after pump connection or after the first few pump strokes.

The Drive Unit

At present, there are three different driving units in clinical use with the Berlin Heart assist device. The Heimes HD 7 (Heimes AG, Aachen, Germany) has served for many years as a very effective driving unit for both univentricular and biventricular long-term support. The IKUS Driving System 2000 (Mediport GmbH, Berlin, Germany) was especially developed for driving extracorporeal blood pumps (Fig. 4). Most recently, the Excor (Mediport GmbH, Berlin, Germany), a wearable driving unit, was designed to make it possible for patients to move freely (Fig. 5).

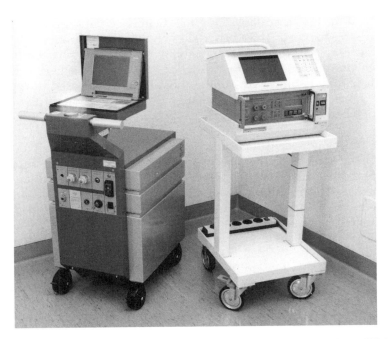

FIGURE 4. Drive systems available for the Berlin Heart assist device. The IKUS 2000 driver (left) is preferred for small children because it can generate high positive and negative pressures and has a variety of drive modes. The lighter Heimes HD-7 driver (right) allows for somewhat greater mobility.

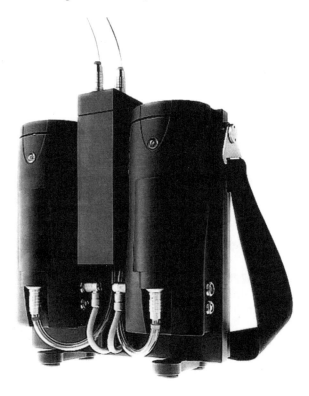

FIGURE 5. The wearable Excor drive unit. The unit can be carried on a cart or in a shoulder holster.

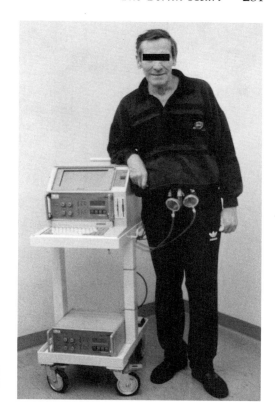

FIGURE 6. Patient on biventricular Berlin Heart support at home with a Heimes drive unit.

The electropneumatic Heimes HD 7 drive unit (Fig. 6) provides an optimal weight/efficiency ratio with maximal security through a redundant compressor system. The low weight, high capacity rechargeable batteries and ability to operate with the standard 12 V electrical current provide patients with a high degree of mobility even when on biventricular support. Several patients at the Deutsches Herzzentrum Berlin have been discharged from the hospital and have spent extended periods at home with their families while on biventricular support with a Heimes driving unit. One patient has been out of hospital with this device for more than 5 months.

The electropneumatic IKUS 2000 provides maximal technical reliability and high efficiency. In principle, the entire drive system consists of three independent drive units (Fig. 7). The safety is based on this double redundancy. Each of these drive units consists of a compressor and electronically controlled pressure and vacuum regulators, which ensure that pressure and vacuum values can be adjusted to obtain optimal operation in the blood pumps. The user operates the entire system through a laptop. The computer responsible for controlling the system is housed in the interior of the drive unit for security reasons, and works independently of the laptop. Like the drive units, the computer system is also redundant, having two identical computers that monitor one another. The safety concept of the IKUS 2000 drive unit is depicted in Figure 7.

The IKUS 2000 drive unit can be operated in four different modes. Normally the left/right-synchronous mode is applied. Then the pump rate and the beginning of systole are identical for the left and right ventricular pump. The pumps can also

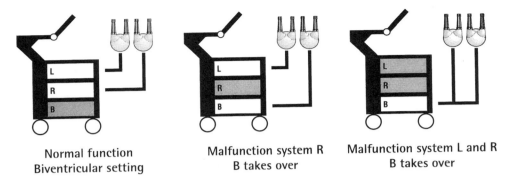

Normal function   Malfunction system R   Malfunction system L and R
Biventricular setting   B takes over   B takes over

FIGURE 7. The security concept of the IKUS 2000 drive unit. A. Normal function B. System 3 takes over for the failing system 1. C. System 3 takes over for failing systems 1 and 2.

be operated in an alternate mode with identical pump rates but alternating left and right filling. This can be advantageous in very small patients, in whom the simultaneous volume shift from the extracorporeal pumps into the chest may lead to problems caused by sharp increases of intrathoracic pressure.

There is a further possibility for setting completely different parameters for the right and left pumps. In cases with recovering native right heart function this option may be needed to prevent pulmonary edema due to a mismatch between right and left ventricular output. Finally, electrocardiogram-triggered operation, set to provide counterpulsation, can be used in patients in whom, after myocardial recovery, weaning from the assist device is attempted.

Most recently, the Excor drive system became available as a wearable drive unit for Berlin Heart assist pumps. Excor is designed as a simple redundant standby feature for univentricular operation. In the biventricular mode, the built-in switching unit automatically ensures that two pumps provide essential support. The system responds to spontaneous changes in blood pressure by adjusting its stroke volume accordingly, thanks to a volume-regulated algorithm that seeks the device's optimum working level. Two plug-in rechargeable batteries guarantee a total service time of 6 hours. Each battery has a display that indicates the current battery charge and which can be checked at a glance at any time. Visual and acoustic alarms warn the patient in the event of unexpected malfunction. Built-in emergency batteries ensure 30 minutes of emergency operation if the rechargeable batteries are completely discharged.

Implantation

The heart is exposed through a midline sternotomy, and cardiopulmonary bypass is instituted.[5] The cannulae are connected to the pulmonary artery, ascending aorta, left atrium, and right atrium. Anastomoses to the great arteries are created at a site close to the heart so as to leave as much of the aorta and the pulmonary artery as possible for future transplantation. The left atrial cannula is placed at the origin of the right upper pulmonary vein with care to avoid venous obstruction. Running 4–0 sutures (polypropylene) are used for arterial anastomosis, while the atrial anastomoses can be either done with multiple pledget-armed 4–0 mattress sutures or two purse-string 3–0 sutures and a few 4–0 mattress sutures. The cannulae are lead through four incisions in the epigastrium. Kinking and tension on the anastomoses must be avoided. The cannulae are then connected to the pumping chambers and the system is carefully de-aired. Support with the Berlin Heart assist device is started as cardiopulmonary bypass is withdrawn. After placement of the mediastinal drains, the chest is closed in the usual fashion. Meticulous attention is paid to hemostasis, particularly around the cannula sites.

The implantation may be carried out with or without the support of a heart-lung machine and cardioplegic arrest. At our institution, we routinely employ cardiopulmonary bypass without cardioplegic arrest for the implantation of the Berlin Heart assist device. In our experience, the majority of patients have been implanted with the Berlin Heart in a biventricular fashion.

Several modifications of the implantation technique have been proposed. In a number of patients in whom myocardial recovery was considered possible, a left atrial cannula was used that could be placed through the mitral valve into the left ventricle. We have used either custom made angled cannulae or a specifically manufactured Berlin Heart cannula. It was expected that more complete unloading of the left ventricle would increase the chance of complete myocardial recovery. However, after prolonged left ventricular support via transvalvular cannulae, substantial damage to the mitral valve was observed. We have since discontinued the use of these cannulae.

Recently, an apical cannula became available that serves the same goal as transmitral drainage. We have used this technique in several patients who have undergone previous cardiac surgery. After the patient was placed on femorofemoral bypass, the device was implanted through a left lateral thoracotomy. The outflow graft was anastomosed to the descending aorta, thereby completely avoiding repeat sternotomy.[6]

Experience with the Berlin Heart Assist Device at the Deutsches Herzzentrum Berlin

The system was first used at our institution in 1988. By February of 1999, the device had been implanted in 346 patients, including 34 children under the age of 16 years. A biventricular support mode was chosen for 281 (81%) patients, isolated left ventricular support was executed in 59 (17%), and isolated right ventricular support in 6 (2%) patients. Indications for mechanical support included bridge to heart transplantation in 203 (59%) patients, post-transplantation cardiac dysfunction in 30 (9%), postcardiotomy heart failure in 51 (15%), pediatric support in 34 (10%) (see below), and others in 28 (8%). The first pediatric system with 12 mL blood pumps was implanted in 1992. Although the Berlin heart remains our most commonly implanted device, our institution has also implanted the Novacor LVAS (Baxter Healthcare Corp., Oakland, CA), the TCI HeartMate (Thermo Cardiosystems, Woburn, MA), and the DeBakey LVAD[7] in an additional 102 patients.

The duration of support has steadily increased over the years. Presently, mean waiting time on Berlin Heart assist devices is 120 days. Overall, the mean duration of mechanical support in Berlin Heart patients has been 63 days. Initially, we tried to transplant patients on mechanical assist devices as soon as possible.[8] However, a growing body of literature has demonstrated the benefits of recovery of end organ dysfunction and physical rehabilitation prior to transplantation.[9,10] At our institution, candidacy for transplantation in mechanically supported patients is withheld in the presence of acute loss of consciousness, oliguria or creatinine greater than 1.5 mg/dL, ventilatory dependency, elevated transaminases (>100 international units per liter), or signs of infection.

Results after heart transplantation have improved over the years.[5] A total of 107 patients have undergone transplantation after bridging with the Berlin Heart assist device, and 79 patients (74%) were discharged after transplantation. Of the 28 early deaths, 17 occurred in patients on mechanical support for less than 3 weeks, supporting the importance of complete recovery from cardiogenic shock before transplantation. Long-term survival after transplantation in bridged patients has been no different from those patients undergoing primary heart transplantation.[11]

The duration of support has further increased due to the ongoing shortage of donor organs in our country. Presently, the longest support with a Berlin Heart has been 525 days on biventricular assistance, and 39 patients have been on Berlin Heart support for more than 90 days. This experience has demonstrated the safety and reliability of the Berlin Heart for extended mechanical support. Significant technical failures have not been encountered and several patients have been discharged home on biventricular support for day trips or permanently.

Our anticoagulation regimen during long-term support is based on warfarin (international normalized ratio of 2.5 to 3.5), aspirin (50 mg per day), and dipyridamole (375 mg per day).[5] The extracorporeal pumps are inspected twice a week for evidence of thrombus formation. If clots are detected, the pumps are cleaned or changed immediately. Given this regimen, thromboembolic events have only occurred in patients with severe septic infections (n = 3). We have maintained the same anticoagulation protocol for patients receiving heparin-coated devices.

The cannulae exit sites are routinely inspected by a specially trained nurse. Major manipulations are omitted and dressings are changed under strictly sterile conditions. Infectious complications have recently been prevented by this standardized approach. With device recipients becoming more active and leaving the hospital, we have encountered minor infections at these exit sites during long-term support. This has caused discomfort and limitation of daily activities in some patients.

Pediatric Assist Device

Until recently, no pulsatile pediatric assist devices have been available. Berlin Heart was the first company to offer such a device, with its miniaturized 25, 15, and 12 mL pumps.[12] Some important design changes had to be included in these new devices. For the smaller blood pumps (12 and 15 mL) an optional modification was introduced by interposing an elastic polyurethane reservoir between the atrial cannula and the inflow chamber port, thus remarkably improving chamber filling (Fig. 2).

Until recently, no custom made pediatric cannulae were available for assist device implantation in small children. We have predominantly used conventional heart-lung machine cannulae, which have several disadvantages. One is substantial obstruction of the small aorta, which may result in an unacceptably high afterload for the heart and delay or absence of myocardial recovery. To overcome this problem we were forced to switch our very small patients from pulsatile ventricular assist devices to extracorporeal membrane oxygenation (ECMO) during the weaning process. More recently, specially designed Berlin Heart pediatric cannulae have become available that can be implanted on the surface of the aorta. This cannula has a flat metal tip and a sewing ring at its 85° angled end that resembles a press-button (Fig. 3). The metal tip is inserted into the arterial lumen and enables secure fixation at the arterial wall by means of the sewing ring. This configuration ensures that there will not be any undue resistance to natural heart output.

Because the resistance of the small-bore cannulae is high during pump operation, positive systolic pressures of up to 350 mm Hg and negative diastolic suction pressures of 100 mm Hg at pumping rates of up to 140 bpm are reached. Therefore, the power requirements are considerably higher than those used in adult pump operation.

A drive unit that fulfills these extraordinary specifications is the IKUS 2000. This driver can be operated by external electrical power as well as by internal batteries for up to 2 hours. It is the preferred system for the first period of assisted circulation because of the wide variety of drive modes possible. In larger children, we have preferred the Heimes HD 7 drive unit because it provides greater mobility.[13] It is, however, limited by less driving power.

Of major concern is the construction of an adequate valve for use in pediatric assist devices. In the pediatric Berlin Heart, a newly developed heparin-coated trileaflet polyurethane valve has been incorporated. In our experience, this valve has proved to be highly reliable and has shown very little evidence of thromboembolic complications.

The implantation technique for pediatric support mimics the procedure outlined above. The patients are routinely placed on extracorporeal circulation. In smaller children, cannulae are secured with purse-string sutures (instead of pledgetted mattress sutures) and tourniquets.

All children are kept on intravenous heparin, aiming at activated clotting times between 140 and 160 seconds. Warfarin and antiplatelet agents are not used in pediatric patients.

Between 1990 and 1999, the Berlin Heart assist device was used in 34 children (18 boys and 16 girls) between the ages of 6 days and 16 years (mean 7.5 years).[2] All were in profound heart failure, 25 had been on a respirator for more than 24 hours, all had signs of acute renal failure exhibited by oliguria-anuria with elevated serum creatinine and urea levels. Twenty-one showed laboratory evidence of hepatic damage.

Six patients presented with acute myocarditis and could not be maintained by conservative means. Four children in this subgroup required cardiopulmonary resuscitation prior to assist implantation and were brought to the operating room under continuous chest massage until extracorporeal circulation could be established.

Duration of mechanical support ranged from 12 hours to 114 days with a mean time duration of 17.3 ± 24.2 days. Nineteen were taken off the assist system either after complete cardiac recovery or at the time of transplantation.

Fifteen patients (44%) died from loss of peripheral circulatory resistance unresponsive to α-receptor agonists, multisystem organ damage, sepsis, or from hemorrhagic complications on the assist system.

Fourteen of the 22 (64%) children supported as a bridge to transplantation reached the goal of recovery from shock sequelae and were judged to be transplantable. Two patients died after transplantation from right heart failure due to high pulmonary vascular resistance and two more patients died from graft failure, one of whom was placed on ECMO after transplantation and succumbed to circulatory failure and sepsis. One patient acquired fungal disease and died from sepsis 3 months post transplant. Ten patients were discharged after transplantation. Presently, nine patients are alive between 10 months and 8.5 years after transplantation with good graft function and uneventful clinical courses.

All six patients implanted for postcardiotomy heart failure died after 12 hours to 8 days of mechanical support, all from causes related to the profoundness of the preceding circulatory failure, ie, multiorgan failure with loss of circulatory resistance, brain death, pulmonary failure, and diffuse hemorrhage.

Of the children implanted for acute myocarditis, two who were brought to the operating room under continuous chest massage died from peripheral circulatory failure, one after 2 and one after 16 days of support. One patient received a transplant after 21 days of support and is alive 1.5 years after the procedure. Three children who were also brought to the operating room under cardiopulmonary resuscitation were supplied with a biventricular system with left ventricular drainage, one with a transmitral tipped cannula, the other two with apical cannulation. All the children recovered and displayed a rapid restoration of their cardiac function. Following recovery from myocarditis, the system was exchanged for short-term ECMO support to facilitate weaning. This approach was taken to avoid obstruction of the ascending aorta due to the relatively large cannulae during the weaning process. The three children have since made an excellent recovery and are fully active with normal heart function after 4 years.

There was no instance of technical failure of the blood pump components or of the drive system. Recovery of end organ function was quite variable. Thirteen of the pediatric patients on the assist system could be taken off the respirator and were mobilized. Out of this group, 11 were transplanted or successfully weaned.

Conclusion

The Berlin Heart assist device has proved to be a highly reliable ventricular support device that addresses a broad variety of patients and clinical conditions. The experience with adult long-term support as well as pediatric assistance has been extremely encouraging. Patients are discharged home and several have now spent far more than 1 year on the biventricular assist device. Fortunately, technical as well as thromboembolic complications have been extremely rare.

The major disadvantage lies in the need for a rather bulky driving unit which limits patient mobility and independence. A new wearable driving unit will address this issue and thereby extend the applicability of the Berlin Heart.

References

1. Hetzer R, Hennig E, Schiessler A, et al. Mechanical support and heart transplantation. *J Heart Lung Transplant* 1992;11:175–181.

2. Hetzer R, Loebe M, Potapov EV, et al. Circulatory support with pneumatic paracorporeal ventricular assist device in infants and children. *Ann Thorac Surg* 1998;66:1498–1506.
3. Kaufmann F, Hennig E, Loebe M, Hetzer R. Improving the antithrombogenicity of artificial surfaces through heparin coating–clinical experience with the pneumatic extracorporeal Berlin Heart assist device. *J Anästhesie Intensivbeh* 1997;4:56–60.
4. Kaufmann F, Hennig E, Weng Y, Hetzer R. Miniaturisierte Blutpumpen für die Kinderherzchirurgie. *Kardiotechnik* 1995;1:7–12.
5. Loebe M, Hennig E, Müller J, et al. Long-term mechanical circulatory support as a bridge to transplantation, for recovery from cardiomyopathy and for permanent replacement. *Eur J Cardiothorac Surg* 1997;11:S11-S24.
6. Pasic M, Bergs S, Hennig E, et al. Simplified technique for implantation of a left ventricular assist system after previous cardiac operations. *Ann Thorac Surg* 1999;67:562–564.
7. Wagner F, Dandel M, Günther G, et al. Nitric oxide in the treatment of right ventricular dysfunction following left ventricular assist device implantation. *Circulation* 1997;96(suppl II):II291-II296.
8. Schiessler A, Friedel N, Weng Y, et al. Mechanical circulatory support and heart transplantation. *ASAIO J* 1994;40:M476-M481.
9. Friedel N, Viazis P, Schiessler A, et al. Recovery of end-organ failure during mechanical circulatory support. *Eur J Cardiothorac Surg* 1992;6:519–523.
10. Ashton RC, Goldstein DJ, Rose EA, et al. Duration of LVAD support affects transplant survival. *J Heart Lung Transplant* 1996;15:1151–1157.
11. Hetzer R, Albert W, Hummel M, et al. Status of patients presently living 9 to 13 years after orthotopic heart transplantation. *Ann Thorac Surg* 1997;64:1661–1668.
12. Ishino K, Loebe M, Uhlemann F, et al. Circulatory support with paracorporeal pneumatic ventricular assist device (VAD) in infants and children. *Eur J Cardiothorac Surg* 1997;11:965–972.
13. Warnecke H, Berdijs F, Hennig E, et al. Mechanical left ventricular support as bridge to cardiac transplantation in childhood. *Eur J Cardiothorac Surg* 1991;5:330–333.

Part II

Available Devices:
B. Intracorporeal Devices

Chapter 22

Intracorporeal Support:

The Intra-aortic Balloon Pump

David N. Helman, MD and Gus J. Vlahakes, MD

Introduction

The intra-aortic balloon pump (IABP) is a mechanical cardiac assist device that was developed in the late 1960s and is used presently to support approximately 100,000 patients annually.[1] Intra-aortic counterpulsation lies at the less complicated, less invasive end of the spectrum of available cardiac assist strategies described in this book; these include extracorporeal membrane oxygenation, ventricular assist devices, and total artificial hearts. The balloon pump has obvious advantages over other mechanical assist devices in terms of ease and rapidity of insertion and removal, but it does not have the capability to provide the level of support of a ventricular assist device or total artificial heart. Another major factor in the utility and popularity of the IABP is that it does not require insertion via a surgical approach and thus may be placed as a means of hemodynamic and/or ischemia stabilization in patients with acute cardiac decompensation, to permit transfer from a facility without cardiac surgical facilities to a tertiary care center.

The IABP, due to these advantages, is the most common cardiac assist device system used today. Prior to surgery, intra-aortic counterpulsation is most frequently used in the settings of cardiogenic shock or ongoing myocardial ischemia refractory to medical therapy, and is also used to provide support during high-risk percutaneous coronary angioplasty. After surgery, the IABP is used in patients who cannot be weaned from cardiopulmonary bypass with the aid of optimized pacing and maximal pharmacologic inotropic support. Finally, balloon pumps are an important means of hemodynamic support in the postoperative period following cardiac surgical procedures for patients with low cardiac output states or persistent ischemia.

From Goldstein DJ and Oz MC (eds). *Cardiac Assist Devices*. Armonk, NY: Futura Publishing Co., Inc.; ©2000.

Development of the IABP

The two principles underlying intra-aortic balloon support, namely diastolic coronary blood flow augmentation and aortic counterpulsation, were first proposed in the 1950s and early 1960s.[2,3] In 1962, Moulopoulos et al[4] reported the use of a latex balloon placed in the descending thoracic aorta that was inflated during diastole and deflated during systole. Experimental studies of the IABP in a canine model were described in 1967 by Schilt et al.[5] Powell and associates[6] found that the IABP increased coronary artery blood flow. Building on laboratory investigations by multiple groups, the first use of the IABP in patients with cardiogenic shock secondary to myocardial infarction was reported by Kantrowitz et al[7] in 1968. In 1973, Buckley and colleagues[8] reported the use of intra-aortic balloon pumping to support patients who could not be weaned from cardiopulmonary bypass. Subsequently, the IABP has undergone technical refinement to the point where it now is the most commonly used mechanical cardiac assist device.

Initially, IABPs were placed surgically either via an open approach to the common femoral artery or directly into the ascending aorta through a median sternotomy. The availability of simple percutaneous systems for IABP placement[9–11] resulted in the widespread use of this technology, with placement now routine in the intensive care unit or cardiac catheterization suite.

There are presently several manufacturers that produce IABP systems in the United States; these include Datascope Corp. (Fairfield, NJ), Arrow International Inc. (Reading PA), and Bard Inc. (Haverhill, MA). The typical IABP is driven from a console with helium as the shuttle gas and with a standard balloon inflation volume of 40 mL for adults. Balloon pumps for smaller adults and pediatric patients are available in smaller sizes. A typical intra-aortic balloon and drive console are shown in Figure 1, panels A and B, respectively.

Physiology of IABP Support

The IABP operates on the principle of intra-aortic counterpulsation. The salutary effects of balloon pumping in the setting of myocardial ischemia or cardiogenic shock are realized in both the systolic and diastolic phases of the cardiac cycle. The balloon, which is positioned in the descending thoracic aorta with its tip just distal to the left subclavian artery, deflates just prior to the beginning of the systolic phase of the cardiac cycle and inflates during the diastolic phase of the cardiac cycle.

By deflating in the aorta immediately prior to the ejection of blood from the left ventricle, the IABP functions to reduce afterload, thereby decreasing left ventricular work and myocardial oxygen consumption. In diastole, the balloon inflates and increases diastolic pressure, resulting in augmented perfusion of the coronary arteries.[6] Coronary artery blood flow during IABP support has been measured in patients by use of transesophageal echocardiography; in one study, peak diastolic coronary flow velocity increased by a mean of 117%, with an increase in mean flow velocity integral of 87%.[12] Moreover, blood flow velocities of 1.5 to 2 times baseline have been measured in the stenosed left anterior descending coronary arteries of patients supported by balloon pumps.[13]

A number of factors determine the effectiveness of balloon pumping, including balloon volume, location in the aorta, rate of inflation and deflation, and timing relative to the events during the cardiac cycle.[14] The latter appears to be the most

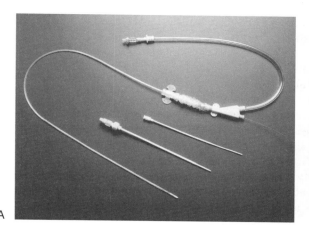

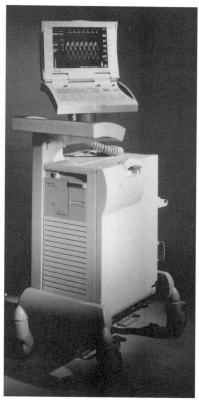

A

B

FIGURE 1. A. Intra-aortic balloon pump catheter. B. Drive console. Courtesy of Datascope, Inc.

important factor for determining the effectiveness of the balloon pump. The optimal inflation/deflation timing has been shown to be with inflation slightly proceeding the dicrotic notch and deflation bordering on isovolumetric systole.[15] Modern IABP controllers have been designed to optimize this timing, not only in the setting of sinus rhythm, but also in the presence of cardiac arrhythmias.

Intra-aortic counterpulsation does not augment cardiac output in the setting of heart failure in the way that a left ventricular assist device augments forward flow. Instead, the IABP provides assistance with its ability to decrease myocardial oxygen consumption by reducing afterload, as well as increasing coronary artery perfusion by augmenting diastolic coronary artery flow. These characteristics make the IABP particularly suited for supporting the patient with myocardial ischemia. In the setting of nonischemic heart failure (ie, dilated cardiomyopathy), the benefits of unloading the left ventricle are still realized even though the augmented coronary flow may not be as valuable as in the setting of ischemia.[16]

The interaction between the IABP and the right ventricle has been investigated. Darrah et al[17] studied the effect of IABP in an experimental model of right heart failure, and found a significant improvement in cardiac function. The authors attributed the improvement to increased left ventricular coronary perfusion with a salutary effect on right ventricular performance realized through a ventricular interdependence mechanism. A clinical case has appeared in the literature, describing the occurrence of right ventricular failure following coronary artery bypass grafting where an IABP facilitated weaning from cardiopulmonary bypass.[18] The authors surmised that right ventricular performance was enhanced by the IABP due to augmented coronary perfusion to a region of myocardium that had possibly been inadequately protected by cardioplegia.

Perfusion to organs other than the heart is also affected by intra-aortic balloon pumping. Reports of altered mental status in patients undergoing intra-aortic counterpulsation have focused attention on studies of the effect of the IABP on cerebral perfusion.[19] Flow reversal in the cerebral arteries in late diastole has been demonstrated in patients on IABPs.[20] Despite the documented reversal of cerebral flow, there were no evident neurologic signs or symptoms and, thus, this flow phenomenon may be of little clinical significance.

Applebaum et al[21] also investigated cerebral blood flow during balloon counterpulsation. These authors found that there was an increase in antegrade carotid flow during diastole but that there was no net increase in flow due to reversal of flow in early systole. Their explanation for this phenomenon was that balloon deflation is typically set to occur on the R wave of the electrocardiogram cycle. They point out, however, that isovolumetric contraction, which begins at approximately the peak of the R wave, has a duration of 40 to 80 milliseconds in healthy patients. The authors state that the duration of isovolumetric contraction can be significantly increased in patients with severe left ventricular dysfunction, to the point where the balloon may deflate prior to ejection of blood into the aorta from the left ventricle. This premature balloon deflation is responsible for the reversal of flow from the cerebral arteries into the aorta.[21]

A situation in which the effect of the IABP on cerebral blood flow is relevant involves the determination of brain death. It has been demonstrated that the IABP may interfere with brain death determination by transcranial Doppler ultrasound measurement; therefore, it may be necessary to discontinue balloon pumping during these measurements.[22]

Indications for IABP Use

The IABP is used in the treatment of patients with myocardial ischemia or hemodynamic instability in the preoperative, intraoperative, and postoperative settings.

Preoperative Placement

Five percent to 10% of patients hospitalized with acute myocardial infarctions will develop cardiogenic shock.[23] In this cohort of patients, as well as those hospitalized patients that exhibit ongoing myocardial ischemia refractory to medical therapy, the IABP is the support device of choice and is often placed by the cardiologist at the time of cardiac catheterization.

At the Massachusetts General Hospital (MGH), between 1980 and 1995, 12.3% of 17,678 patients undergoing cardiac surgery were supported with an IABP perioperatively.[24] Notably, 70.6% had the IABP placed before surgery. This is in contrast to two other large IABP series in which 18.4%[25] and 35.7%[26] of perioperative IABPs were placed preoperatively. Preoperative IABP placement allows for stabilization of the patient with an acute coronary syndrome prior to proceeding to the operating room for revascularization. A study of 163 consecutive patients with ejection fractions

≤25% who were undergoing coronary artery bypass grafting was undertaken to investigate the effects of preoperative IABP placement.[27] This study found that the 30-day mortality in patients with preoperative IABP placement was 2.7% compared with 11.9% for patients not having a preoperative IABP. These findings argue for liberal use of preoperative IABPs in patients with poor heart function coming to cardiac surgery.

Intraoperative Placement

The IABP is used intraoperatively when weaning from cardiopulmonary bypass is not possible despite pacing and maximal pharmacologic inotropic support. In this setting, the balloon is inserted with the goal of obtaining hemodynamic support that will allow for recovery of native myocardial function postoperatively. The decision to place an IABP while in the operating room is often based on fairly subjective criteria and trends rather than a fixed algorithm. Factors that are considered include anticipated difficulty of balloon pump insertion and the clinical trend in terms of gradual improvement versus gradual deterioration in the operating room.

Postoperative Placement

IABPs are valuable in the postoperative period in situations in which a low cardiac output state is present. In several large clinical series, postoperative IABP placement has been reported to be much less frequent than either preoperative or intraoperative insertion.[24-26] In the postoperative setting, simultaneous evaluation for causes of hemodynamic deterioration (eg, cardiac tamponade) is essential.

IABP Placement

When the IABP was first introduced, it was placed through an open approach to the common femoral artery with the tip of the balloon positioned in the descending thoracic aorta just distal to the left subclavian artery. A prosthetic graft was anastomosed to the common femoral artery, through which the balloon was inserted. A technique for avoiding possible infectious complications associated with prosthetic material involves constructing a tube to the common femoral artery with a piece of pericardium.[28] These techniques for the surgical approach to the common femoral artery, however, are no longer in use.

The development of a percutaneous approach to IABP insertion was an important milestone in the history of intra-aortic counterpulsation that allowed for its widespread use by nonsurgeons.[9-11] A randomized trial of percutaneous versus surgical IABP insertion found that both methods had similar insertion success rates.[29] During the period from 1991 to 1995 at the MGH, 96.5% of all IABPs were placed percutaneously.[24]

While percutaneous placement is preferable, on occasion it is necessary to place the balloon directly into the ascending aorta in the operating room in patients in whom atherosclerotic disease or extreme tortuosity of the aortoiliac system does not allow passage of the balloon catheter from the femoral vessels.[30,31] Transthoracic IABP placement initially required balloon removal with an open chest, but subsequent balloon removal techniques under local anesthesia with the chest closed have been described.[32]

Nunez et al[33] described a technique, prior to the introduction of percutaneous balloon catheters, for use in the setting of an aorta that is too crowded to apply a partial occlusion clamp. The approach involved the sewing of a prosthetic graft to the aorta with partial thickness sutures placed only into the aortic media. The aortotomy for balloon insertion was then made through the lumen of the graft. The graft with the balloon catheter was then brought out of the chest through the right second intercostal space.

With the advent of the percutaneous balloon pump catheter, it became possible to insert the device directly into the ascending aorta with the chest open in the operating room without the use of a prosthetic graft as an introducer.[34] To minimize the risk of embolization of thrombus that may have formed around the catheter, the innominate and left common carotid arteries are occluded for approximately 10 seconds while the catheter is removed.[34] Alternatively, temporary manual compression of the carotid arteries can be performed by the anesthesiologist at the time of balloon removal.

A strategy that can greatly facilitate the placement of an IABP via the common femoral artery in the high-risk patient that cannot be weaned from cardiopulmonary bypass is the preoperative placement of a femoral arterial monitoring line. This is easily accomplished prior to starting cardiopulmonary bypass when the femoral arterial pulse is palpable, rather than attempting to locate the common femoral artery while on cardiopulmonary bypass. The line provides subsequent guidewire access for an insertion sheath and IABP placement.

It is of utmost importance to insert the IABP into the common femoral artery rather than one of its branches. Puncture of either the superficial femoral artery or the profunda femoris artery leads to a high incidence of complications. The percutaneous balloon pump inserted in the groin should penetrate the common femoral artery just at the inguinal ligament. In some patients, the common femoral artery may be short, and there may be little room for error.

An important consideration that must be evaluated prior to inserting a balloon pump in the groin relates to a history of previous prosthetic grafts to the common femoral artery. The primary concern about puncturing a prosthetic graft is the risk of introducing infection. Shahian and Jewell[35] reported balloon pump placement through a 6 mm polytetrafluoroethylene (PTFE) sidearm graft anastomosed to an aortobifemoral graft. IABP removal was accomplished by excision of excess sidearm graft and oversewing. More recently, LaMuraglia and colleagues[36] reported their experience at the MGH with percutaneous IABP insertion in the setting of aortofemoral or aortoiliac prosthetic grafts. The authors recommend that a careful physical examination be performed prior to insertion to rule out an anastomotic false aneurysm. With a "mature" aortofemoral graft and in the absence of an aneurysm, the authors concluded that percutaneous insertion is acceptable. In this study, patients considered to have a mature graft were those greater than 2 years out from placement, although a strict cutoff was not defined. The authors recommended that patients with immature aortofemoral grafts should undergo surgical IABP placement. In the patient with an aortoiliac graft, either percutaneous or surgical approaches were acceptable; however, fluoroscopy should be used to minimize an injury at the anasto-moses. Fluoroscopy may be particularly useful in patients who have a side-to-end proximal aortic graft anastomosis; knowledge of the operative details of the original vascular operation or distal aortography may be helpful.

A number of reports of IABP insertion through sites other than the common femoral arteries or the ascending aorta have been presented in the literature. The insertion of the balloon catheter into the subclavian artery when the femoral approach is not feasible has been reported.[37,38] One subclavian artery placement technique involves IABP insertion through an 8 mm PTFE graft anastomosed to the left subcla-vian artery under local anesthesia.[38]

IABP insertion via the right or left axillary arteries has been described as a means of providing improved patient mobility with the device in place.[39] This insertion technique involves a transverse infraclavicular incision from the deltopectoral groove to the mid clavicle. The pectoralis major muscle is split in the direction of its fibers and the clavipectoral fascia is divided to expose the axillary artery and brachial plexus. Device removal is performed in the operating room.

An alternative insertion technique that was devised to allow increased patient mobility is the suprainguinal insertion of the IABP under local anesthesia.[40] The IABP is placed through a PTFE sheath in the external iliac artery with a skin exit site adjacent to the anterior superior iliac spine. This group has reported IABP support durations up to 86 days with this particular placement technique that allows patients to ambulate.

Anticoagulation During Balloon Pumping

In general, when the balloon pump is used preoperatively, intravenous heparin is mandated not only by the presence of the balloon and introducer sheath, but also by the nature of the patient's underlying heart disease, which is generally ischemic. In patients who have IABPs placed for heart failure, anticoagulation is also used, and the degree of anticoagulation is generally dictated by the degree of heart disease. With regard to the IABP system, anticoagulation is used primarily to prevent throm-bosis in the artery where the balloon has been inserted and, to a lesser extent, to prevent thromboemboli from the balloon itself.

Patients who leave the operating room with an IABP in place after having under-gone conventional cardiopulmonary bypass are not maintained on heparin, but are given intravenous low molecular weight dextran at a rate of 20 mL/h that is initiated after chest tube output rates have decreased to acceptable rates. In the small subset of patients that may require extended postoperative IABP support, consideration might be given to changing over from low molecular weight dextran to heparin after 4 or 5 days. Because of the risk of anaphylaxis, it is recommended that a small test dose of dextran be given prior to initiation of full strength low molecular weight dextran.

IABP Timing: Synchronization with the Cardiac Cycle

IABP timing is based on the relationship of balloon inflation and deflation to the dicrotic notch of the cardiac cycle.[41] The IABP should be synchronized so that

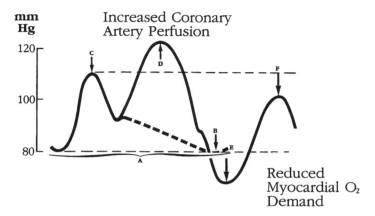

FIGURE 2. Arterial pressure waveform with correct intra-aortic balloon pump timing. Courtesy of Datascope, Inc. A = one complete cardiac cycle; B = unassisted aortic end-diastolic pressure; C = unassisted systolic pressure; D = diastolic augmentation; E = reduced aortic end-diastolic pressure; F = reduced systolic pressure.

it deflates at the onset of systole and inflates in diastole. This provides the desired effects of reducing afterload during systole while enhancing coronary artery flow during diastole. The guide to analyzing the correct synchronization of the balloon pump to the cardiac cycle is the arterial pressure waveform. Figure 2 shows an example of an arterial pressure tracing with correct balloon pump timing. Correct timing is confirmed by observation of augmentation of the diastolic pressure, reduction of pressure immediately prior to ejection, and attainment of a peak diastolic pressure that is greater than the peak systolic pressure.

There are three potential sources of a balloon pump synchronization signal: 1) R wave sensing from an electrocardiogram; 2) arterial pulse detection from by an arterial tracing; and 3) R wave sensing of implanted atrial and/or ventricular pacing wires. The detection of the R wave initiates balloon deflation such that the balloon will be fully deflated during mechanical systole.

Electrical noise in the operating room from the surgical cautery system can cause interference with balloon pump timing and makes the use of alternative, nonelectrical sources of sensing important. We have used a system that employs photoelectric detectors placed over the pacemaker light-emitting diodes. This system allows for balloon pump timing based on the atrial and ventricular pacing light-emitting diodes, as well as the sense light-emitting diode, while accomplishing filtration of electrical noise.

Arrhythmias increase the complexity of the timing of inflation and deflation of the intra-aortic balloon, but can be overcome by modern electronic control techniques. In the setting of a tachyarrhythmia, the balloon pump may be set at a 1:2 ratio instead of 1:1 ratio, resulting in every-other-beat augmentation.

IABP Weaning and Removal

The removal technique for percutaneously placed IABPs in the common femoral artery involves withdrawal of the device and application of manual pressure over the insertion site for at least 30 minutes. Recent advances in catheter technology may allow sealing of the arterial entrance site of the balloon catheter as the device is removed. Following removal, monitoring of distal perfusion of the leg is performed by manual or Doppler pulse examination intermittently over 48 hours. In addition, the patient is not allowed to ambulate for 48 hours following IABP removal, to ensure good sealing of the insertion site. The site is monitored for bleeding, as well as for the possible formation of a retroperitoneal hematoma or false aneurysm.

Prior to removing the balloon catheter, it is necessary to determine that the patient will tolerate its removal from a hemodynamic standpoint. Different weaning protocols have been applied in this regard. One such protocol dictates that the pump be switched from a 1:1 augmentation frequency to 1:2, then to 1:4, and finally to 1:8 as tolerated while following the patient's hemodynamic parameters. The duration of time spent in the 1:4 and the 1:8 modes should be minimized, as there is an increased risk of thrombosis on the balloon surface in these modes, in which inflation and deflation occur less frequently. Once hemodynamic stability is ensured, the IABP should be placed back in the 1:2 mode to lower the likelihood of thrombosis until it can be removed.

If heparin is being administered, it should be discontinued with sufficient time prior to IABP removal in order to permit normalization of the partial thromboplastin time. In general, coagulation function should be normal prior to balloon removal, with a platelet count greater than $50,000/mm^3$ and prothrombin time not exceeding 15 seconds.

Results of IABP Support in Cardiac Surgical Patients

Torchiana et al[24] reported an analysis of 2175 perioperative IABP placements at MGH from 1980 to 1995 that revealed a mortality rate of 16.3%. Two other large series of patients undergoing cardiac surgical procedures with perioperative IABP support have reported mortality rates of 28.7%[26] and 44.0%.[25] In the MGH series, multivariate predictors of death in medical and surgical patients receiving IABPs included insertion in the operating room or intensive care unit, transthoracic insertion, advanced age, procedures other than coronary artery bypass grafting or percutaneous transluminal coronary angioplasty, and insertion for cardiogenic shock.[24] In this series, predictors of death with intraoperative IABP placement were age, mitral valve replacement, prolonged cardiopulmonary bypass, urgent or emergent operation, preoperative renal dysfunction (creatinine >1.5 mg/dL), complex ventricular ectopy, right ventricular failure, and emergency resumption of cardiopulmonary bypass.

A report from St. Louis University Medical Center identified the following independent predictors of mortality in cardiac surgical patients supported with IABPs: preoperative New York Heart Association class, transthoracic IABP insertion, use of preoperative intravenous nitroglycerin, age, female gender, and preoperative IABP insertion.[25]

Baldwin et al[42] developed a model for predicting postcardiotomy IABP survival by studying 322 patients who required IABP support to be weaned from cardiopulmonary bypass. The overall mortality rate in their series was 48.4%. They identified the following variables that, if present before or within 10 minutes of the first attempt at weaning from cardiopulmonary bypass, were predictive of mortality: 1) complete heart block (need for pacing at weaning); 2) advanced age; 3) elevated preoperative blood urea nitrogen; and 4) female gender.

Christenson et al[43] reported a 47.9% mortality rate among 169 patients undergoing IABP placement for postcardiotomy heart failure. They identified preoperative myocardial ischemia and combined cardiac surgical procedures as risk factors for perioperative mortality.

Complications of IABP Use

Vascular Complications

Vascular complications represent the most frequent serious morbidity associated with IABP placement and use, with reported complication rates for percutaneous IABPs ranging from 9% to 36%.[44] The most common insertion site for the balloon is the common femoral artery, which can be associated with peripheral ischemia secondary to vascular occlusion, thrombosis, or embolism. Shahian et al[45] have pointed out the importance of cannulating the common femoral and not the superficial femoral artery in order to minimize vascular complications. Factors associated with higher rates of lower extremity ischemia include female gender, diabetes mellitus, and preexisting peripheral vascular disease.[46]

Injury to the aorta, such as the development of an intramural hematoma, has been reported with the use of balloon pumps.[47] An autopsy study performed on 45 patients expiring after balloon counterpulsation found a total of 19 vascular complications, including dissection of the aorta or its distal branches, arterial perforation, arterial thrombi, arterial emboli, and limb ischemia, although only four of these complications were suspected prior to the patients' deaths.[48]

In addition to vascular injury, arterial occlusion has been reported in association with IABP use. A case of occlusion of the left internal mammary artery caused by malpositioning of the tip of the balloon in the left subclavian artery has been reported.[49] Lower-body ischemia has been found to result from sustained intra-aortic balloon inflation that was believed to have resulted from kinking of the balloon.[50] The balloon could not be deflated, and its puncture with a guidewire was needed to allow for removal.

The question arises as to how patients do in the long term following the need for IABP use. A prospective trial found that ipsilateral lower limb ischemia occurred in 18% of patients 12 to 20 months following IABP use.[51] The patients at greatest risk for long-term ischemic complications were those with the following characteristics: 1) occurrence of acute limb ischemia; 2) cardiogenic shock as the indication for IABP use; and 3) history of smoking.

With the knowledge that peripheral vascular complications are not infrequent as a result of IABP use, careful monitoring of lower extremity perfusion is required. Several options exist in the case in which peripheral ischemia is present. Of course, if hemodynamically tolerated, the IABP can be removed. In the setting in which the balloon pump is required for continuing support in the presence of peripheral ischemia, an IABP can be placed on the contralateral side immediately following the removal of the original IABP. Thrombectomy and repair of the arterial puncture site with a vein patch may be required. Another therapeutic option is placement of a prosthetic femoral-femoral bypass graft to relieve limb ischemia.[52,53]

Intra-abdominal Complications

In addition to complications of ischemia involving the peripheral vasculature in the setting of IABP use, complications involving the intra-abdominal organs have been reported. It is not difficult to envision the disruption of atheromatous material in the aorta during IABP insertion and pumping. Allen et al[54] analyzed their experience with patients undergoing cardiopulmonary bypass and found that the IABP use was one of the risk factors associated with the development of mesenteric ischemia following cardiac surgery.

A case of a small bowel infarction secondary to occlusion of the superior mesenteric artery by the balloon tip in the setting of IABP placement via the ascending aorta has been reported.[55] Acute pancreatitis temporally related to IABP placement has been described and is thought to result from atheroemboli or compromise of pancreatic blood flow due to IABP insertion.[56]

Splenic infarction necessitating splenectomy following IABP insertion has been reported.[57] Analysis of this pathology specimen revealed infarction secondary to cholesterol emboli to the splenic vessels.

Neurologic Complications

Neurologic complications of IABP support are much less frequent than vascular complications, but they do occur. Cases of paraplegia associated with IABP use have been reported.[58–66] The mechanisms proposed to account for these complications include spinal cord infarction secondary to aortic dissection or adventitial hematoma and occlusion of the artery of Adamkiewicz with plaque emboli.[64]

Stroke has been reported following balloon rupture with cerebral helium embolization, although this occurrence is very rare.[67,68] Hyperbaric oxygen therapy has been found to minimize the severity of the resultant neurologic deficit.[67]

Balloon Rupture

Balloon rupture is a phenomenon that has been reported and attributed to calcified aortic plaques causing abrasive destruction of the balloon.[69–75] Balloon rupture is heralded by the appearance of blood in the catheter and has been reported in 0.5% to 6% of patients.[1] Nishida et al[73] reported an overall balloon rupture rate of 1.7% in 2803 patients supported with balloons from five manufacturers. It has been suggested that reducing the balloon size used in smaller patients may minimize the likelihood of balloon rupture.[71] The reported sequelae of balloon rupture include helium embolization, as mentioned above, infection, and hemodynamic instability.[76] Balloon rupture has also been reported to cause balloon entrapment, which results from leakage of blood into the balloon and clot formation that blocks complete balloon deflation.[77] In one study, surgical removal was required in 10 of 11 patients with balloon entrapment caused by clot formation inside the catheter.[73] It has been suggested that using intraluminal streptokinase with heparinized saline flushing to dissolve clot and allow balloon removal may be an alternative to surgical removal.[78] However, the argument has been made that the lumen of the balloon is not sterile and the instillation of streptokinase and heparinized saline might cause intra-arterial injection of nonsterile contents through the perforation in the balloon.[79]

Infectious Complications

Infectious complications are quite rare with percutaneous IABP placement. The rate of infection in over 3000 percutaneously inserted balloons at MGH was reported as 0.1%, while in approximately 1500 surgically placed balloons, the rate of infection was 1.4%.[24]

IABP Support in Pediatric Patients

Long-term left ventricular assist devices are not yet widely available for smaller adult and pediatric patients with body surface area less than 1.5 m^2. For this reason, IABPs are important devices for the support of pediatric patients with heart failure. IABP use in children has been reported by some centers.[80–82] One factor that makes IABP use less effective in children than adults is the elasticity of the pediatric aorta.[80] Balloon insertion in pediatric patients via the external iliac artery has been reported by del Nido et al[83] as a means of minimizing the risk of limb ischemia.

Conclusion

The IABP, developed over 30 years ago, has become the most frequently used mechanical cardiac assist device. The ability to insert the balloon pump percutaneously has broadened its application from the initial designs that required surgical placement. The IABP now plays an important role in the support of the cardiac surgical patient from the preoperative to the postoperative period. Thresholds for balloon pump insertion vary between institutions and among individual surgeons, and take into account risks versus benefits of support. Aggressive balloon pump placement strategies preoperatively have been shown to reduce perioperative mortality in patients undergoing cardiac surgery. Prophylactic balloon pump placement in high-risk patients who are anticipated to require support in the perioperative period may improve outcomes.

Vascular complications remain the major morbidity of femoral balloon pump insertion, and careful attention to lower extremity perfusion is required. Complication rates should continue to decrease as advances in catheter technology are realized.

As the field of mechanical cardiac assist devices continues to advance, it is likely that the IABP will continue to maintain an important role due to its ease of insertion and its capacity to unload the left ventricle while augmenting coronary blood flow.

References

1. Bolooki H. *Clinical Application of the Intra-Aortic Balloon Pump.* 3rd ed. Armonk, NY: Futura Publishing Company, Inc.; 1998.
2. Kantrowitz A. Experimental augmentation of coronary flow by retardation of the arterial pressure pulse. *Surgery* 1953;34:678–687.
3. Clauss RH, Birtwell WC, Albertal G, et al. Assisted circulation. I. The arterial counterpulsator. *J Thorac Cardiovasc Surg* 1961;41:447–458.
4. Moulopoulos SD, Topaz O, Kolff WJ. Diastolic balloon pumping (with carbon dioxide) in the aorta. A mechanical assistance to the failing circulation. *Am Heart J* 1962;63:669–675.
5. Schilt W, Freed PS, Khalil G, Kantrowitz A. Temporary non-surgical intraarterial cardiac assistance. *Trans Am Soc Artif Intern Organs* 1967;13:322–327.
6. Powell WJJ, Daggett WM, Magro AE, et al. Effects of intra-aortic balloon counterpulsation on cardiac performance, oxygen consumption, and coronary blood flow in dogs. *Circ Res* 1970;26:753–764.
7. Kantrowitz A, Tjonneland S, Freed PS, et al. Initial clinical experience with intraaortic balloon pumping in cardiogenic shock. *JAMA* 1968;203:113–118.
8. Buckley MJ, Craver JM, Gold HK, et al. Intra-aortic balloon pump assist for cardiogenic shock after cardiopulmonary bypass. *Circulation* 1973;48(1 suppl):III90-III94.
9. Subramanian VA, Goldstein JE, Sos TA, et al. Preliminary clinical experience with percutaneous intraaortic balloon pumping. *Circulation* 1980;62:I123-I129.
10. Bregman D, Nichols AB, Weiss MB, et al. Percutaneous intraaortic balloon insertion. *Am J Cardiol* 1980;46:261–264.
11. Leinbach RC, Goldstein J, Gold HK, et al. Percutaneous wire-guided balloon pumping. *Am J Cardiol* 1982;49:1707–1710.
12. Katz ES, Tunick PA, Kronzon I. Observations of coronary flow augmentation and balloon function during intraaortic balloon counterpulsation using transesophageal echocardiography. *Am J Cardiol* 1992;69:1635–639.
13. Hutchison SJ, Thaker KB, Chandraratna PA. Effects of intraaortic balloon counterpulsation on flow velocity in stenotic left main coronary arteries from transesophageal echocardiography. *Am J Cardiol* 1994;74:1063–1065.
14. Barnea O, Moore TW, Dubin SE, Jaron D. Cardiac energy considerations during intraaortic balloon pumping. *IEEE Trans Biomed Eng* 1990;37:170–181.
15. Zelano JA, Li JK, Welkowitz W. A closed-loop control scheme for intraaortic balloon pumping. *IEEE Trans Biomed Eng* 1990;37:182–192.
16. Rosenbaum AM, Murali S, Uretsky BF. Intra-aortic balloon counterpulsation as a 'bridge' to cardiac transplantation. Effects in nonischemic and ischemic cardiomyopathy. *Chest* 1994;106:1683–1688.
17. Darrah WC, Sharpe MD, Guiraudon GM, Neal A. Intraaortic balloon counterpulsation improves right ventricular failure resulting from pressure overload. *Ann Thorac Surg* 1997;64:1718–1723.
18. Kopman EA, Ramirez-Inawat RC. Intra-aortic balloon counterpulsation for right heart failure. *Anesth Analg* 1980;59:74–76.
19. Sanders KM, Stern TA, O'Gara PT, et al. Delirium during intra-aortic balloon pump therapy. Incidence and management. *Psychosomatics* 1992;33:35–44.
20. Brass LM. Reversed intracranial blood flow in patients with an intra-aortic balloon pump. *Stroke* 1990;21:484–487.
21. Applebaum RM, Wun HH, Katz ES, et al. Effects of intraaortic balloon counterpulsation on carotid artery blood flow. *Am Heart J* 1998;135:850–854.
22. van der Naalt J, Baker AJ. Influence of the intra-aortic balloon pump on the transcranial Doppler flow pattern in a brain-dead patient. *Stroke* 1996;27:140–142.
23. Mueller HS. Role of intra-aortic counterpulsation in cardiogenic shock and acute myocardial infarction. *Cardiology* 1994;84:168–174.
24. Torchiana DF, Hirsch G, Buckley MJ, et al. Intraaortic balloon pumping for cardiac support: Trends in practice and outcome, 1968 to 1995. *J Thorac Cardiovasc Surg* 1997;113:758–764.
25. Naunheim KS, Swartz MT, Pennington DG, et al. Intraaortic balloon pumping in patients requiring cardiac operations. Risk analysis and long-term follow-up. *J Thorac Cardiovasc Surg* 1992;104:1654–1660.

26. Creswell LL, Rosenbloom M, Cox JL, et al. Intraaortic balloon counterpulsation: Patterns of usage and outcome in cardiac surgery patients. *Ann Thorac Surg* 1992;54:11–18.

27. Dietl CA, Berkheimer MD, Woods EL, et al. Efficacy and cost-effectiveness of preoperative IABP in patients with ejection fraction of 0.25 or less. *Ann Thorac Surg* 1996;62:401–408.

28. Zapolanski A, Weisel RD, Goldman BS, et al. Pericardial graft for intraoperative balloon pump insertion. *Ann Thorac Surg* 1982;33:516–517.

29. Goldberg MJ, Rubenfire M, Kantrowitz A, et al. Intraaortic balloon pump insertion: A randomized study comparing percutaneous and surgical techniques. *J Am Coll Cardiol* 1987;9:515–523.

30. Gueldner TL, Lawrence GH. Intraaortic balloon assist through cannulation of the ascending aorta. *Ann Thorac Surg* 1975;19:88–91.

31. Shirkey AL, Loughridge BP, Lain KC. Insertion of the intraaortic balloon through the aortic arch. *Ann Thorac Surg* 1976;21:560–561.

32. Salerno TA. Insertion of the intra-aortic balloon through the ascending aorta and its removal under local anesthesia. *Can J Surg* 1983;26:69.

33. Nunez L, Aguado MG, Iglesias A, Larrea JL. Transaortic cannulation for balloon pumping in a "crowded aorta." *Ann Thorac Surg* 1980;30:400–402.

34. Bonchek LI, Olinger GN. Direct ascending aortic insertion of the "percutaneous" intraaortic balloon catheter in the open chest: Advantages and precautions. *Ann Thorac Surg* 1981; 32:512–514.

35. Shahian DM, Jewell ER. Intraaortic balloon pump placement through Dacron aortofemoral grafts. *J Vasc Surg* 1988;7:795–797.

36. LaMuraglia GM, Vlahakes GJ, Moncure AC, et al. The safety of intraaortic balloon pump catheter insertion through suprainguinal prosthetic vascular bypass grafts. *J Vasc Surg* 1991;13:830–835.

37. Mayer JH. Subclavian artery approach for insertion of intra-aortic balloon. *J Thorac Cardiovasc Surg* 1978;76:61–63.

38. Rubenstein RB, Karhade NV. Supraclavicular subclavian technique of intra-aortic balloon insertion. *J Vasc Surg* 1984;1:577–578.

39. McBride LR, Miller LW, Naunheim KS, Pennington DG. Axillary artery insertion of an intraaortic balloon pump. *Ann Thorac Surg* 1989;48:874–875.

40. Buchanan SA, Langenburg SE, Mauney MC, et al. Ambulatory intraaortic balloon counterpulsation. *Ann Thorac Surg* 1994;58:1547–1548.

41. Plummer PM. Biomedical engineering fundamentals of the intra-aortic balloon pump. *Biomed Instrum Technol* 1989;23:452–459.

42. Baldwin RT, Slogoff S, Noon GP, et al. A model to predict survival at time of postcardiotomy intraaortic balloon pump insertion. *Ann Thorac Surg* 1993;55:908–913.

43. Christenson JT, Buswell L, Velebit V, et al. The intraaortic balloon pump for postcardiotomy heart failure. Experience with 169 intraaortic balloon pumps. *Thorac Cardiovasc Surg* 1995;43:129–133.

44. Busch T, Sirbu H, Zenker D, Dalichau H. Vascular complications related to intraaortic balloon counterpulsation: An analysis of ten years experience. *Thorac Cardiovasc Surg* 1997; 45:55–59.

45. Shahian DM, Neptune WB, Ellis FHJ, Maggs PR. Intraaortic balloon pump morbidity: A comparative analysis of risk factors between percutaneous and surgical techniques. *Ann Thorac Surg* 1983;36:644–653.

46. Alderman JD, Gabliani GI, McCabe CH, et al. Incidence and management of limb ischemia with percutaneous wire-guided intraaortic balloon catheters. *J Am Coll Cardiol* 1987;9: 524–530.

47. Vilacosta I, Castillo JA, Peral V, et al. Intramural aortic hematoma following intra-aortic balloon counterpulsation. Documentation by transesophageal echocardiography. *Eur Heart J* 1995;16:2015–2016.

48. Isner JM, Cohen SR, Virmani R, et al. Complications of the intraaortic balloon counterpulsation device: Clinical and morphologic observations in 45 necropsy patients. *Am J Cardiol* 1980;45:260–268.

49. Rodigas PC, Bridges KG. Occlusion of left internal mammary artery with intra-aortic balloon: Clinical implications. *J Thorac Cardiovasc Surg* 1986;91:142–143.

50. Ferrell MA, Doherty M, Zusman RM, Nash IS. Total aortic occlusion caused by sustained

balloon inflation: A previously unreported complication of intraaortic balloon counterpulsation. *Cathet Cardiovasc Diagn* 1993;30:211–213.

51. Funk M, Ford CF, Foell DW, et al. Frequency of long-term lower limb ischemia associated with intraaortic balloon pump use. *Am J Cardiol* 1992;70:1195–1199.

52. Gold JP, Cohen J, Shemin RJ, et al. Femorofemoral bypass to relieve acute leg ischemia during intra-aortic balloon pump cardiac support. *J Vasc Surg* 1986;3:351–354.

53. Friedell ML, Alpert J, Parsonnet V, et al. Femorofemoral grafts for lower limb ischemia caused by intra-aortic balloon pump. *J Vasc Surg* 1987;5:180–186.

54. Allen KB, Salam AA, Lumsden AB. Acute mesenteric ischemia after cardiopulmonary bypass. *J Vasc Surg* 1992;16:391–395.

55. Jarmolowski CR, Poirier RL. Small bowel infarction complicating intra-aortic balloon counterpulsation via the ascending aorta. *J Thorac Cardiovasc Surg* 1980;79:735–737.

56. Rizk AB, Rashkow AM. Acute pancreatitis associated with intra-aortic balloon pump placement. *Cathet Cardiovasc Diagn* 1996;38:363–364.

57. Busch HMJ, Cogbill TH, Gundersen AE. Splenic infarction: Complication of intra-aortic balloon counterpulsation. *Am Heart J* 1985;109:383–385.

58. Tyras DH, Willman VL. Paraplegia following intraaortic balloon assistance. *Ann Thorac Surg* 1978;25:164–166.

59. Singh BM, Fass AE, Pooley RW, Wallach R. Paraplegia associated with intraaortic balloon pump counterpulsation. *Stroke* 1983;14:983–986.

60. Scott IR, Goiti JJ. Late paraplegia as a consequence of intraaortic balloon pump support. *Ann Thorac Surg* 1985;40:300–301.

61. Harris RE, Reimer KA, Crain BJ, et al. Spinal cord infarction following intraaortic balloon support. *Ann Thorac Surg* 1986;42:206–207.

62. Rose DM, Jacobowitz IJ, Acinapura AJ, Cunningham JN Jr. Paraplegia following percutaneous insertion of an intra-aortic balloon. *J Thorac Cardiovasc Surg* 1984;87:788–789.

63. Riggle KP, Oddi MA. Spinal cord necrosis and paraplegia as complications of the intra-aortic balloon. *Crit Care Med* 1989;17:475–476.

64. Stavridis GT, O'Riordan JB. Paraplegia as a result of intra-aortic balloon counterpulsation. *J Cardiovasc Surg* 1995;36:177–179.

65. Hurle A, Llamas P, Meseguer J, Casillas JA. Paraplegia complicating intraaortic balloon pumping. *Ann Thorac Surg* 1997;63:1217–1218.

66. Beholz S, Braun J, Ansorge K, et al. Paraplegia caused by aortic dissection after intraaortic balloon pump assist. *Ann Thorac Surg* 1998;65:603–604.

67. Frederiksen JW, Smith J, Brown P, Zinetti C. Arterial helium embolism from a ruptured intraaortic balloon. *Ann Thorac Surg* 1988;46:690–692.

68. Myers GJ, Landymore RW, Leadon RB, Squires C. Fracture of the internal lumen of a Datascope Percor Stat-DL Balloon, resulting in stroke. *Ann Thorac Surg* 1994;57:1335–1337.

69. Price C, Briffa NP, Lynn MA. Perforation of an intraaortic balloon twice in one patient. *J Cardiovasc Surg* 1992;33:44–45.

70. Mayerhofer KE, Billhardt RA, Codini MA. Delayed abrasion perforation of two intra-aortic balloons. *Am Heart J* 1984;108:1361–1363.

71. Cox PMJ, Kellett M, Goran SF, et al. Plaque abrasion and intra-aortic balloon leak. *Chest* 1995;108:1495–1498.

72. Rajani R, Keon WJ, Bedard P. Rupture of an intra-aortic balloon. A case report. *J Thorac Cardiovasc Surg* 1980;79:301–302.

73. Nishida H, Koyanagi H, Abe T, et al. Comparative study of five types of IABP balloons in terms of incidence of balloon rupture and other complications: A multi-institutional study. *Artif Organs* 1994;18:746–751.

74. Alvarez JM, Brady PW, Wilson RM. Intra-aortic balloon rupture. An increasing trend? *ASAIO J* 1992;38:862–863.

75. Sutter FP, Joyce DH, Bailey BM, et al. Events associated with rupture of intra-aortic balloon counterpulsation devices. *ASAIO Trans* 1991;37:38–40.

76. Stahl KD, Tortolani AJ, Nelson RL, et al. Intraaortic balloon rupture. *ASAIO Trans* 1988; 34:496–499.

77. Aru GM, King JTJ, Hovaguimian H, et al. The entrapped balloon: Report of a possibly serious complication. *J Thorac Cardiovasc Surg* 1986;91:146–149.

78. Lambert CJ. Intraaortic balloon entrapment. *Ann Thorac Surg* 1987;44:446.

79. Milgalter E, Mosseri M, Uretzky G, Romanoff H. Intraaortic balloon entrapment: A complication of balloon perforation. *Ann Thorac Surg* 1986;42:697–698.
80. Pollock JC, Charlton MC, Williams WG, et al. Intraaortic balloon pumping in children. *Ann Thorac Surg* 1980;29:522–528.
81. Veasy LG, Blalock RC, Orth JL, Boucek MM. Intra-aortic balloon pumping in infants and children. *Circulation* 1983;68:1095–1100.
82. Webster H, Veasy LG. Intra-aortic balloon pumping in children. *Heart Lung* 1985;14:548–555.
83. del Nido P, Swan PR, Benson LN, et al. Successful use of intraaortic balloon pumping in a 2-kilogram infant. *Ann Thorac Surg* 1988;46:574–576.

Chapter 23

Intracorporeal Support:

Thermo Cardiosystems Ventricular Assist Devices

Daniel J. Goldstein, MD

Historical Perspective

In 1965 Thermo Electron, the parent company of Thermo Cardiosystems Incorporated (TCI; Woburn, MA), submitted a proposal to the National Heart Lung Blood Institute for the development of an artificial heart. Six companies, including TCI, were awarded research grants and, 1 year later, Thermo Electron developed its first axisymmetric left ventricular pump (Fig. 1). In 1970, the concept of textured biocontacting surfaces was developed—an idea that proved to be one of the most important contributions to the field of mechanical support.[1] The ensuing years were marked by the development of the first implantable left ventricular assist device (LVAD) pump and pneumatic driver, as well as the application of textured surfaces to the blood contacting surfaces of the LVAD pump. In 1975, the first integrated implantable electric LVAD was produced and the first LVAD system with tissue valves was created. Based on the success of the initial clinical trials of LVAD support conducted in the late 1970s, the Food and Drug Administration (FDA) awarded Thermo Electron an investigational device exemption for the pneumatic pusher-plate HeartMate device. The first clinical implant of this device took place at the Texas Heart Institute in 1986. In the meantime, ongoing research with the electric version of the HeartMate culminated with an investigational device exemption in 1990 and its first clinical application shortly thereafter. Concerns regarding patient quality of life and interest in outpatient support sparked the development of a portable, wearable driver that reached the clinical arena in 1995 (Sweden). That same year, the FDA approved the Randomized Evaluation of Mechanical Assistance for the Treatment of Congestive Heart Failure (REMATCH) trial, which aims to compare LVAD technology with maximal medical therapy for the treatment of patients with end-stage heart disease

From Goldstein DJ and Oz MC (eds). *Cardiac Assist Devices*. Armonk, NY: Futura Publishing Co., Inc.; ©2000.

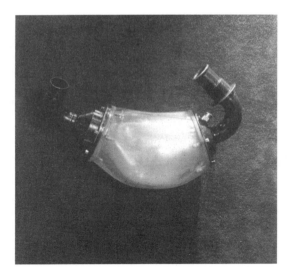

FIGURE 1 The first axisymmetric left ventricular assist device developed by Thermo Electron.

who are not candidates for transplantation.[2] The first patient discharge to home with implantable LVAD support occurred in 1997 and marked the dawn of the era of successful outpatient mechanical support as a bridge to transplantation.

Device Description

The HeartMate LVAD is an implantable pulsatile blood pump that is available in pneumatically driven (implantable pneumatic, or IP) or electrically powered (vented electric, or VE) models. The IP device is fabricated from sintered titanium and houses a flexible, textured, polyurethane diaphragm (Fig. 2) bonded to a rigid pusher-plate that is actuated pneumatically from a portable external console. The VE model, available since 1991, uses the same pusher-plate mechanism and has similar flow characteristics, but it features a low-speed torque motor (composed of a stator, a magnet assembly, and an electronic commutator) that drives a pair of nested helical cams. Two lines (contained in a single conduit in the most recent VE model) lead from the implanted LVAD, through the skin, to the external environment. One line contains the electric cable to the bedside console (IP) or external portable battery pack (VE), while the second line acts as an air vent, allowing air transfer in and out of the motor chamber. Air transfer is necessary in order to maintain the pressure in the chamber near atmospheric conditions[3]; in essence, for every beat, a volume of air equivalent to the volume of blood pumped must be accommodated. To reduce the possibility of infection, the line/s is/are covered with polyester velour to encourage tissue bonding at the skin line.

Like the natural left ventricle, both the IP and VE models are equipped with inflow and outflow valves—25 mm porcine xenograft valves (Medtronic-Hancock, Minneapolis, MN) within inlet and outlet Dacron® graft conduits. Both pumps can generate a maximum stroke volume of 85 mL and a maximum pump output of 11 L/min. The pumps can be operated in fixed rate or automatic modes. In the latter and more physiologic mode, an eject cycle begins only after the blood pump is at

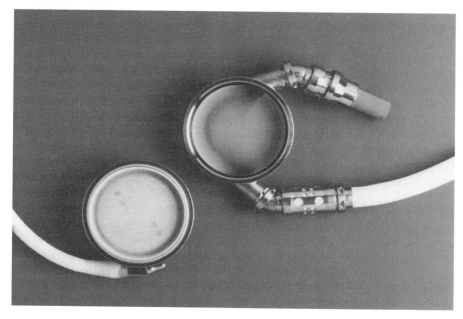

FIGURE 2. The HeartMate pump opened. The device is made of sintered titanium housing a flexible, textured, polyurethane diaphragm (left).

least 90% filled; this mode automatically maximizes the amount of blood pumped by the system and is responsive to circulatory demand. A schematic representation of the HeartMate VE LVAD is depicted in Figure 3.

The most unique property of the HeartMate devices lies in the design for the blood contacting portions of the device. To encourage the formation of a biologic lining, the blood contacting portion of the titanium housing incorporates titanium microspheres and the flexible diaphragm is covered with integrally textured polyurethane. These textured surfaces promote the adherence of cellular blood elements (Fig. 4) and the formation of a pseudointimal layer.[1,4] It is the feeling of some investigators that this unique surface may be responsible for the low thromboembolic risk associated with this device despite the avoidance of systemic anticoagulation.[5]

The current HeartMate wearable devices have external back-up mechanisms so that in the event of device failure, support is continued without the need for reoperation. If the device should fail, the native heart would usually be able to provide systemic support until the device can be examined. Because the electronic control unit resides outside the body, it can be easily repaired should failure of the software, chip, or electronics occur. Finally, if the motor device fails, the single pusher-plate mechanism can be pneumatically activated with a hand-held portable pump (Fig. 5).

Implantation Technique

Most of the mortality associated with device support occurs in the early postoperative period and may be impacted by implantation technique. Over our 8-year

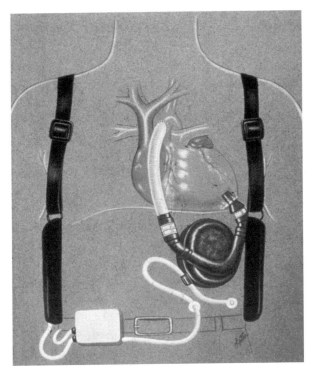

FIGURE 3. Schematic representation of the HeartMate VE LVAD.

clinical experience with LVAD support, our implantation technique has been modified to address the morbidity associated with different aspects of the operation. Particular attention has been devoted to 1) development of the preperitoneal pocket and drive line tunnel; 2) outflow graft positioning and length; 3) creation of the apical cuff and inflow cannula passage; 4) intraoperative management of bleeding sites, de-airing, and separation from cardiopulmonary bypass; and 5) other surgical considerations.[6]

Preperitoneal Pocket

Significant morbidity associated with intra-abdominal placement of the LVAD led us to abandon this approach and favor the preperitoneal location. The latter offers several advantages including 1) avoidance of excessive heat and fluid loss from the abdominal cavity; 2) prevention of internal organ erosion, bowel obstruction, or intra-abdominal adhesions; and 3) greater ease in dealing with pocket infections.

Following midline sternotomy, the incision is extended to 2 cm above the umbilicus, and dissecting of the preperitoneal fat away from the undersurface of the rectus sheath (Fig. 6) creates a preperitoneal pocket. Superiorly, it is extended to the undersurface of the diaphragm until the apex of the heart can be palpated just lateral to the inferior phrenic vessels. The pocket is extended laterally and inferiorly. If there is difficulty with the development of the desired plane, the rectus sheath is entered and the posterior rectus sheath is left as a patch overlying the peritoneum. This is

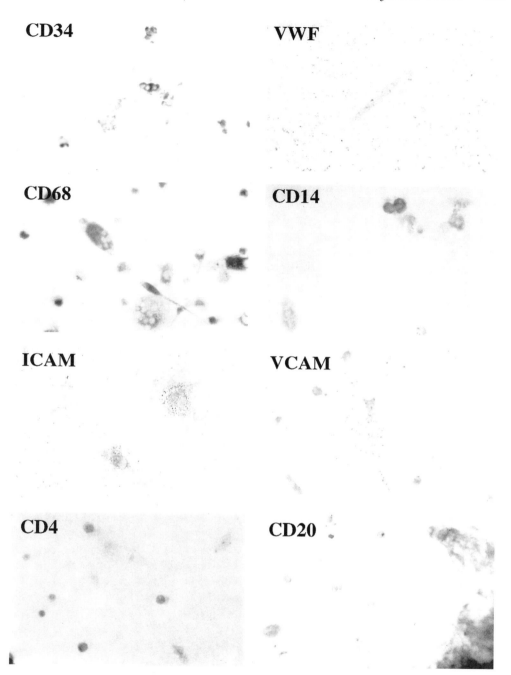

FIGURE 4. Cellular blood elements and molecules arising on the surface of the HeartMate textured surface. CD34 = marker for pluripotent stem cell; CD68 = marker for activated macrophage; VWF = von Willebrand factor; CD14 = marker for monocyte; ICAM = intercellular adhesion molecule; VCAM = vascular cell adhesion molecule; CD4 = marker for T cells; CD20 = marker for activated B cells. Courtesy of Talia Spanier, MD, Columbia University. See for color plate.

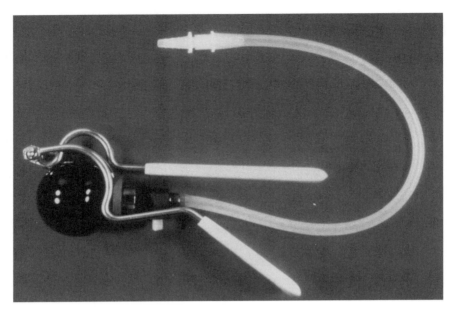

FIGURE 5. Hand-held pump that allows the HeartMate device to be activated manually should the device fail catastrophically.

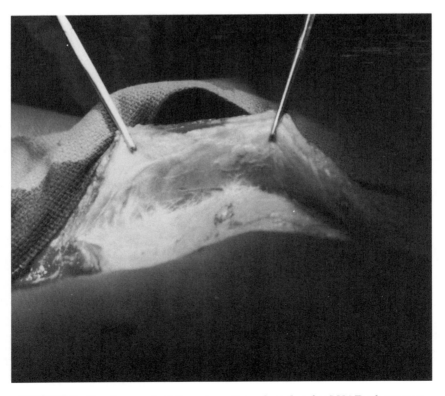

FIGURE 6. Development of the preperitoneal pocket for LVAD placement.

particularly necessary inferiorly, near the umbilicus. A plastic model of the device can be inserted into the pocket to tailor the size of the pocket.

Drive Line Tunnel

The HeartMate VE possesses a single drive line, which is made to exit in the right mid to lower quadrant area. A 1.5 cm incision is made in the right midabdomen, about halfway between the costal margin and the superior iliac spine, approximately 6 to 7 cm lateral to the umbilicus. A special device with a screw tip is passed tunneled through the incision, along a curve that passes just below the umbilicus and back in semilunar fashion toward the inferior border of the preperitoneal pocket. The screw tip of the device is then screwed onto the distal end of the drive line (which has a plastic applicator to accept the screw tip), and the drive line is then pulled through the created tunnel and out the small right abdominal incision (Fig. 7). Efforts should be made to make the subcutaneous tunnel as long as possible to ensure maximal coating and tissue ingrowth onto the drive line, and to reduce the risk of infection.

Outflow Graft Anastomosis

A partial occluding clamp is placed on the right lateral surface of the ascending aorta and a longitudinal aortotomy tailored to the diameter of the outflow graft

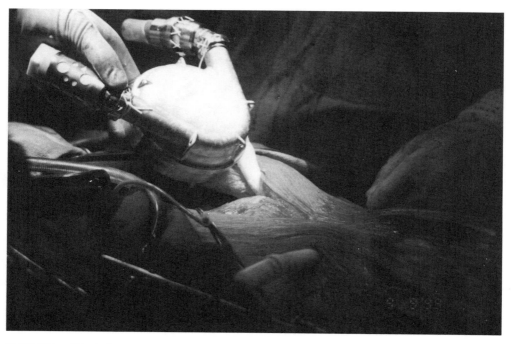

FIGURE 7. The left ventricular assist device drive line is passed subcutaneously around the umbilicus and made to exit in the right lower quadrant through a small stab wound incision.

is made. The outflow graft is then cut the appropriate length—usually 12 to 15 cm—keeping in mind that a graft that is too long will kink as the chest is closed (Fig. 7). We have favored two anastomotic techniques: one involves the use of interrupted pledgetted 3-0 prolene mattress sutures and the second entails the use of two running 3-0 prolene sutures (heel-to-toe and toe-to-heel) with two buttressing strips of bovine pericardium on the aortic aspect of the anastomoses. Meticulous technique must be followed and perfect hemostasis ensured, as this represent the most common site of postoperative bleeding; furthermore, less than perfect anastomoses can lead to late disruption and dissection.

Apical Cuff and Inflow Cannula Passage

With the outflow anastomoses in place, the LVAD pump is comfortably placed in the preperitoneal pocket. The previously vented left ventricular apex is elevated and a sling is made with a towel to keep the apex in optimal position. A circular coring knife is then used (passed over the vent—usually a Foley catheter with the balloon inflated inside the ventricular cavity) to create the apical defect (Fig. 8). Residual muscle or scar that may impinge on the cannula is removed, as is any loose endocardial thrombus. Pledgetted horizontal mattress sutures of 2-0 ethibond are placed deep into the myocardium in order to gather it, and through the sewing cuff

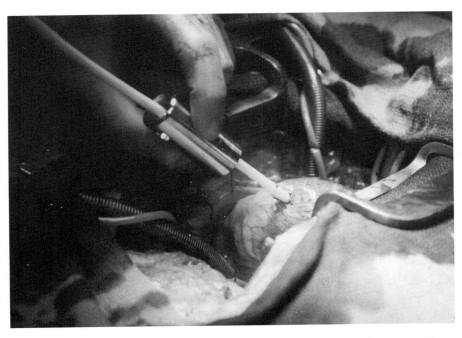

FIGURE 8. A Foley catheter has been placed into the left ventricle via the apex, and a coring knife is used to create a defect.

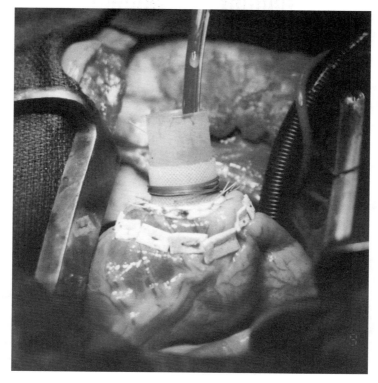

FIGURE 9. The tissue has been gathered with pledgetted tevdek sutures.

(Fig. 9). Meticulous hemostasis at the edges and epicardial surface must be obtained at this time, as it is virtually impossible to visualize this area after the inflow has been attached. Once the cuff is secure, the diaphragm is taken down from medial to lateral until enough space has been created to allow passage of the LVAD inflow into the chest (Fig. 10). Following this, and with the LVAD sitting comfortably in the preperitoneal pocket, the inflow cannula is inserted through the silicone sewing cuff until the entire titanium surface is within the cuff.

De-aring Protocol

Several precautions are taken to minimize the chance of air embolism. First, once the inflow is connected, the LVAD is filled with blood and the device is allowed to serve as a left ventricular vent. Second, the patient is placed in steep Trendelenburg position, he or she is volume-loaded and ventilated in order to search for air under transesophageal echocardiographic guidance. Third, a vascular clamp is kept on the outflow graft and the outflow graft connectors are screwed together, ensuring a water- and air-tight seal. Fourth, a needle hole is placed on the outflow graft as the device is manually actuated. Fifth, a 14 g aortic root cannula (DLP Inc., Grand Rapids, MI) is inserted into the ascending aorta (or outflow graft) and placed on suction to evacuate air. Finally, the surgical field (and in particular the inflow cannula) is kept

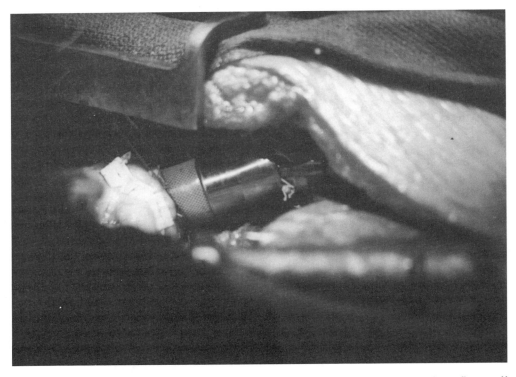

FIGURE 10. Surgeon's view. The inflow to the LVAD has been connected to the inflow cuff in the left ventricular apex. Note how the diaphragm has been partly divided from medial to lateral to allow comfortable passage of the LVAD inflow. The pump is seen sitting in the preperitoneal pocket.

under fluid while cardiopulmonary bypass flow is reduced to minimize the chance of the device sucking air.

Concluding Maneuvers

As cardiopulmonary bypass is weaned, the device is activated at a fixed rate of 40 bpm. Appropriate inotropic support is instituted as the patient is separated from bypass. We almost routinely employ Primacor (Sanofi Winthrop, New York, NY), Dobutrex (Eli Lilly & Co., Indianapolis, IN), and pressor support with low-dose Levophed (Sanofi Winthrop) and Pitressin (Parke-Davis, Morris Plains, NJ) as necessary (see Chapter 9 for details on the use of this latter agent).

The graft is positioned on the right lateral side of the heart to prevent kinking and to reduce the chance of injury at reoperation (for transplantation). The mediastinum is drained with anterior and posterior chest tubes, and a Jackson-Pratt-type bulb suction device is placed in the preperitoneal pocket.

Other Surgical Considerations

Four particular scenarios merit separate discussion.

Ventricular Aneurysm

Ventricular aneurysms are not uncommon in patients with end-stage ischemic cardiomyopathy. Small aneurysms are left intact. A large aneurysm, however, can be sucked into the inflow cannula with devastating consequences. Hence, in the presence of such an aneurysm, the aorta is cross-clamped (to avoid embolization of endocardial thrombus), the heart is arrested, and the aneurysm is plicated or excised.

Coronary Artery Disease

If the patient has had previous bypass grafting, efforts are made to preserve open grafts. Occasionally, we have bypassed coronary lesions at the time of LVAD implantation to reduce the theoretical risk of perioperative ischemia, right heart dysfunction, and arrhythmias. Furthermore, in the rare event of device failure, a revascularized heart may provide better back-up support until the device can be examined. Moreover, revascularization in the setting of left ventricular rest may provide the ideal milieu for ventricular recovery and allow for future device weaning and explantation.

Aortic Valve Regurgitation

The presence of aortic valve regurgitation limits LVAD performance and jeopardizes organ perfusion.[7] The reduction in left ventricular end-diastolic pressure afforded by LVAD assistance increases the transvalvular gradient and systolic backflow into the left ventricle, thus diminishing effective left-sided output. As the severity of aortic regurgitation increases, the net forward flow and end organ perfusion can be severely compromised. Therefore, if the calculated aortic regurgitant flow (difference between LVAD flow and right-sided thermodilution cardiac output) is greater than 2 L/min, we suture the aortic valve closed or insert a bioprosthesis.

Bleeding

We routinely use Trasylol (Bayer Corporation, West Haven, CT) during LVAD implantation, as it has been shown to decrease blood loss, blood use, right-sided circulatory failure, and perioperative mortality in patients with bleeding.[8] At the time of transplantation, we again administer Trasylol but do not give the test or loading dose until we are ready for institution of cardiopulmonary bypass in the rare event of severe anaphylaxis.[9]

Criteria Selection, Contraindications, and Limitations

In general, potential LVAD recipients must be candidates for transplantation and, hence, the presence of any contraindication to transplantation negates candidacy for long-term LVAD support (except as part of the aforementioned REMATCH study). Cardiac and noncardiac factors that are carefully scrutinized are outlined in Table 1.

While the major causes of perioperative mortality following LVAD insertion—hemorrhage and right heart failure—have been reduced with increasing experience and with use of Trasylol[8] and inhaled nitric oxide,[10,11] additional major improvements can only result from improved patient screening. A scoring system based on criteria easily obtainable at the time of first evaluation has been predictive of successful early outcome after LVAD implantation. The clinically usable scale pre-

---

Table 1

Factors that Contraindicate or Require Correction Prior to Consideration for LVAD Support

---

Cardiac factors
1. Hemodynamic criteria:
   Systolic blood pressure <80 mm Hg
   Cardiac index <2.0 L/min/m^2
   Pulmonary capillary wedge pressure >20 mm Hg
   Inotropic and/or intra-aortic balloon support
2. Right ventricular failure
3. Valvular lesions
   Aortic regurgitation
   Mitral stenosis
   Coronary artery disease
   Arrhythmias
   Septal defects

Noncardiac factors
1. Central nervous system
   Significant neurologic deficit
   Psychiatric disorder that will impede independent LVAD management
   Compliance issues
2. Pulmonary
   Severe obstructive or restrictive disease
   Decreased diffusion capacity in common in heart failure and is not considered a contraindication
3. Renal
   Need for dialysis
4. Hepatic
   Insufficiency resulting in inability to synthesize clotting factors
5. Peripheral vascular disease
   Bilateral iliofemoral occlusions
6. Infectious disease
   Active sepsis
7. Other
   Small body surface area (<1.5 m^2)
   Independent comorbidities that are life-threatening—metastatic cancer, etc.

LVAD = left ventricular assist device.

dicts which patients are unlikely to survive device insertion and on whom intervention would likely be futile. According to this statistical analysis, predictive factors for perioperative mortality include 1) oliguria (urine output <30 mL/h); 2) elevated central venous pressure (>16 mm Hg); 3) need for mechanical ventilation; 4) elevated prothrombin time (>16 sec); and/or 5) prior mediastinal operation.[12]

Institutional Experience and Worldwide Registry

Between 1990 and April 1999, 150 patients underwent placement of a HeartMate LVAD (53 IP, 17 VE-1, 80 VE-2) as a bridge to transplantation at our institution. Details of this experience are summarized in Table 2. Sixty-eight percent of patients were successfully bridged to transplantation, 27% expired, and 4% underwent device explantation as a bridge to recovery. Causes of death included multisystem organ failure (n=9), sepsis (n=8), right heart failure (n=4), cerebrovascular accident (n=4), unknown (n=4), pulmonary embolism/hypoxia (n=3), air embolism (n=2), aortic tear/dissection (n=2), and one case each of gastrointestinal bleeding, small bowel obstruction, drive line rupture, and massive intraoperative bleeding.

As of June 1999, 1837 patients have undergone implantation of a HeartMate device (1152 IP, 685 VE) in over 120 institutions worldwide, with success rates (excluding 30-day perioperative mortality) that approximate 90%. Average duration of support has been 89 days for IP devices and 117 days for VE devices. The total experience amounts to 484 cumulative patient-years (394 patient-years in the US, 90 patient-years internationally). Data from the Thermo Cardiosystems Worldwide Registry are summarized in Table 3 and Figure 11.

Table 2	
LVAD Experience at Columbia Presbyterian Medical Center	
	n = 150
Age (yrs)	
Range	11–65
Mean	49±14
M/F	117/33
Diagnosis	
Ischemic cardiomyopathy	76 (51%)
Idiopathic dilated cardiomyopathy	59 (39%)
Other	15 (10%)
Length of support (days)	
Range	0–605
Mean	93±92
Outcome	
Transplanted	102 (68%)
Expired prior to transplant	40 (27%)
Explanted	8 (4%)
Ongoing mechanical support	2 (1%)

LVAD = left ventricular assist device.

Table 3

Worldwide Thermo Cardiosystems LVAD Experience

	USA	International
Institutions		
Participating institutions	90	33
Number of implants	1550	287
Cumulative patient-years	374	90
Clinical profile		
% Female	15	12
Ischemic cardiomyopathy (%)	43	22
Idiopathic cardiomyopathy (%)	48	64
Myocardial infarction (%)	5	7
Other (%)	4	7
Length of support		
Patients supported >90 days	697	118
Patients supported >180 days	208	59
Patients supported >360 days	37	22
Number of patients ongoing	158	41

LVAD = left ventricular assist device.

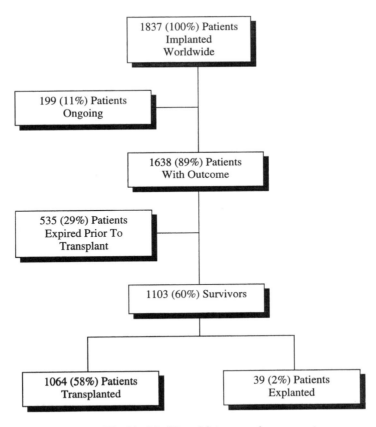

FIGURE 11. Worldwide HeartMate experience—outcomes.

Summary

The Thermo Cardiosystems LVAD systems were the first mechanical circulatory support devices to be approved by the FDA for bridging to transplantation. The models in current use have been proven to be safe, effective, and reliable tools for the treatment of end-stage heart disease. In several patients, the devices have functioned well in excess of 2 years. These successes have sparked interest in the use of these devices as alternatives, rather than bridges to transplantation.

Perhaps the greatest contribution of the Thermo Cardiosystems devices rests on their unique design for the blood contacting surfaces that has resulted in a very low incidence of thromboembolic events despite the fact that most of its recipients do not receive systemic anticoagulation. Furthermore, investigations into the mechanisms underlying this protective effect have unearthed fascinating interactions between host (patient) and device that have led to a greater understanding of systemic immune responses.

We must keep in mind that these devices represent only the first generation of reliable mechanical support devices. Flaws exist and modifications are constantly being made to address these flaws. We will only advance the technology by pushing it to failure and modifying the devices as we learn from their shortcomings. Failure must be viewed as the road to progress.

References

1. Rose EA, Levin HR, Oz MC, et al. Artificial circulatory support with textured interior surfaces: A counterintuitive approach to minimizing thromboembolism. *Circulation* 1994; 90(uppl II):II87-II91.
2. Rose EA, Moskowitz AJ, Packer M, et al. The REMATCH Trial: Rationale, design and endpoints. *Ann Thorac Surg* 1999;67:723–730.
3. Frazier OH. The development of an implantable portable electrically powered left ventricular assist device. *Semin Thorac Cardiovasc Surg* 1994;6:181–187.
4. Dasse KA, Chipman SD, Sherman CN, et al. Clinical experience with textured blood-contacting surfaces in ventricular assist devices. *ASAIO Trans* 1987;10:418–425.
5. Slater JP, Rose EA, Levin HR, et al. Low thromboembolic risk without anticoagulation using advanced-design left ventricular assist devices. *Ann Thorac Surg* 1996;62:1321–1327.
6. Oz MC, Goldstein DJ, Rose EA. Preperitoneal placement of ventricular assist devices: An illustrated stepwise approach. *J Card Surg* 1995;10:288–294.
7. Goldstein DJ, Oz MC, Rose EA. Implantable left ventricular assist devices. *N Engl J Med* 1998;339:1522–1533.
8. Goldstein DJ, Seldomridge JA, Chen JM, et al. Use of aprotinin in LVAD recipients reduces blood loss, blood use, and perioperative mortality. *Ann Thorac Surg* 1995;59:1063–1067.
9. Goldstein DJ, Choudhri A, Argenziano M, et al. Repeat administration of aprotinin for staged cardiac transplantation. *J Circ Support* 1998;1:27–30.
10. Argenziano M, Choudhri A, Moazami N, et al. Randomized, double-blind trial of inhaled nitric oxide in LVAD recipients with pulmonary hypertension. *Ann Thorac Surg* 1998;65: 340–345.
11. Salamonsen RF, Kaye D, Esmore DS. Inhalation of nitric oxide provides selective pulmonary vasodilation, aiding mechanical cardiac assist with the Thoratec left ventricular assist device. *Anaesth Intensive Care* 1994;22:209–210.
12. Oz MC, Goldstein DJ, Pepino P, et al. Screening scale predicts patients successfully receiving long term implantable left ventricular assist devices. *Circulation* 1995;92(suppl II):II169-II173.

Chapter 24

Intracorporeal Support:

The Novacor Left Ventricular Assist System

Narayanan Ramasamy, PhD, Rita L. Vargo, MSN, RN,
Robert L. Kormos, MD, and Peer M. Portner, PhD

The Novacor Left Ventricular Assist System: System Evolution

The Novacor left ventricular assist system (LVAS) was the first electrically powered heart assist device designed as an integrated, ultimately totally implantable system intended for definitive treatment of end-stage heart disease.[1-3] This solenoid-actuated dual pusher-plate blood pump uses a smooth polyurethane pump sac with bioprosthetic valved conduits and polyester (PET) inflow cannula and outflow extension. A unique feature of the Novacor LVAS is its complete symmetry. The system uses a high-efficiency linear motor—a pulsed solenoid energy converter with two identical, pivoted armature assemblies. When energized, the balanced solenoid closure drives the dual pusher-plates through identical load decoupling springs, resulting in freedom from reaction forces or torques, gyroscopic effects, or momentum transfer to conduits, leads, or adjacent body tissues.[3]

The totally implantable initial design of the Novacor system (Fig. 1) had a fully autonomous implant that comprised the pump/drive unit, an electronic controller with rechargeable battery, a subcutaneous belt skin transformer secondary for transcutaneous power transfer across the intact skin, and a variable volume compensator. Externally worn components included the belt skin transformer primary and wearable battery packs.

Components of this totally implantable system have been under development since 1970.[1,2,4,5] Experimental studies of individual components or subsystems, and subsequently of the total system, have been reported.[6,7] Table 1 summarizes preclinical animal studies, initially in the bovine and canine models and, since 1984, in

From Goldstein DJ and Oz MC (eds). *Cardiac Assist Devices.* Armonk, NY: Futura Publishing Co., Inc.; ©2000.

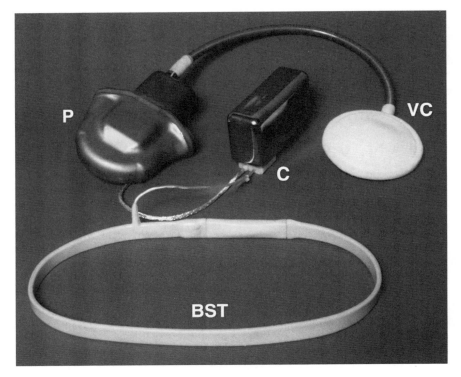

FIGURE 1. Totally implantable Novacor LVAS (N120), implanted components. BST = belt skin transformer; C = controller/battery; P = pump/drive unit; VC = volume compensator.

the ovine model. The totally implantable system (N120) configuration successfully completed a 2-year National Institutes of Health (NIH)-sponsored and audited device readiness testing (DRT) program. From 1986 to 1989, 12 complete systems (excluding bioprosthetic valves) were tested at 37°C in physiologic saline for periods up to 3 years, each system completing the mandated 2-year in vitro test, without any system failures.[8,9] The bioprosthetic valves were life-tested separately, in conventional accelerated test fixtures at LVAS loads, without failure, for the equivalent of 3 years. The

	Table 1			
	Summary of Preclinical Animal Studies			
Subsystem	Animal Model	# Implants	Cumulative Duration (yrs)	Longest Duration (days)
LVAS	Bovine	75	7	161
	Ovine	129	27	359
Belt skin transformer	Canine	66	36	898
	Ovine	5	7	1148
Volume compensator	Ovine	8	5	767
Totally implantable LVAS	Ovine	4	1	260

LVAS = left ventricular assist system

Novacor LVAS was the only system (of four tested) to successfully complete the NIH DRT protocol.

During the same period, a partially implantable Novacor LVAS configuration, intended for short-term support, was developed to evaluate clinical viability and to gain a better understanding of the biologic interfaces. This configuration used the same implanted solenoid-actuated dual pusher-plate blood pump, but exteriorized the other components via a percutaneous vent tube containing power and control leads connected to an extracorporeal electronic control and power system. The first clinical use of this bedside console-based system took place at Stanford University Medical Center in 1984 in the first (successful) bridge to transplant. A 51-year-old male recipient with ischemic heart disease on intravenous inotropes and balloon pump was supported for 8.5 days.[10] To improve patient mobility, independence, and quality of life, the bedside console was replaced in 1993 by a wearable controller and battery packs; the controller employed components developed and tested for the totally implantable LVAS.[11] The early clinical experience with these configurations (console-based and wearable) is summarized in Table 2.

The current configuration of the Novacor LVAS, the valved-conduit system (N100PC), was developed in 1991 and was first used clinically in 1993. The principal differences between this and the prior configuration (N100P) are: 1) sealed bearings in the solenoid actuator to improve durability; 2) modifications to reduce acoustic noise (N100PCq, not available in the US); 3) custom designed, integrally sinused, externally stented, porcine-valved conduits to improve flow around the valves; 4) sealed outflow conduit extension, initially Hemashield® (Boston Scientific, Natick, MA) (collagen-coated PET), more recently Vascutek (gelatin-sealed PET; Gelseal®, Vascutek, Renfrewshire, Scotland); and 5) knitted, uncrimped gelatin-sealed Vascutek (PET) inflow conduit and cannula, integrally supported to resist deformation, creasing, and radial motion.

Anatomic placement of this wearable system is illustrated in Figure 2 and a cut away view of the implanted pump/drive unit with valved conduits, inflow conduit/cannula, outflow extension, and percutaneous vent tube is shown in Figure 3.

Real time in vitro reliability testing has been carried out, to failure, for the N100PC system.[12] Twelve systems completed a 3-year continuous test before continuing on to failure with a "most probable" lifetime (based on a Weibull model) of 4.34 years. The results of in vitro testing of the systems are presented in Table 3.

Table 2

System Evolution: Global N100P Clinical Results

	Bedside Console	Wearable System I	N100P Cumulative Experience
Implant	1984–1995	1993–1997	1984–1997
Application	BTT	BTT/BTR	BTT/BTR
# Recipients	182	174	356
Implant duration (days)	39 (1–370)	75 (1–795)	57 (1–795)
Transplanted	113 (62%)	104 (60%)	217 (61%)
Weaned	0	4 (2%)	4 (1%)
Implant years	19	36	55

BTT = bridge to transplant; BTR = bridge to recovery.

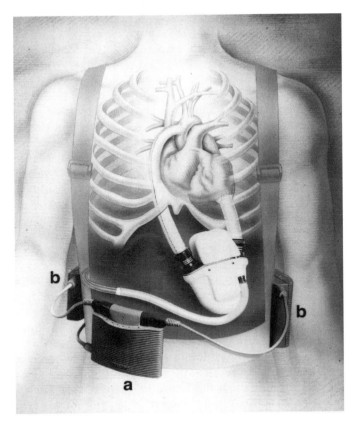

FIGURE 2. Novacor N100PC. Anatomic placement with external wearable controller (a) and power packs (b).

The first clinical implant of the valved-conduit system took place in 1993 at Henri Mondor Hospital, University of Paris. A 46-year-old male with idiopathic cardiomyopathy was supported for 103 days prior to successful transplantation. In the same year, regulatory approval was received in Europe for the N100PC wearable system. A multicenter clinical study was conducted in the US during the years 1996 to 1998 to support Food and Drug Administration (FDA) premarket approval. The

Table 3
Reliability of Novacor LVAS Systems: In Vitro Test Results

System	Mission Time (yrs)	Duration of Testing (yrs)			# Units	# Failures
		Cumulative	Mean	Longest		
N120[1]	2	28.6	2.2	3	12	0
N100P[2]	2	14.8	3	3	5	0
N100PC[3]	3	50.4	4.2	5.6	12	0

[1] Totally implantable system, NIH audited testing; [2] system with wearable controller and batteries; [3] current clinical system. LVAS = left ventricular assist system.

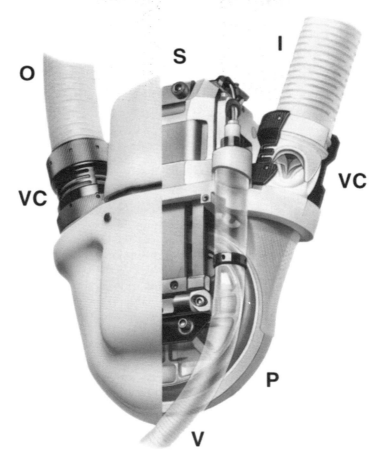

FIGURE 3. Novacor N100PC implanted components (cut away section). I = inflow cannula/ graft; O = outflow extension; P = pump sac; S = solenoid actuator; V = percutaneous vent/ leads; VC = porcine valved conduits.

premarket approval submission, which included 156 LVAS recipients and 35 controls from 21 US centers, was approved in 1998 for the bridge-to-transplant indication. The N100PC system has also been approved for use in Canada (1999) and in Japan (1999).

Patient Selection

Successful LVAS outcome depends on optimal patient selection and timing of implantation. The primary determinant of outcome is patient status at implant and early intervention before onset of hepatic, renal, or respiratory failure. It is also important to evaluate infection, right ventricular status, and dysrhythmia during the selection process, because these conditions may influence long-term bridge outcomes.

In the US, the FDA multicenter bridge-to-transplant study protocols described both inclusion and exclusion criteria for LVAS implantation. Inclusion and exclusion criteria for cardiac transplantation were an integral part of this study protocol. The bridge-to-transplant population was a subset of in-hospital acutely decompensated patients on intravenous inotropic support and/or balloon pump support. Additional device-specific exclusion criteria included documented blood dyscrasia, presence of a prosthetic aortic valve, and recipient body surface area less than 1.5 m². Clinical experience has demonstrated that preoperative hepatic and renal failure are predictors of unfavorable outcome after LVAS placement.[13-15]

Implant Technique

The original implant technique has been described previously,[16] although widespread experience has led to variations in technique.[17-19] A median sternotomy is performed, with the skin incision extended below the umbilicus. The right rectus muscle is mobilized off the posterior sheath approximately 4 to 5 cm from the midline, to allow the outflow conduit to pass easily under the sternum and to facilitate subsequent closure of the incision. The left rectus muscle is mobilized between the left costal margin and left iliac crest and laterally beyond the rectus sheath in a plane between the external and internal oblique muscles, to fashion the pump pocket. The outflow conduit is sized to length and anastomosed to the partially cross-clamped aorta. If the patient is unstable, the conduit can be anastomosed following institution of cardiopulmonary bypass. The percutaneous vent tube is tunneled from the pump pocket, subcutaneously, to exit midway between the right costal margin and the anterosuperior iliac crest. The inflow cannula is placed into the left ventricle through a ventriculotomy at the left ventricular apex. Alternatively, the anastomoses may be performed in antegrade fashion, with left ventricular cannulation performed first. Once the conduits are positioned, the pump/conduit system is de-aired through a needle hole in the outflow extension. The pump is started at a low fixed rate and, as the pump output increases, the patient is weaned from bypass and the LVAS operating mode is switched to fill-to-empty. Right heart failure can be unmasked at the time LVAS pumping is initiated. Transesophageal echocardiogram visualization of the right ventricle is critical to diagnose deteriorating right ventricular function and to determine the need for additional right ventricular support.

Perioperative Management

Risks and complications of circulatory support are multifactorial in nature. Bleeding may result from impaired synthesis of coagulation factors and coagulopathy due to hepatic dysfunction, and by activation of fibrinolysis secondary to blood contact with foreign surfaces. Excessive blood loss and transfusion of blood products can lead to an increase in pulmonary vascular resistance and exacerbation of right heart failure. Aprotinin (Trasylol, Bayer Corporation, West Haven, CT) has been used to reduce perioperative blood loss and need for blood products. Some clinicians reserve the use of Trasylol to the transplant operation to limit the risk of anaphylactic response to a second exposure. Cardiac tamponade requiring surgical exploration is one of the complications of perioperative bleeding.

Right ventricular failure is primarily an intraoperative or perioperative phenomenon. Right ventricular dysfunction may be increased by the effects of cardiopulmonary bypass and volume overload—often in the setting of intraoperative bleeding and multiple transfusions—on occasion requiring additional right ventricular mechanical support. Centrifugal pumps (Chapter 17) and, more recently, ABIOMED (Danvers, MA) and Thoratec (Berkeley, CA) right ventricular assist devices (RVADs) (see Chapters 18 and 19, respectively) have been used for short duration (typically <7 days) to manage right ventricular failure in LVAS recipients. In the cumulative experience of more than 1000 Novacor LVAS recipients, one had a post-implant right ventricular infarction and required an RVAD; another, over a postoperative period of 1 year, experienced progressive right ventricular dysfunction and exertional angina due to progressive right coronary artery stenosis, but was managed medically.

While some investigators favor biventricular assist systems to reverse end organ dysfunction, there has been a decrease in RVAD use in Novacor LVAS recipients, from greater than 12% in the late 1980s to a current rate of less than 6%. The need for RVAD support is usually short and transient. Recently, the use of inhaled nitric oxide in high-risk patients has, through pulmonary vasodilation, further reduced the need for right ventricular mechanical support (See Chapter 7). There is currently no reliable predictor of post-implant right ventricular dysfunction. Some investigators have suggested that a pre-implant right ventricular stroke work index of less than 7 is associated with post-implant right ventricular dysfunction. Others have noted that LVAD recipients with pulmonary edema on chest x-ray, and fever without elevation in white blood cell count, tend to have a higher incidence of hemodynamically significant right ventricular dysfunction.[20] A few instances of prolonged RVAD use in Novacor LVAS recipients have been reported, the attributed reason being intractable ventricular arrhythmias (Kormos RL, personal communication, March 1998).

Antithrombotic Therapy

Management of anticoagulation and antiplatelet therapy has evolved since the start of clinical trials in 1984. The current recommended guideline is early induction of antiplatelet therapy (perioperative period) and heparin when chest tube bleeding has diminished to less than 60 mL/h, to maintain an activated partial thromboplastin time of 1.5 times control. Conversion to warfarin is usually accomplished when the patient is fully mobilized and stable, with liver function restored to near normal (usually within 3 weeks post implant). The target international normalized ratio (INR) is 2.0 to 3.0, and periodic INR monitoring is recommended to adjust for dietary change and to keep anticoagulation in the therapeutic range. Some centers manage the patient with heparin and aspirin for prolonged periods. There has been a wide intercenter variability in the management of antithrombotic therapy,[21] and no single antithrombotic regimen has prevailed.

Outpatient Support

Once the patient is stable, fully ambulatory, and properly trained, there is little reason for in-hospital stay. Discharge from the hospital also requires an appropriate out-of-hospital setting, usually home. The first recipient transferred to an outpatient setting was a 15-year-old with idiopathic cardiomyopathy who was discharged in 1990 on a console-based system to the University of Pittsburgh Medical Center "Family House."

Since 1993, with the availability of the wearable Novacor LVAS, an increasing proportion of LVAS recipients have been discharged from the hospital. This has allowed a better quality of life, reduced risk of infection, and greatly reduced financial burden to the family and to society. Typically, the recipient can be discharged home in 4 to 6 weeks post implant, with medical therapy reduced to antithrombotic management similar to that for a patient with a mechanical heart valve.

Results

The American Bridge-to-Transplant Experience

The US multicenter bridge-to-transplant study included 156 LVAS recipients (129 core, 27 noncore) and 35 controls. Core patients satisfied all the inclusion and exclusion criteria of the investigational protocol and had no missing data. While 77% of the core group LVAS recipients survived to transplant, only 37% of the control group was transplanted ($P<0.0001$). Survival to transplant for the noncore patients was 57%. Data on recipient survival are presented in Table 4, and Table 5 summarizes the core patient characteristics. Actuarial survival for the core and control groups is presented in Figure 4.

Of the 24 (23%) recipients who did not survive to transplant, half died within 30 days of device implant (operative deaths). The predominant reason for early mortality was patient-centered, and included cardiac arrhythmias, sepsis, and multiorgan failure. Late mortality (>30 days after implantation) was mainly due to sepsis (7 patients, 58%) while two patients died of multiorgan failure and two secondary to cerebrovascular events.[22] Early morbidity included bleeding and right ventricular,

Table 4
United States Premarket Approval Results

LVAS recipients, core (satisfy all entry criteria)	
# patients	129
Mean support duration (days)	80
Transplanted	81 (77%)
Died on LVAS support	24
Remaining on LVAS support	24
LVAS Recipients, noncore	
# patients	27
Transplanted	12 (57%)
Remaining on LVAS support	6
Controls	
# patients	35
Transplanted	13 (37%)

LVAS = left ventricular assist system.

Table 5

US Premarket Approval Study: Core Patient Characteristics

Number of patients	129
Age, mean (range), years	49 (16–65)
Body surface area, mean (range), m^2	1.9 (1.5–2.5)
% Male	84
Etiology of heart failure	
Nonischemic cardiomyopathy	67 (52%)
Ischemic cardiomyopathy	46 (35%)
Acute myocardial infarction	14 (11%)
Other	2 (2%)
Pre-implant balloon pump use	64%
Transfer from another hospital	55%
Diabetes	23%
Smoking history	42%
Renal disease	7%
Prior myocardial infarction	42%
Preimplant ventilatory support	23%

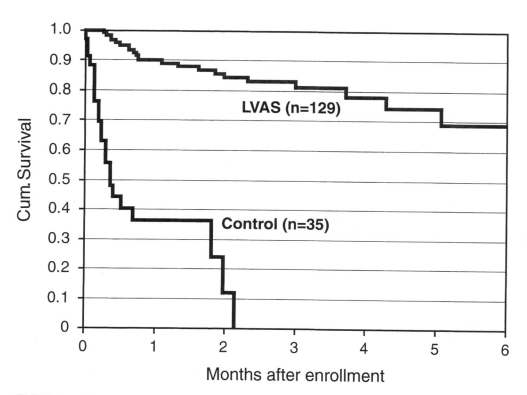

FIGURE 4. Novacor N100PC recipient survival to transplant comparison of left ventricular assist system recipients (77% transplanted) and control patients (35% transplanted), $P<0.0001$.

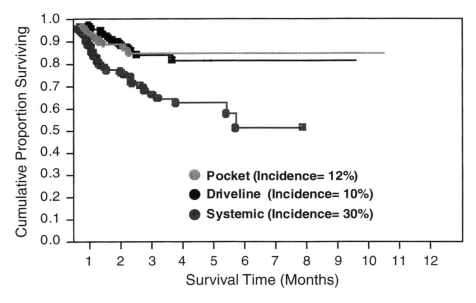

FIGURE 5. Freedom from infection (N100PC core recipients, n = 129).

renal, hepatic, and respiratory dysfunction—factors attributable to advanced heart failure exacerbated by the surgical intervention. There was a 20% incidence of postoperative management-related bleeding, a 30% incidence of systemic infection, and a 26% incidence of embolic stroke. The actuarial freedom from infection is presented in Figure 5. The impact of bacteremia on neurologic events is illustrated in Figure 6.

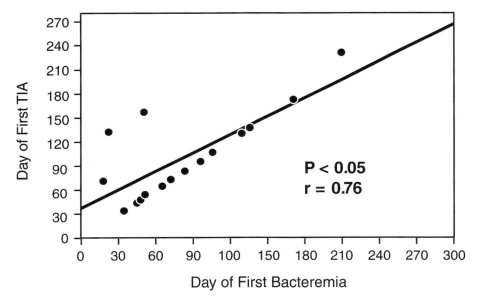

FIGURE 6. Incidence of (first) TIA, relationship to bacteremia (N100PC core recipients, n = 129).

Global Experience

Since 1984, more than 1000 (1040 to date) recipients have been supported by the Novacor LVAS in centers in the US and Europe as well as Argentina, Australia, Canada, Japan, Russia, and Taiwan. Of these, 655 (63%) have received the N100PC device. The current cohort of 88 recipients has been supported for an average duration of 254 days and 60% of these recipients are at home. The indication for implantation for the majority of the recipients (93%) has been as a bridge to transplantation. The rest were implanted as bridge to recovery or as definitive (or destination) therapy (Table 6).

Since the introduction of the N100PC wearable system in 1993, both the duration of support and the proportion of recipients discharged from the hospital have progressively increased (Fig. 7). In 1998, half of the Novacor LVAS recipients were supported for more than 6 months and 60% were discharged home. The most common reason for a recipient to stay in the hospital was the absence of adequate family support for discharge.

Recent European experience with recipients discharged for more than 1 year has been described.[23] The median hospital stay, duration of home discharge, and total LVAS support time are listed in Table 7. Four of these long-term recipients returned to work while on device support, and one went back to school. During this out-of-hospital period, nearly half (48%) were readmitted, primarily for treatment of infection (mostly percutaneous lead exit site) or for readjustment of antithrombotic therapy. There were no pump failures in this 76-year cumulative period of home discharge. While the US experience has been limited by FDA-mandated caregiver restrictions (during the investigational phase), the overall results have been similar. This increasing experience demonstrates dependable system reliability and manageable recipient morbidity in the outpatient setting.

A total of eight (0.8%) pump replacements have been carried out in an experience of more than 1000 implants and cumulative support of greater than 300 patient-years. Extensive in vitro testing has identified a single failure mode, bearing wear.[12] A reliable signature of approaching bearing failure provides adequate time (3 months) for elective device replacement. Two recipients (0.2%) required device re-

Table 6

Novacor LVAS: Global Experience

Number of recipients	1040
Application:	
Bridge to transplant	972 (93.4%)
Bridge to recovery	45 (4.3%)
Destination therapy (alternative to transplant)	23 (2.3%)
Cumulative experience	297 patient-years
Currently supported	88
Support duration, mean, days (longest)	254 (1500+)
Recipients >1 yr support	19
Out of hospital (%)	60+
Duration out of hospital (%)	85+

LVAS = left ventricular assist system.

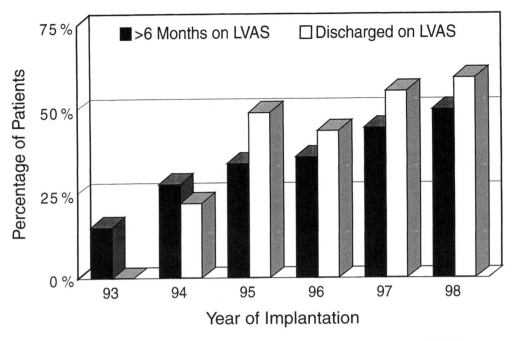

FIGURE 7. Novacor N100PC recipients, home discharge experience (global).

placement for bearing wear-out, one at 3.8 years and the other, prematurely, at 8 months. Two pump replacements were precipitated by damage to the external cable and two were secondary to patient management (perioperative connector short circuit by electrolyte immersion in one, and urine aspiration through the vent tube in the other). One pump was replaced for valvular endocarditis and one, early postoperatively (<24 hours), following an encapsulation leak. Patient outcome was unaffected in all of these device replacements.

A modified (gelatin-sealed, integrally supported, uncrimped, knitted PET) inflow cannula/conduit was introduced in 1998. By preventing distortion and improving wall shear rate, this conduit has resulted in a significant reduction (>50%) in

Table 7	
European Experience with Extended (>1 Year) Outpatient Support	
Number of recipients discharged home for >1 yr	17
Total LVAS support time, median (range)	1.6 (1.1–3.4) years
Hospital stay prior to discharge, median (range)	61 (29–150) days
Stay outside hospital, median (range)	1.4 (1.0–3.1) years
Cumulative	29.4 patient-years
% LVAS support	88

LVAS = left ventricular assist system.

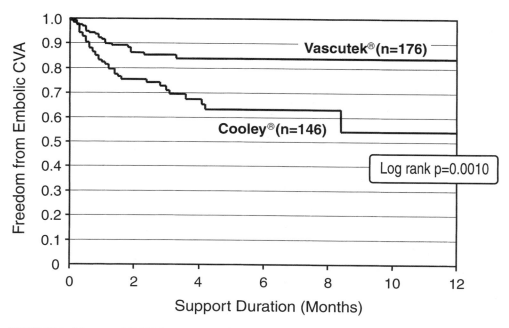

FIGURE 8. Novacor N100PC recipients, freedom from cerebral embolism (global) with Cooley® and Vascutek inflow conduits.

morbidity due to cerebral embolism.[24] The embolic stroke rate of 12% in a recent 176-recipient (43 centers, 56 patient-years) experience with this inflow conduit contrasts favorably with a prior cohort of 146 US recipients with the earlier (unsupported, crimped, woven PET) conduit, and a 26% stroke rate (odds ratio 0.39, $P = 0.001$). A comparison of actuarial freedom-from-event for these two cohorts is presented in Figure 8. Explanted conduits show a smooth, thin pseudoneointima with no distortion for the integrally supported conduit, in contrast to the creased, patchy, and loose pannus of the earlier conduit (Fig. 9). This suggests that the dominant mechanism for embolic complications has been of a particulate (pannus) rather than thrombotic origin. The majority of embolic events occur early (<30 days after implantation) with both conduit designs, and the median time for these events is similar. There is substantial intercenter variability in this and other complications,[25] suggesting variability in patient selection and management. The relationship between embolic events, infection, and early postoperative antiplatelet management has been emphasized.[21,22,26] Ongoing device refinement and aggressive treatment of infection should result in further reduction in overall morbidity as well as late mortality.

European Bridge-to-Recovery Experience

A reduction in cardiac size and improved contractility in some patients with dilated cardiomyopathy on extended LVAS support has led to the hypothesis that

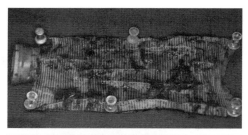

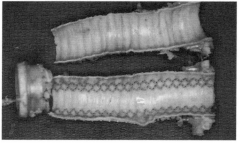

FIGURE 9. Woven uncoated polyester (top, explanted at 126 d) and gelatin-sealed PET (bottom, explained at 154 d) inflow cannula/conduits at explant.

circulatory support can cause "reverse remodeling."[27-30] Endpoints of this experience include sustained correction of the neurohormonal responses to heart failure, structural changes in myocyte function, and improvement and maintenance of cardiac contractility after device weaning and removal.[31] The optimal time required for recovery is unclear. Much of the Novacor BTR experience comes from a single center, the Deutches Hertzcentrum in Berlin.[28,32] This experience is discussed in detail in Chapter 21. The management strategy for these patients (most with idiopathic dilated cardiomyopathy) has included maximum left ventricular unloading during the early inflammatory phase together with optimized antifailure therapy. Evaluation of recovery was performed during pump-off echocardiographic studies of ventricular function. Patients were weaned and pumps removed when cardiac recovery was observed. At a duration of 6 months after weaning, 78% of the patients were alive without transplant and, at 24 months, 59% were alive without transplant. As yet,

Table 8
European Experience with Bridge to Recovery

Recipients with cardiac recovery and device explant	25 (22M, 3F)
Age, mean (range), years	40 (18–61)
Etiology of heart failure	
Cardiomyopathy	22 (88%)
Acute myocarditis	2 (8%)
Coronary artery disease	1 (4%)
LVAS support, mean (range), days	176 (30–795)
Follow-up (postexplant)	
Early mortality, <30 days	2 (8%)
Transplanted	3 (12%[1])
Postexplant survival average (range), days	625 (9–1487 +)

[1] Transplanted 45 to 216 days after explantation. LVAS = left ventricular assist device.

there are insufficient data to determine the viability of this promising therapy. Table 8 summarizes the current experience with bridge to recovery. A multicenter study protocol is under development for further prospective evaluation of bridge to recovery.

Definitive or Destination Therapy

The Novacor LVAS was developed, from the outset, as a "permanent" system for long-term, definitive (destination) therapy. More than 50 Novacor LVAS recipients have been supported for longer than 1 year (longest >4 years), most as a bridge to transplantation. The outcomes in this long-term cohort have been encouraging,[23,33]; all recipients have been discharged from the hospital and are enjoying an improved quality of life, and many have been able to return to their previous occupation. Twenty-three patients have received implants as definitive therapy. Multinational (Europe) and multicenter (US) protocols are under development for controlled studies.

Quality of Life

The measurement of health-related quality of life is becoming more important as health care providers assess treatment in terms of cost and value to patients (This

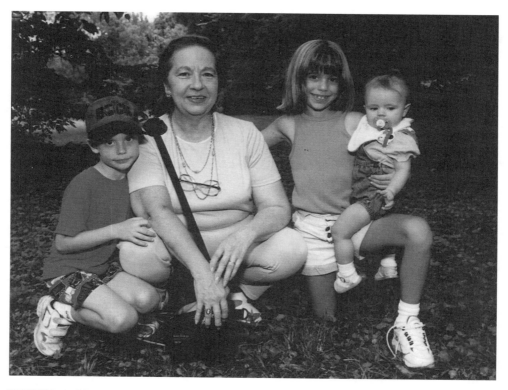

FIGURE 10. Novacor N100PC, quality of life: Novacor LVAS recipient discharged home (US).

topic is developed in Chapter 15). Quality-of-life studies in LVAS patients using the Index of Life Satisfaction Scale, report comparable high ratings between Novacor LVAS outpatients and transplant recipients at 7 months post transplant.[34] Overall, discharged LVAS patients more closely resemble transplant recipients than patients waiting for transplant. In contrast to the much poorer quality of life reported by patients awaiting transplantation, outpatient LVAS support provides relief of symptoms of heart failure (Fig. 10) and allows the recipient a choice of living arrangements.

Summary

Substantial progress has been made over the past decade with mechanical support of the failing heart. Systems have not only demonstrated short- to intermediate-term efficacy as a bridge to transplantation, but also promise as a bridge to recovery and an elective alternative to transplant. Measurements of functional capacity and physiologic parameters have shown that biochemical markers of heart failure normalize and heart failure symptoms resolve with extended support, improving exercise tolerance and allowing a return to activities of daily living. The long-term experience with the Novacor system demonstrates device reliability and safe operation for extended periods outside the hospital setting. This supports its use as definitive therapy in patients who cannot receive a transplant.

Wide intercenter variability in morbidity and mortality shows that patient selection and management are important factors in a positive outcome. The transformation of mechanical circulatory support from an emerging therapeutic option for end-stage heart failure to an established alternative to transplant can also become a reality through a multidisciplinary approach.

References

1. Portner PM, Oyer PE, Jassawalla JS, et al. An implantable permanent left ventricular assist system for man. *Trans Am Soc Artif Intern Organs* 1978;24:98–102.
2. Portner PM, Oyer PE, Jassawalla JS, et al. An alternative in end-stage heart disease: Long-term ventricular assistance. *Heart Transplant* 1983;III:47–59.
3. Portner PM, Jassawalla JS, Oyer PE, et al. A totally implantable ventricular assist system for terminal heart failure. In Kantrowitz A (ed): *ASAIO Primers in Artificial Organs: Left Ventricular Assist Devices*. Philadelphia: JB Lippincott; 1988:57–76.
4. Portner PM, Dong E Jr, Jassawalla JS, LaForge DH. Performance of an implantable controlled solenoid circulatory assist system. *Trans Am Soc Artif Intern Organs* 1973;19:235–238.
5. Portner PM, Griepp RB, Jassawalla JS, et al. An intrathoracic solenoid drive system for chronic left ventricular bypass. *Trans Am Soc Artif Intern Organs* 1976;22:297–314.
6. Ramasamy N, Phillips L, Chen H et al. Long-term in vivo evaluation of volume compensator for a left ventricular assist system. *Trans Fifteenth Ann Soc Biomaterials* 1989;12:37.
7. Ramasamy N, Chen H, Miller P, et al. Chronic ovine evaluation of a totally implantable electrical left ventricular assist system. *Trans Am Soc Artif Intern Organs* 1989;25:402–404.
8. Jassawalla JS, Daniel MA, Chen H, et al. In vitro and in vivo testing of a totally implantable left ventricular assist system. *ASAIO Trans* 1988;34:470–475.
9. Daniel MA, Lee J, LaForge D, et al. *In Vitro Testing of a Totally Implantable Left Ventricular Assist System*. Presented at the 1990 Annual ASAIO Meeting. Abstract.
10. Portner PM, Oyer PE, McGregor CGA, et al. First human use of an electrically powered implantable ventricular assist system. *Artif Organs* 1985;9(A):36.

11. Miller PJ, Billich TJ, LaForge DH, et al. Initial clinical experience with a wearable controller for the Novacor left ventricular assist system. *ASAIO J* 1994;40:M464-M470.
12. Lee J, Miller PJ, Chen H, et al. Reliability model from the in vitro durability tests of a left ventricular assist system. *ASAIO J* 1999. In press.
13. Oz MC, Goldstein DJ, Pepino P, et al. Screening scale predicts patients successfully receiving long-term implantable left ventricular assist devices. *Circulation* 1993;92 (suppl II): II169-II173.
14. Kormos RL, Murali S, Dew MA, et al. Chronic mechanical circulatory support: Rehabilitation, low morbidity, and superior survival. *Ann Thorac Surg* 1994;57:51–58.
15. Farrar DJ and Thoratec Investigators. Preoperative predictors of survival in patients with Thoratec ventricular assist devices as a bridge to heart transplantation. *J Heart Lung Transplant* 1994;13:93–101.
16. Portner PM, Oyer PE, Pennington G, et al. Implantable electrical left ventricular assist system: Bridge to transplantation and the future. *Ann Thorac Surg* 1989;47:142–150.
17. Loisance D, Cooper GJ, Deleuze PH, et al. Bridge to transplantation with the wearable Novacor left ventricular assist system: Operative technique. *Eur J Cardiothorac Surg* 1995; 9:95–98.
18. Scheld HH, Hammel D, Schmid C, et al. Beating heart implantation of a wearable Novacor left ventricular assist device. *Thorac Cardiovasc Surg* 1996;44:62–66.
19. Vigano M, Martinelli L, Minzioni G, et al. Modified method for Novacor left ventricular assist device implantation. *Ann Thorac Surg* 1996;61:247–249.
20. Kormos RL, Gasior TA, Kawai A, et al. Transplant candidate's clinical status rather than right ventricular function defines need for univentricular versus biventricular support. *J Thorac Cardiovasc Surg* 1996;111:773–783.
21. Hunt BJ, Parmar K, Jansen PGM, et al. A prospective study of haemostatic changes after implantation of the Novacor LVAS. *J Heart Lung Transplant* 1999;18:143. Abstract.
22. Kormos RL, Rasmasamy N, Sit S, et al. Bridge to transplant experience with the Novacor left ventricular assist system: Results of a multicenter US study. *J Heart Lung Transplant* 1999;18:163. Abstract.
23. Jansen PGM, Wheeldon DR, Portner PM. Long-term home discharge support with Novacor LVAS. *J Heart Lung Transplant* 1999;18(1):67. Abstract.
24. Ramasamy N, Jansen P, Wheeldon D, et al. Inflow conduit in implantable left ventricular assist device (LVAD): Influence on outcomes. *Artif Organs* 1999;23:7. Abstract.
25. El-Banayosi A, Deng M, Loisance DY, et al. The European experience of Novacor left ventricular assist (LVAS) therapy as a bridge to transplant: A retrospective multi-centre study. *Eur J Cardiothorac Surg* 1999;15:835–841.
26. Copeland JG, Arabia FA, Banchy ME, et al. The CardioWest total artificial bridge to transplantation: 1993 to 1996 National trial. *Ann Thorac Surg* 1998;66:1662–1669.
27. Dipla K, Mattiello JA, Jeevanandum V, et al. Myocyte recovery after mechanical circulatory support in humans with end-stage heart failure. *Circulation* 1998;97:2316–2322.
28. Mueller J, Wallukat G, Weng YG, et al. Weaning from mechanical cardiac support in patients with idiopathic dilated cardiomyopathy. *Circulation* 1997;96:542–549.
29. Westaby S, Jin XY, Katsumata T, et al. Mechanical support in dilated cardiomyopathy: Signs of early left ventricular recovery. *Ann Thorac Surg* 1997;64:1303–1308.
30. Frazier OH, Myers TJ, Radovancevic B. The HeartMate left ventricular assist system: Overview and 12-year experience. *Texas Heart Inst J* 1998;25:265–271.
31. Cohn JN, Bristow MR, Chien KR, et al. Report of the National Heart, Lung, and Blood Institute Special Emphasis Panel on Heart Failure Research. *Circulation* 1997;95:766–770.
32. Hetzer R, Mueller JH, Weng YG, et al. *Mid-term Follow-up of Patients Who Had LVAD Removal Following Cardiac Recovery in End-stage Dilated Cardiomyopathy.* Presented at 79th Annual American Association for Thoracic Surgery Meeting, New Orleans, LA; 1999.
33. Loisance DY, Jansen PGM, Wheeldon DW, Portner PM. *Long-term Mechanical Circulatory Support with the Wearable Novacor LVAS.* Presented at the 13th Annual Meeting European Association for Cardio-thoracic Surgery, Glasgow, Scotland; 1999.
34. Dew MA, Kormos RL, Winowich S, et al. Quality of life outcomes in left ventricular assist system: Inpatients and outpatients. *ASAIO J* 1999;45:218–225.

Chapter 25

Intracorporeal Support:

The CardioWest Total Artificial Heart

Jack Copeland, MD, Francisco Arabia, MD, Richard Smith, MSEE, and Paul Nolan, PhD

Introduction

The total artificial heart (TAH), now known as the CardioWest TAH, was the product of the pioneering work of Dr. Willem Kolff at the University of Utah. The device made its clinical debut in the early 1980s as a permanent device,[1] the Jarvik-7 TAH. In the ensuing years, it was used successfully as the Symbion TAH.[2–4] Despite documented safety and efficacy, regulatory issues led to the loss of its investigational device exemption in January of 1991. Subsequently, all implants were halted in the United States and were markedly reduced in Europe.

Because of our strong belief in the merits of the device as a short-term bridge to transplant and as a longer term circulatory support device, a new investigational device exemption study was begun in 1993 and a multicenter trial was undertaken.[5] In this chapter, we describe the CardioWest TAH device, outline the implantation technique, review the indications and limitations of the device, and examine the results of the recently completed clinical trials.

Device Description

The CardioWest TAH is a pneumatic biventricular pulsatile pump that is implanted in the orthotopic position. It consists of two ventricles connected to the respective native atria and greater vessels. An air hose or drive line covered with double velour material passes from each ventricle transcutaneously to a console that

From Goldstein DJ and Oz MC (eds). *Cardiac Assist Devices*. Armonk, NY: Futura Publishing Co., Inc.; ©2000.

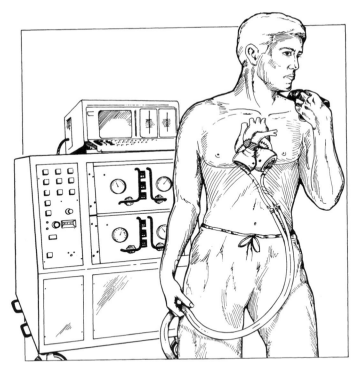

FIGURE 1. Schematic illustration depicting the position and relative size of the CardioWest TAH and its console.

pulses pressurized air and monitors pump function (Fig. 1). The maximal blood volume of the ventricular chamber is 70 mL. The two ventricles and adjacent intraventricular space displace a total of 1500 mL.

Cardiac outputs with the CardioWest TAH generally run in the 6 to 8 L/min range. Blood returning to the heart enters the native atria and passes across an inflow ''quick-connect'' cuff that has been anastomosed to the atrium at the level of the atrioventricular valve annulus. This cuff attaches to the rigid pump housing via a 27 mm Medtronic-Hall inflow valve, allowing the blood to enter a spherical polyurethane chamber. One half of the chamber lining is immobile, anchored to the chamber wall, while the other half is a mobile four-layered polyurethane diaphragm. A steel reinforced drive line exits from this latter half of the ventricle. Pulses of air pressure from the console, delivered via the drive line, push the diaphragm and thus the blood through a 25 mm Medtronic-Hall valve into an outflow Dacron™ graft anastomosed to a great vessel (Figs. 2 and 3). Once the device is implanted and de-aired, cardiopulmonary bypass is discontinued, allowing the device to fully support the circulation. Initially, a central venous pressure of 15 mm Hg is helpful in obtaining adequate device filling. Later, when the chest is closed, vacuum (-10 to 15 cm H_2O) is added to the device in diastole, resulting in improved ventricular filling at lower venous pressures.

The systolic pressure controls are set 30 to 40 mm Hg higher than current or anticipated great vessel systolic pressures. This provides a margin of safety in case

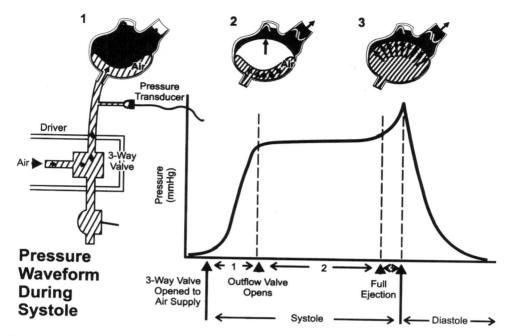

Pressure Waveform During Systole

FIGURE 2. Pressure waveform during systole. During systole, there is a progressive rise in pressure until the valve opens as indicated by phase 1. After the valve opens, air enters on the diaphragm side driving blood out the outflow valve. The diaphragm then reaches its maximal excursion and there is an isovolumic peak of pressure indicated by phase 3 and the peak at the end of the pressure wave. The outflow valve then closes and diastole begins.

of sudden increases in systemic and/or pulmonary vascular resistance. The laptop computer on the console continuously displays systemic and pulmonary pressure curves for the pulses of air delivered to the ventricles, such as the curve shown in Figure 2. As a ventricle fills with a systolic pulse of pressurized air and the diaphragm moves to maximal excursion, the ventricle is emptied ("full eject"). The pressure curve generated by this pneumatically systole rises rapidly (dp/dt is approximately 4000 mm Hg/sec on the left side, and 2000 mm Hg/sec on the right side) as displayed in Figure 2 (phase 1 of systole). During the plateau phase (Fig. 2, phase 2 of systole), blood is ejected as a result of the movement of the diaphragm. A peak at the end of the pressure curve represents an isovolumic pressure rise after full excursion of the diaphragm (full ejection of the ventricle). If the systolic pressure control on the console is dialed down to the point that the full ejection peak disappears, the device pressure will approximate the patient's systolic pressure. If the systolic pressure on the device is reduced further, cardiac output falls and venous pressure rises.

The basic concept of running the CardioWest TAH may be simply stated: "Never full fill, always full eject." Indeed, full ejection is necessary to provide optimal flow and adequate end organ perfusion. Full displacement of the diaphragm with each beat in addition prevents blood stasis within the device, hence decreasing the possibility of thrombus formation. To ensure full ejection, the console is set to a pressure of 30 to 40 mm Hg higher than the great vessel pressure. Seldom is it necessary to manipulate the pressure controls after initial stability has been attained.

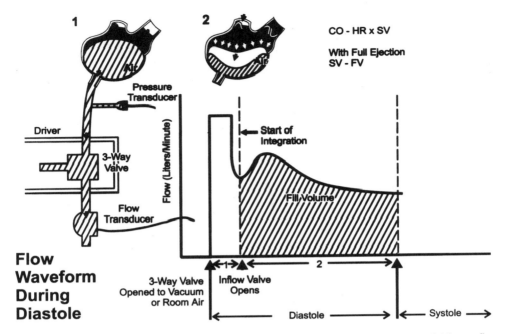

FIGURE 3. Flow waveform during diastole. There is an initial peak during which no flow occurs, indicated by phase 1. The inflow valve opens at the onset of phase 2 and flow, in liters per minute, is traced. The computer calculates the area under the flow curve that is equal to the volume.

The "never full fill" part of our philosophy is based on Starling curve physiology and is accomplished with the aid of three other settings: heart rate, percent systole, and vacuum. Figure 3 shows the "cushion of air" on the air side of the diaphragm during diastole (represented by the second drawing of the ventricle). By providing this space for additional filling that is not used while the patient is stable, the venous return may increase, resulting in a higher stroke volume. For example, during exercise, cardiac output can increase without the need to change console settings. This "reservoir" acts to receive increasing venous return provided it is not fully filled. Hence, as long as volume overload is avoided, the device can act along a Starling curve with venous return translated into increased cardiac output.

The fill volume display on the console laptop computer is derived from pneumo-tachometers that measure the flow of air out of the ventricles. A curve such as that shown in Figure 3 is continuously generated for each ventricle. The initial part of the curve represents flow prior to opening of the inflow valve (indicated by 1). The inflow valve opens early in diastole. The computer measures the area under the flow curve during diastole which equals the stroke volume of the ventricle. This number multiplied by the heart rate provides the device cardiac output, which is also displayed continuously for both ventricles.

Full filling on the type of display shown in Figure 3 is represented by an abrupt mid-diastolic drop of flow rate to zero, which corresponds to a volume in mL equal to the capacity of the ventricle. The CardioWest ventricles are 70 mL in volume, and full fill volumes are slightly lower than this amount.

In cases of excess volume as indicated by full filling, increasing the device pulsation rate can be very helpful. The cardiac output increases, the ventricles cease filling fully, and the central venous pressure drops. Assuming a heart rate of 150 bpm and a fill volume of 60 mL, a 9 L/min output can be obtained without full filling. In practice, efforts are made to maintain the heart rate below 130 to 140 bpm because of the tendency for hemolysis at higher heart rates. Commonly, we maintain cardiac outputs in the 6 to 8 L/min range.

Further fine tuning can be achieved by manipulation of the percent systole control setting. As the name suggests, it controls the amount of time that the device cardiac cycle will occupy with systole. Thus, if the percent systole is set at 45%, systole will occupy 45% and diastole will occupy 55%. Changes in this parameter can be used to optimize filling time of the ventricle. In the presence of full filling, the percent systole can be lengthened; this will lead to a reduction in filling (diastolic) time, thereby preventing full filling. Naturally, this strategy can reduce cardiac output and increase central venous pressure, but it might be helpful in a normovolemic patient. The percent systole control is most valuable in the patient with low filling volumes and a relatively fast heart rate, in whom a shortening in the percent systole will result in increased diastolic filling and improved cardiac output. Finally, the vacuum control provides a third method to influence ventricular filling; by increasing negative diastolic pressure, filling can be increased.

Intravascular volume status is of paramount importance in patients with this device. A central venous pressure of 6 to 14 mm Hg is most often observed with the following settings: heart rate of 120 to 140 bpm, percent systole 45%, and vacuum -10 cm H_2O. Following the "never full fill" dictum from the outset, and in the absence of dramatic changes in intravascular volume, we have found little need to make console control changes over long periods.

Our policy for post-implant patients includes the removal of all intravascular lines within 7 to 10 days of implantation. This goal is often achieved because the console provides continuous real-time parameters that allow assessment of ventricular filling, namely, fill volume and fill pressure curves, digital stroke volume readouts, ventricular outputs, as well as trends that plot ventricular outputs over time.

Anticoagulation is instituted as follows. Aspirin (81 mg daily) and dipyridamole (Persantine, Boehringer Ingelheim Pharm. Inc., Ridgefield, CT) (100 mg every 6 hours) are started 6 hours after implantation. Heparin (500 U/h) is begun once the chest tube output has dropped to 10 mL/h, and is adjusted to maintain the partial thromboplastin time in the 40- to 50-second range. Once the patient can tolerate oral medications, warfarin is administered with a goal of obtaining an international normalized ratio (INR) of 2.5 to 3.5, and a significant prolongation of the "r" phase of the thromboelastogram. This endpoint is often lower in the early postoperative period because of coexisting thrombocytopenia and hypocoagulable state. In addition, pentoxyphilline (Trental, Hoechst Marion Roussel Inc., Kansas City, MO) (400 mg three times a day) is begun at this time.

Commonly, by the second or third postoperative day, the TAH recipient is off heparin and receiving aspirin, warfarin, Persantine, and Trental. INR, platelet count, bleeding time, platelet aggregation studies, and thromboelastogram are routinely checked. As a rule, we administer 325 mg of aspirin for each 100,000 platelets (up to 3 aspirins per day). If more antiplatelet effect is desired, clopidogrel (Plavix, Sanofi Winthrop Pharmaceuticals, New York, NY and Bristol Myers Squibb, Princeton, NJ) (75 mg daily) is added. Bleeding time is kept at 15 to 20 minutes (upper normal is

10 minutes), and efforts are taken to decease in vitro platelet response to epinephrine, adenosine diphosphate, and arachidonic acid while maintaining normal responsiveness to collagen. The thromboelastogram is used as an overall assessment of coagulation and platelet function: the "r" component is used as a guide for anticoagulant effect with heparin or coumadin; the "MA" component is used as an estimate of platelet function and interaction with fibrinogen; the TPI (thrombodynamic potential index) is employed as a guide to the patient's coagulability. Patients are maintained in the normocoagulable range represented by a TPI of 5 to 15. A typical adult male chronically receives coumadin 5 to 8 mg daily, aspirin 650 to 975 mg daily, Persantine 1600 mg daily, and Trental 1200 mg daily.

Once the patient is stable, phlebotomies and bleeding times are reduced to twice per week. All blood testing is performed with "micro" techniques, minimizing the amount of blood needed. In the presence of local or systemic infection, the patients are rendered more hypercoagulable and, hence, we monitor infected patients more frequently.

Implantation Technique

The primary goals of implantation are perfect hemostasis and excellent fit.[6] The latter requires more planning, experience, and care. Proper fitting is less dependent on technique than it is on choosing a recipient with adequate intrathoracic space to accommodate the TAH.

Fitting criteria guidelines are presented in Table 1. Most normal sized adult males and many adult females with dilated cardiomyopathies have adequate space to receive a CardioWest TAH. Not all of the listed criteria need to be met. For instance, patients with ischemic cardiomyopathy and slight cardiac enlargements can be fitted with the device if they have a large anteroposterior chest dimension. Patients with body surface area less than 1.7 m², thin chests, or near normal cardiac silhouette are at increased risk of "fit problems" such as inferior vena cava or left pulmonary vein compression.

Having chosen a suitable candidate, the implantation goal of perfect hemostasis is attainable in most instances. The patient's chest should not be closed until the operative field is dry. Perioperative bleeding and mediastinal hematomas may not only cause atrial cuff tamponade, but may also lead to mediastinal infection, sepsis, hypercoagulability, and eventual stroke.[7]

An important adjunct to the surgical technique is the inhibition of fibrinolysis.[8,9]

Table 1

Fitting Criteria Guidelines for Placement of the CardioWest TAH

Body surface area ≥1.7 m²
Cardiothoracic ratio >0.5
Left ventricular diastolic dimension >66 mm
Anteroposterior distance (sternum to T-10, on CT scan) >10 cm
Combined ventricular volume (on CT scan) >1500 mL

CT = computed tomography; TAH = total artificial heart.

We originally used the serine protease inhibitor aprotinin (Trasylol, Bayer Corporation, West Haven, CT) at device implantation. While excellent hemostasis was achieved, several profound anaphylactic reactions were observed during readministration of Trasylol at the time of transplantation. Hence, we now employ the plasminogen inhibitor epsilon-aminocaproic acid (Amicar, Immunex Corp., Seattle, WA) in high doses (100 mg/kg bolus followed by 60 mg/kg/h infusion for 4 hours, rarely exceeding a total dose of 30 g) at implant and reserve Trasylol (not exceeding 6 million units) for the subsequent transplant procedure.

In brief, the technique involves creating atrial and great vessel anastomoses that will not leak. Equally important is mastering the "quick connectors" and realizing that the orientation created by coupling the quick connectors determines the final position of the ventricles.

Prior to the incision, we cut the atrial connectors to size. We always cut these in circular fashion, approximately 6 mm from the connector (Fig. 4). Next, a median sternotomy is performed with care not to enter the pleural spaces, since adhesions from the lung to the device must be avoided. The drive lines are then tunneled to the left epigastrium, with care taken to keep them at least 5 cm apart. To facilitate passage, the tunnel is dilated with Heggar dilators followed by a pull through with a 2" Penrose drain; the inside of the drive line is kept completely dry. At least 3 to 4 cm of Dacron-covered drive line should lie outside the skin. The ventricles are then covered with a sterile towel outside the wound to the left of the retractor.

The heart is prepared for total bypass. Prior to heparinization, blood is aspirated from the right atrium for preclotting the outflow conduits. After preclotting three times using 60 mL per aspiration, the grafts are stretched and left covered to dry.

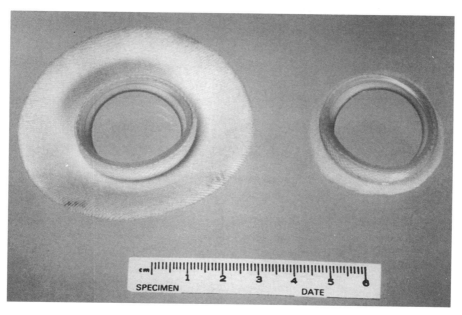

FIGURE 4. Atrial quick connectors. On the left is the atrial quick connector as it is removed from the package. On the right, the connector has been cut and readied for implantation leaving a 5 to 6 mm cuff.

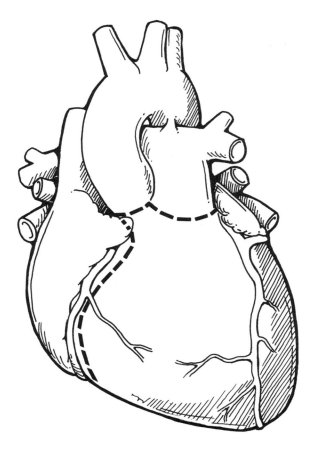

FIGURE 5. Cardiectomy. Dotted lines indicate the approximate sites of incision for removal of native ventricles.

Care is taken to ensure the absence of debris within the grafts' lumen. Cardiopulmonary bypass with bicaval cannulation is instituted, electrical fibrillation is induced, and aortic cross-clamping is performed. The principles of cardiectomy are to obtain maximal great vessel length by transecting the vessels at the sinotubular junction. The line of excision for the ventricles starts on the ventricular side of the atrioventricular groove (Fig. 5). Ventricular tissue is then trimmed away to create atrial cuffs at the level of the atrioventricular annuli. Valve leaflets are removed, leaving a 1 to 2 mm rim of valvular tissue to strengthen the anastomoses.

Further preparations include oversewing the coronary sinus inside the right atrium (large needle 4–0 polypropylene suture) and mobilization of the proximal ends of the great vessels for approximately 2 to 3 cm. Next, the circumference of the atrial cuffs is buttressed with strips of Teflon felt (Fig. 6). This maneuver strengthens the quick connector anastomosis, preventing bleeding from the cut edge of the very vascular atrioventricular groove. To complete this step, several Teflon felt strips (1 cm × 15 cm) are cut, and a running stitch of 3–0 polypropylene (large MH needle) secures the strips to the outer wall of the atrial cuffs while obliterating the entire raw surface of the atrioventricular groove.

Subsequently, the atrial quick connector anastomoses are created. The left atrial quick connector is anastomosed first. The connector is inverted before the anastomo-

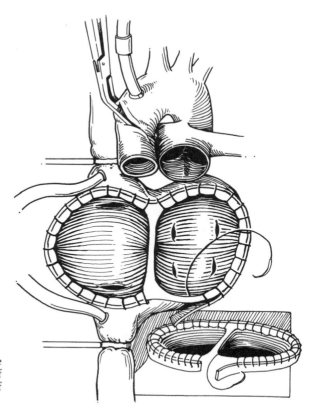

FIGURE 6. Strips of Teflon are whipped-stitched to the outside of the atrial cuff prior to placement of quick connectors.

ses are begun. We use 3–0 polypropylene suture with a large needle and take small bites to tailor the smaller connector to the larger atrium (Fig. 7). The atrial septum is sutured twice, once from the suture line of each connector. After completion of both atrial connector anastomoses, the ventricles are momentarily placed in the chest to determine the length of outflow graft needed for each ventricle. The lengths required are usually 3 to 5 cm for the left outflow and 5 to 6 cm for the right. A simple end-to-end anastomosis for each great vessel is made with 4–0 polypropylene suture (Fig. 8). At this point, we check for anastomotic leaks with "testers," plastic fittings for the atrial and outflow connectors. After we attach the tester to the quick connector in question, we inject saline under pressure to detect leaks in the anastomosis. Suture closure and rechecking follows.

Next, the ventricles are connected. First, the atrial connector of the left ventricle is snapped on to the left atrial quick connector (Fig. 9). This is done after careful assessment of the optimal position for the ventricle. A fairly posterior position for the left ventricular outflow valve keeps it out of the path for the right ventricular outflow graft. One of the advantages of the quick connectors is that repositioning is easy, provided it is done at this time. The ventricle is then filled with saline and the aortic connection is made. A similar approach is made with the right ventricle, connecting the atrium first and the outflow conduit later. De-airing the right side is easy and consists of removing the caval tapes just before connecting the outflow conduit. The appearance at completion of implantation is depicted in Figure 10.

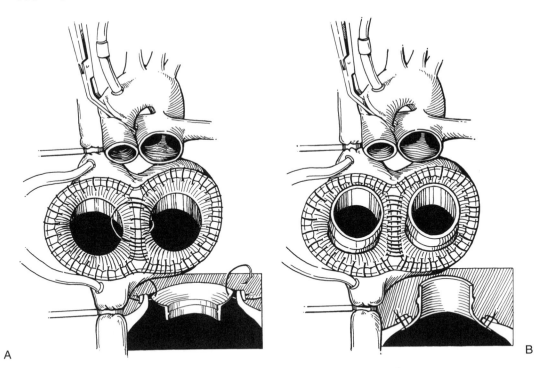

A

B

FIGURE 7. The quick connectors are now sewn in place.

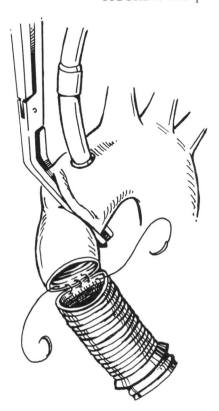

FIGURE 8. Great vessel anastomosis to outflow conduits is performed.

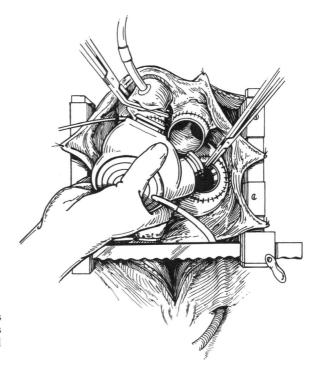

FIGURE 9. After all anastomoses are completed, the left ventricle is placed first by attaching the atrial connector.

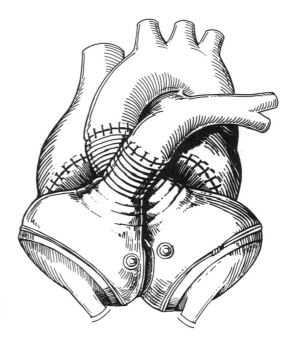

FIGURE 10. Appearance after completion of the implantation of the CardioWest TAH.

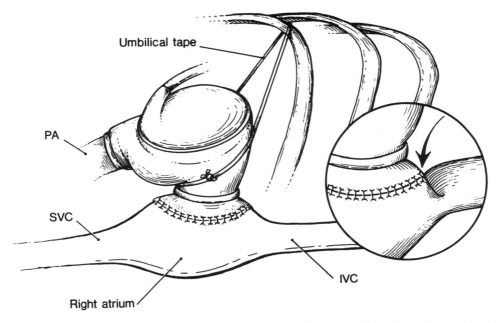

FIGURE 11. Decompression of the inferior vena cava can be accomplished by right ventriculo-pexy to the anterior chest wall using umbilical tape or heavy suture attached to the body of the right ventricle or the rigid part of the air tubing.

De-airing is performed with the patient in the deep Trendelenburg position. The ascending aorta is vented, the aortic cross-clamp is removed, the caval tapes are removed, and console pumping is started immediately, but at a slow rate. Mechanical ventilation is restarted and rapid transfer from cardiopulmonary bypass to CardioWest support is performed. De-airing is continued until all vestiges of air by transesophageal echocardiography are gone.

Following protamine administration and return of the patient to the flat supine position, meticulous examination for surgical hemostasis is undertaken. Under echo-cardiographic guidance, the TAH is positioned with great care to avoid any gradients at the inferior vena cava or left pulmonary veins with the chest closed. Trial closures are made before a final position is chosen. Before the sternum, is closed, a Goretex membrane is sewn to the edge of the pericardium, completely covering the device and facilitating reentry into the anterior mediastinum.

Maneuvers that facilitate positioning include changes in the intrathoracic drive line length, use of the Velcro connection between the two ventricles, and, if necessary, ventriculopexy to the chest wall using either the body of the right ventricle (Fig. 11) or the drive line take-off to move the ventricle anterior and leftward.

Indications for TAH Support

In our opinion, the CardioWest TAH is the device of choice for bridge to trans-plantation in patients with rapid decompensation involving biventricular failure that

Table 2

Characteristics of 24 Patients Undergoing
CardioWest TAH Implantation at the
University of Arizona Health Science Center

NYHA Class IV
Mean inotropic support:
   Dopamine 6.4 μg/kg/min
   Dobutamine 16 μg/kg/min
   Epinephrine 0.4 μg/kg/min
Central venous pressure 19 ± 6 mm Hg
Pulmonary vascular resistance 2.53 Woods units
Serum creatinine 1.4 mg/dL
Total bilirubin 1.9 ± 1.2 mg/dL

NYHA = New York Heart Association; TAH = total artificial heart.

is unresponsive to maximal medical therapy.[5] As emphasized previously, only appropriately sized patients can receive the device (Table 1). In our experience[10] with 24 patients (mean age 46 years, 83% male), all were functional Class IV and inotrope-dependent (Table 2). Two patients underwent TAH implantation in the operating room after failure to wean from cardiopulmonary bypass at the time of primary operation. Two patients had pre-implantation extracorporeal membrane oxygenation. Four patients had pre-implantation cardiac arrests. Eleven patients were ventilator-dependent and two were receiving intra-aortic balloon pump support prior to implantation.

Availability and clinical experience with the Novacor LVAS (Baxter Healthcare Corp., Oakland, CA) and Thoratec BiVAD (Thoratec Laboratories, Berkeley, CA) systems at our institution has given us a better perspective on the optimal indications and clinical scenarios for placement of the TAH. We use the device in patients who are less than 67 years of age who meet the size criteria previously outlined and who are deemed to be suitable transplant candidates. In addition, patients must have hemodynamic and clinical signs of significant right heart failure. Patients may have pulmonary edema, elevated pulmonary vascular resistance, elevated serum creatinine without need for dialysis, and hepatic failure with bilirubin as high as 6 mg/dL, as long as the etiology is felt to be passive hepatic congestion. Large patients and those who need a high cardiac output (in the 8 L/min range) because of vasoplegic conditions are likely to attain equivalent outputs with the TAH. Rapidly decompensating patients usually respond well. Arrhythmias are not a problem, and rarely do we need to institute inotropic therapy other than renal dose dopamine. Most anuric patients have return of normal renal function following TAH implantation.

Limitations

The major disappointing limitation of this device is that it does not fit into all patients. Until future smaller ventricles are available, the stringent sizing guidelines must be followed carefully. Furthermore, at the time of implant, transesophageal echocardiography and great care and patience must be exercised to attain a perfect lie during chest closure.

Because of the need for strict anticoagulation regimens post implantation, patients with contraindications to systemic anticoagulation cannot be considered candidates for TAH placement.

At this time, patients are tethered to a large console (Fig. 1) that requires special care, including pressurized air outlets and air tanks. Battery power and air tanks can provide 2 hours of out-of-room time for walks and exercise. Until a portable driver becomes available (one is nearly ready for trials), out-of-hospital existence is not practical.

Clinical Results and Outcomes

Results of the national trial of the CardioWest TAH have recently been published.[5] Four centers contributed 27 implants and 18 matched retrospective controls. There were 1411 implant-days with an average of 52 ± 42 days of support (range 12 to 186 days). Twenty-five (93%) patients underwent heart transplantation, and 24 (89%) were discharged home with survivals extending up to 5 years. In the control group, 10 patients (56%) died while awaiting transplantation, 8 (44%) were transplanted, and 7 were discharged with 6 (33% of total) long-term survivors. Survival of TAH recipients was significantly greater ($P<0.00001$) than that of controls.

All 27 implanted patients had at least one adverse event (median 5 events per patient; range 1 to 22). Most adverse events were not device-related and most (59%) occurred within the first 2 weeks following implantation. "Serious" adverse events were defined as those contributing to or causing death or delaying transplantation. Of a total of 175 adverse events, only 13 were deemed to be serious. The most common sources of morbidity were infection (nearly 90% of patients had an infection but only in 10% was it considered serious), reoperation (31 procedures including eight chest reexplorations), bleeding (10 events), hepatic dysfunction, and renal insufficiency. No serious neurologic events occurred; nonserious events included 9 transient ischemic attacks, 3 seizures, 2 episodes of impaired state of consciousness secondary to anoxia or metabolic derangement, 1 retinal hemorrhage, 1 retinal embolus, and 1 cerebrovascular accident. The latter occurred in the perioperative period and consisted of a hemiplegia that resolved in 3 months. The linearized rate for stroke was 0.97% per patient-year and the linear rate for all emboli was 12.7%. None of the thromboembolic events affected clinical outcome.

Two patients died during TAH support. One patient succumbed to sepsis and multisystem organ failure after 21 days of support. The second death occurred on the 124th post-implant day secondary to device failure from diaphragmatic rupture. Twenty-five of 27 (89%) patients survived to discharge.

Internationally, as of June 1998, there were 114 implants with a 69% transplantation rate and a 92% discharge rate for transplanted patients.[11,12] The international experience differs from that in the US in that the percentage of patients surviving to transplant is lower, presumably due to less stringent selection criteria. However, the survival rate after transplantation for both the national and international cohorts exceeds the reported survival after primary heart transplantation in the International Registry. This strongly suggests that the CardioWest allows selected dying patients to survive and to become superior candidates for transplantation.

The clinical results have been dramatic, converting unstable dying patients into stable convalescing TAH recipients. By the end of the first week, patients begin cardiac rehabilitation. They care for themselves, walk within the confines of the hospital campus, and exercise daily. They become more independent from hospital staff in a 2-room apartment with cooking facilities. Tethered by 8' drive lines to a large console on wheels, however, they cannot leave the hospital. A portable console, slightly larger than a shoe box, is nearly ready for clinical trials and should significantly improve the quality of life of future TAH recipients.

References

1. Devries WC, Anderson JH, Joyce LD, et al. Clinical use of the total artificial heart. *N Engl J Med* 1984;310:273–278.
2. Johnson KE, Prieto M, Joyce LD, et al. Summary of the clinical use of the Symbion total artificial heart: A registry report. *J Heart Lung Transplant* 1992;11:103–116.
3. Cabrol C, Gandjbakhch I, Pavie A, et al. Total artificial heart as a bridge to transplantation: La Pitie 1986 to 1987. *J Heart Transplant* 1988;7:12–17.
4. Copeland JG, Smith R, Icenogle TB, et al. Orthotopic total artificial heart bridge to transplantation: Preliminary results. *J Heart Transplant* 1989;104:569–578.
5. Copeland JG, Arabia FA, Banchy ME, et al. The CardioWest total artificial heart bridge to transplantation: 1993 to 1996 national trial. *Ann Thorac Surg* 1998;66:1662–1669.
6. Arabia FA, Copeland JG, Pavie A, Smith RG. Implantation technique for the CardioWest total artificial heart. *Ann Thorac Surg* 1999;68:698–704.
7. Arabia FA, Copeland JG, Smith RG, et al. Infections with the CardioWest total artificial heart. *ASAIO J* 1998;44:M336-M339.
8. Copeland JG. Aprotinin and the artificial heart. In Pifare R (ed): *Blood Conservation with Aprotinin*. Philadelphia: Hanley & Belfus; 1995:325–330.
9. Szefner J, Cabrol C. Control and treatment of hemostasis in patients with a total artificial heart: The experience at La Pitie. In Pifare R (ed): *Anticoagulation, Hemostasis, and Blood Preservation in Cardiovascular Surgery*. Philadelphia: Hanley & Belfus; 1993:237–264.
10. Copeland JG, Arabia FA, Smith RG, et al. Arizona experience with CardioWest Total Artificial Heart bridge to transplantation. *Ann Thorac Surg* 1999;68:756–760.
11. Arabia FA, Copeland JG, Smith RG, et al. International experience with the CardioWest total artificial heart as a bridge to heart transplantation. *Eur J Cardiothorac Surg* 1997; 11(suppl):S5-S10.
12. Copeland JG, Pavie A, Duveau D, et al. Bridge to transplantation with the CardioWest total artificial heart: The international experience 1993 to 1995. *J Heart Lung Transplant* 1996;15:94–99.

Part III

Future Devices

Chapter 26

Axial Flow Pumps

Joseph J. DeRose, Jr., MD and Robert K. Jarvik, MD

Introduction

The encouraging results with pulsatile outpatient left ventricular assist devices (LVADs)[1–3] have led to the development of smaller and more compact support systems. The existing long-term implantable systems are presently too large for patients with a body surface area less than 1.5 m^2, rendering them unsuitable for children and most small adults. Moreover, implantation of present long-term devices remains plagued by perioperative bleeding complications, and device explantation at the time of transplant is technically cumbersome.

Axial blood flow pumps that will overcome the size constraints imposed by present pulsatile systems are currently under development. These devices are simple in design with few moving parts, small blood contacting surfaces, and no valves. Ease of insertion promises to obviate the technical problems of device explantation. Although several devices are presently in the developmental stage, the Jarvik 2000® axial flow impeller pump (Jarvik Heart Inc., New York, NY), the United States Surgical axial flow cannula pump, the Nimbus/University of Pittsburgh (UOP) axial flow system, and the DeBakey/NASA axial flow pump are the four devices that are closest to clinical application.

Pulsatile versus Nonpulsatile Flow

Cardiopulmonary Bypass

Circulatory support using cardiopulmonary bypass (CPB) has been the most readily available setting for the evaluation of the physiologic effects of nonpulsatile flow. Nonpulsatile flow during CPB is associated with progressive arterial vasoconstriction, increased cardiac afterload, and reduced visceral perfusion.[4,5] A decrease in carotid baroreceptor discharge has been proposed as a possible mechanism for

From Goldstein DJ and Oz MC (eds). *Cardiac Assist Devices*. Armonk, NY: Futura Publishing Co., Inc.; ©2000.

the observed vasoconstriction in the setting of nonpulsatile bypass.[6] Studies have shown a partial improvement in the neurohumoral reflexes elicited by baroreceptor discharge when pulsatile CPB is compared to nonpulsatile CPB.[6] A loss of pulsatile flow in the renal arteries during CPB increases renin release, and subsequent angiotensin II-induced vasoconstriction provides another mechanism for vasoconstriction.[7,8] Reductions in platelet-derived thromboxane A_2[9] and an increase in endothelial production of nitric oxide[10] have also been noted when pulsatile CPB is compared with nonpulsatile CPB.

The well documented peripheral vasoconstriction observed during nonpulsatile CPB results in reduced tissue perfusion and potential end organ damage. Animal studies have provided evidence that nonpulsatile systems result in a state of abnormal function of the hypothalamic-pituitary-adrenal axis.[11] The anterior pituitary remains unresponsive to thyrotrophin-releasing hormone and adrenocorticopic hormone during CPB and this effect is reversed within 30 minutes of the termination of CPB.[11,12] Comparable results have been reported in relation to the posterior pituitary and its secretion of vasopressin.[13] Liver dysfunction, ischemic pancreatitis, and reductions in gastric pH also appear to be blunted when pulsatile CPB systems are compared with nonpulsatile systems.[14–16] However, although measurable changes in organ perfusion can be demonstrated in nonpulsatile CPB, gross clinical organ function remains intact and capable of sustaining homeostasis. A prospective randomized study of patients undergoing bypass grafting comparing pulsatile and nonpulsatile perfusion demonstrated no significant differences in cell counts, cytokine milieu, or hemodynamics.[17]

Ventricular Assist Systems

Bioengineering considerations make nonpulsatile flow pumps much more attractive than pulsatile systems. The need for moving flexible diaphragms, unidirectional valves, and seams for the valves to connect to the pump housing increases the risk of altered pump function, thrombosis, and component failure with pulsatile pumps. A single moving part is all that is necessary to provide nonpulsatile flow. The potential for enhanced durability of nonpulsatile support devices is an attractive feature when considering them for chronic circulatory support. Furthermore, the compact design, ease of insertion, and lower energy requirements of these systems pose significant advantages over pulsatile assist systems.

Given these bioengineering advantages, an understanding of the chronic effects of nonpulsatile flow remains critically important. Experiments comparing pulsatile and nonpulsatile CPB are difficult to apply to acute and chronic ventricular assist device support. The limitation of the CPB data is related to coexisting factors including systemic hypothermia, bypassing of the pulmonary circulation, extracorporeal oxygenation, the concomitant administration of anesthetic agents, and the use of CPB for short-term circulatory support.

More recent animal data suggest that complete circulatory support with nonpulsatile devices is associated with minimal clinical alterations in end organ function.[17–19] Early work with prolonged centrifugal pump support revealed that a period of adaptation to nonpulsatile flow occurs. Exaggerated levels of catecholamines, fluid overload, electrolyte imbalance, and anemia which occurs over the first week of support normalizes over the ensuing 2 months of chronic support.[20] Further laboratory studies have documented that chronic centrifugal left ventricular support does not affect cerebral blood flow,[21] cerebral autoregulation,[22] pulmonary function,[23] oxygen transport and use,[24] and autonomic nerve reflex control.[25] Despite reductions in cortical renal blood flow during acute left ventricular nonpulsatile assistance, no change in renal function has been clinically demonstrated in these experimental models.[26] Moreover, long-term support with axial flow pumps in various animal models has failed to demonstrate significant clinical, biochemical, or microscopic end organ damage for up to 6 months of nonpulsatile support.[27,28]

Myocardial Unloading with Axial Flow Support

The advantages of left ventricular bypass have been demonstrated in the setting of CPB, and include marked reductions in myocardial oxygen consumption and left ventricular work.[29,30] Pierce et al[29] showed that significant reductions in myocardial oxygen demand are achieved only when complete left ventricular unloading occurs during nonpulsatile left ventricle-to-aortic bypass. Similar findings have been obtained in studies of left heart unloading with axial flow pump assist devices.[31,32] Both pressure and volume unloading are most profound in the failing ventricle. Figure 1 demonstrates the reduction in the pressure rate product (pressure unloading) and the left ventricular external work (volume unloading) with increasing pump speed under both normal and (β-blocked conditions. In the completely unloaded state, a 15% to 20% reduction in myocardial oxygen consumption is achieved (Fig. 2). Furthermore, an increase in mean aortic pressure and a concomitant decrease in left ventricular end-diastolic pressure results in an increase in coronary perfusion pressure. Such unloading establishes a favorable hemodynamic and physiologic milieu for left ventricular recovery.

Jarvik 2000 Axial Flow Pump

Device Description

The Jarvik 2000 ventricular assist system is an axial flow impeller pump under development through a collaboration of the Texas Heart Institute, the Oxford Heart Center, and Transicoil Inc. (Valley Forge, PA). It measures 2.5 cm in diameter and 5.5 cm in length with a weight of 85 g and a displacement volume of 25 mL (Fig. 3). A pediatric model is also under design that is one fifth the size of the larger model and weighs 18 g with a displacement volume of 5 mL.

The pump's only moving part is the rotor, which is housed in a titanium casing and is supported by ceramic bearings that are immersed in the bloodstream. The impeller is powered by an electromagnetic field across the motor air gap through which the blood flows. Power is delivered by a small percutaneous cable and is regulated by a brushless direct-current motor that determines motor speed. The present adult size design operates at fixed rate motor speeds that are determined by the controller (8000 to 12,000 rpm). Designs for a permanently implantable human

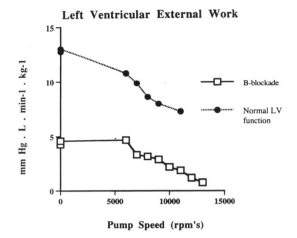

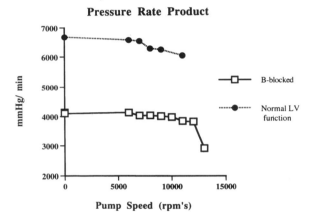

FIGURE 1. Linear left ventricular unloading is achieved by axial flow pumping in both esmolol ((β-blockade) and baseline conditions. Both volume unloading as measured by left ventricular work (top) and pressure unloading as measured by the pressure rate product (bottom) are maximally affected when complete unloading occurs.

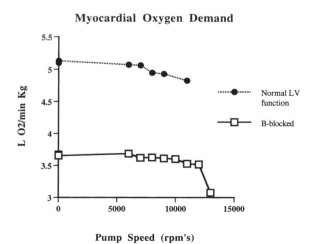

FIGURE 2. Myocardial oxygen demand (MVO_2) as measured by the pressure work index is only minimally reduced in the baseline ventricle secondary to volume but not pressure unloading. In the esmolol-depressed ventricle, the combination of volume and pressure unloading results in a marked decrease in MVO_2. Notice that this effect is achieved only when complete unloading is accomplished.

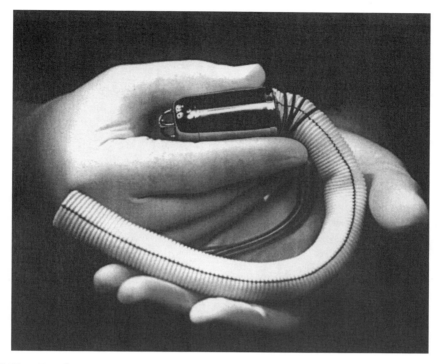

FIGURE 3. Jarvik 2000 axial flow impeller pump showing ventricular sewing cuff, power cable, and Dacron outflow graft.

model employ a motor rate that will be responsive to heart rate and adjustable by the patient according to activit level.

Device Implantation

Implantation of the device in experimental ovine models does not require CPB. After systemic heparinization (1 mg/kg), outflow is established to the descending aorta with a preclotted woven Dacron™ graft (Fig. 4, panel A). Inflow into the device is established via left ventricular apical cannulation.

In the sheep model of device implantation, power cables are tunneled subcutaneously from the left chest cavity to the neck, where they exit the skin and are attached to direct-current or rechargeable batteries. Extensive clinical experience with current implantable pulsatile LVADs has demonstrated that the thick, stiff drive line penetrating mobile skin and subcutaneous tissue contributes to the risk of drive line infection. In order to alleviate this problem, the Jarvik 2000 system was developed with a percutaneous titanium button that is screwed to the skull. With use of an exit site through highly vascular scalp skin, and by fixing of the cables in relation to the overlying skin, prompt healing occurs. In animal studies, the titanium pedestal resulted in no drive line infections versus a 20% infection rate when the power cables were merely tunneled subcutaneously and delivered through the skin.[33] A

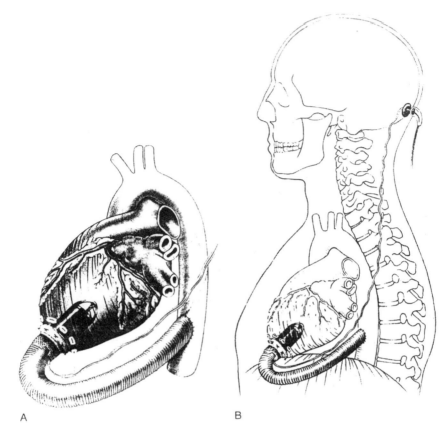

A   B

FIGURE 4. A. Implantation of the Jarvik 2000 with apical left ventricular inflow, and outflow via Dacron graft anastomosed to the descending thoracic aorta. Electrical cables are delivered percutaneously through the abdominal wall and attached to the power supply B. Proposed design for the permanently implanted human device. The electrical power cable is transmitted to the skin by way of a titanium pedestal screwed to the outer table of the skull to prevent movement.

subcutaneous exit site for the power cables will be employed when the device is used as a bridge to transplantation. However, for long-term permanent patient use, a percutaneous pedestal will be screwed to the outer table of the temporal bone. A discrete, detachable electric wire will pass behind the neck and then under the patient's jacket or clothing and below the shirt to a battery and controller system worn on the belt or in a vest (Fig. 4, panel B).

Experimental Results

The performance of the Jarvik 2000 has been extensively studied in ovine models with normal cardiac function. No chronic implantations to date have been performed in animal models of heart failure or in humans. However, acute experiments have been performed in β-blocked animals.

Kaplon et al[34] at the Columbia Presbyterian Medical Center reported the earliest experimental results with a smaller prototype of the Jarvik 2000 in seven long-term sheep. Device support ranged from 3 to 123 days with no evidence of extensive hemolysis or end organ damage. Despite anticoagulation with warfarin to an international normalized ratio of 1.5, there was one device failure from inflow thrombus. Four other failures occurred at varying time points from broken electric power cables. Macris et al[35] at the Texas Heart Institute have reproduced similar results with long-term implantation of the present, larger device in more than 20 calves. Six animals have been supported for more than 5 months, with the longest support time being more than 8 months. Pump speed in this study was maintained at approximately 10,000 rpm with flows of 5 to 6 L/min. Continuous axial flow resulted in a blunted arterial pressure contour, which varied based on the animal's degree of exercise. All animals received warfarin, aspirin, and dipyridamole. There was no significant hemolysis or end organ damage in any of the supported animals as measured by plasma free hemoglobin and post mortem examination. The most common cause of early termination was broken electrical wires. More recent implantations have resolved this problem with a new cable strain relief system that can withstand 10 times the force of the previous cable design.

With modifications of the housing and rotor/stator junction, the most recent Jarvik 2000 has been tested in 17 adult sheep at the Oxford Heart Center, with a goal to develop a device for destination therapy.[28,36] In this experience, Westaby and colleagues again demonstrated the pump's ability to flow 5 to 6 L/min at low power requirements. At maximal pump output, total capture of the arterial pressure tracing was also possible with flow rates of 8 to 9 L/min. Although five of the sheep in this study died of perioperative complications, 12 survived between 3 and 198 days (mean 44 days) with functioning devices. Modifications of the electrical cables resulted in few wire complications and both hemolysis and end organ damage were undetectable. One animal experienced thrombus inflow occlusion in the setting of endocarditis. All other devices were free of pannus ingrowth and thrombus at the time of sacrifice, with virtually no bearing wear within the device.

Parnis et al[37] have recently tested a rate-responsive controller, which has been incorporated into the latest Jarvik 2000. By detecting rotational speed alteration with varying heart rates, the rate-responsive controller is capable of automatically changing pump speed based on level of activity as assessed by heart rate. Full support of β-blocked animals was also demonstrated with complete capture of the arterial tracing (mean aortic pressure -70 mm Hg, pump flow 6 L/min). Although not planned as a component of the bridge-to-transplant device, it is hoped that the rate-responsive controller will become an integral part of the permanently implanted model to be employed as an alternative to transplantation.

Future Developments

Two developmental arms of the Jarvik 2000 continue to move forward. The previous animal work at the Texas Heart Institute has provided the framework for an investigational device (IDE) application. This device will most likely employ an external set rate controller, subcutaneous drive line exit sites, and power supply via a wall plug unit, lead acid batteries (2 hours), or lithium batteries (6 to 8 hours).

Limited implantation of this device under an IDE as a bridge to transplantation is expected within the next year. Simultaneously, continued efforts are aimed at developing a version of the Jarvik 2000 that would be used as an alternative to transplantation under the National Institutes of Health (NIH) Innovative Ventricular Assist System (IVAS) program. Rate-responsive controller systems and transcutaneous energy transmission systems are all components of the system that are under continuing development.

Nimbus/UOP Axial Flow System

Device Description

Since 1995, Nimbus and the UOP have been developing a totally implanted axial blood flow pump under the NIH IVAS program. The actual device design is still undergoing changes, but the basic pump elements have remained the same. The current prototype (Fig. 5) employs an electromagnetically driven axial rotor and matching stator incorporated within the pump housing. The pump/rotor is the only moving part. The 14 mm inner diameter titanium device weighs 176 g and has a displacement volume of 62 mL. The inflow cannula is a wire-reinforced right angle cannula with a felt sewing cuff for insertion into the left ventricular apex. The outflow cannula is connected to a 14 mm polytetrafluoroethylene graft which is anastomosed

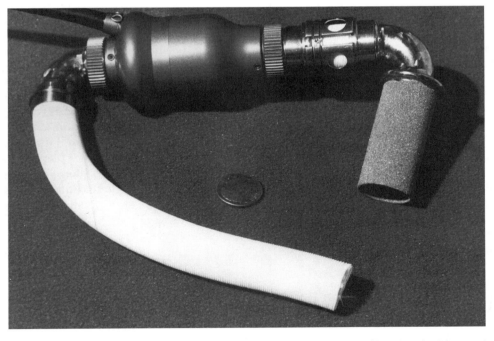

FIGURE 5. Nimbus/University of Pittsburgh axial blood flow pump. (Reprinted with permission from Nimbus, Inc., Rancho Cordova, CA.)

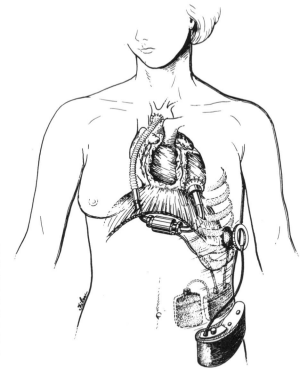

FIGURE 6. Design for proposed Nimbus/University of Pittsburgh left ventricular assist system. The device is placed in a properitoneal space below the diaphragm and is powered by either compact batteries or through a transcutaneous energy transmission system. (Reprinted with permission from Nimbus, Inc., Rancho Cordova, CA.)

to the thoracic aorta (Fig. 6). A single electrical drive line exits the skin to a controller that adjusts pump speed in response to physiologic demand. Speed control is established by interpreting the level and dynamics of the current drawn by the motor. In order to eliminate the need for percutaneous drive lines, a transcutaneous energy transmission system is under development. It uses two coils, one implanted and one external, which act as a transformer to pass energy across the skin.

Device Implantation

The current animal implantation design does not require CPB. Through a left lateral thoracotomy and after heparinization, the outflow polytetrafluoroethylene graft is anastomosed to the descending thoracic aorta. In the human model, the outflow graft may alternatively be sewn to the ascending aorta. The left ventricular apex serves as the inflow site. In a calf model of implantation, the pump is placed in a subcutaneous pocket below the diaphragm. Anticoagulation is administered with coumadin to an international normalized ratio of 3.0 to 4.0.

Experimental Results

In vitro tests have been promising, with minimal bearing wear after 6 months of continuous pump operation in a recirculating bench loop.[38,39] To date, chronic implantations have been reported in six calves with normal cardiac function.[40,41] Pump speed was maintained at an average of 10,100 rpm with a flow rate of 5 L/min. Maximal flow rates of 8 L/min were possible at the highest pump speed. Support times in the study ranged from 6 to 181 days (mean of 57 days). Hemolysis was minimal and no laboratory evidence of end organ damage could be recorded. Despite anticoagulation with coumadin, however, 5 of the 6 animals had thrombus present at the time of sacrifice. In two experiments, gross examination of the blood contacting surfaces revealed the presence of thrombus within the pump chambers. In three additional experiments, small amounts of thrombus were noted in areas joining the pump inlet and outlet ports to the cannulae. At necropsy, the only evidence for emboli that could be found were small renal cortical infarcts in several animals.

Future Developments

A new motor with increased efficiency and decreased blood trauma and diamond-coated biomaterials to decrease heat transfer are under development to reduce thrombotic complications. Continued advances in computer-assisted controllers and transcutaneous energy transfer systems promise to make the Nimbus/UOP ventricular assist system an elegant device for long-term permanent implantation. At present, its development remains experimental with no immediate plans for investigational human use.

DeBakey/NASA Axial Flow Ventricular Assist System

A small axial flow ventricular assist device has been under development since 1993, by a cooperative effort between the Baylor College of Medicine and the NASA/Johnson Space Center. The device measures 3" long and 1" in largest diameter, with a weight of 53 g and a displacement volume of 15 mL.

A three-stage development strategy has been adopted in order to produce a small device for long-term implantation. An atraumatic pump for 2 days of paracorporeal implantation in calves has been developed in phase I studies.[42] Pump running times have averaged 78 minutes with no evidence of hemolysis or end organ damage. The pump speed has been maintained at approximately 11,000 rpm with flow rates of 3.6 to 5.2 L/min. With modifications of the cylindrical outflow tube, phase II experiments have been undertaken in an attempt to decrease thrombogenicity for a 2-week implantation period.[43,44] More than 20 pumps have been tested in paracorporeal implantation with continuous heparin to maintain activated clotting times greater than 250 seconds. Minimal hemolysis has been noted with no end organ damage detected. At explantation following 2 weeks of uninterrupted support, very slight thrombus in the hub areas of some pumps has been found.

The last stage of development of the DeBakey/NASA axial flow ventricular device aims to focus on establishing a durable, fully implantable, long-term blood pump. Intracorporeal implantation will most likely employ left ventricular apical inflow with descending thoracic aorta outflow. Thrombus formation appears to be minimal with full oral anticoagulation. Continued device design changes are ongoing with hopes to provide a long-term implantable device within the next 2 years. Detailed description of this device along with initial clinical experience are described in Chapter 27.

United States Surgical Corporation Axial Flow Cannula Pump

The well known systemic inflammatory response that occurs following CPB has resulted in renewed efforts to perform off-bypass coronary artery bypass grafting (CABG). The use of LVADs for left heart bypass has been employed as an adjunct to such off-bypass revascularization in high-risk patients.[45] The United States Surgical Corporation (USSC) is presently developing an axial flow cannula pump to be used for left or right heart unloading during routine and high-risk beating heart CABG.

Device Description and Implantation

The pump is a disposable modification of the Jarvik 2000 that is connected in line with standard venous and arterial cannulae (Fig. 7). Inflow is established via cannulation of either the left ventricular apex or the left atrium and outflow is via standard ascending aortic cannulation (Fig. 8). In experimental models, systemic heparinization has been carried out (3 mg/kg), but lower dose heparin may also be feasible. The entire bypass loop fits comfortably on the operating table with a single electrical cable and a pressure monitoring line passed off to the controller. An electromagnetic flow probe can be attached around the outflow tubing, allowing continuous pump flow to be displayed on a light-emitting diode readout on the controller. The

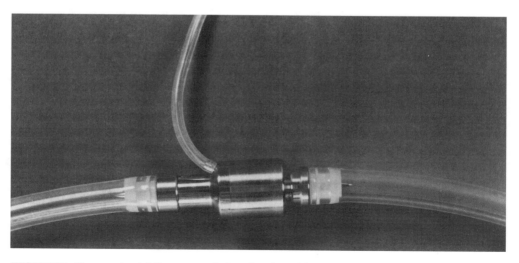

FIGURE 7. Compact axial flow pump being developed by the United States Surgical Corporation. Standard cannulae are attached to either end of the device and provide isolated left heart bypass.

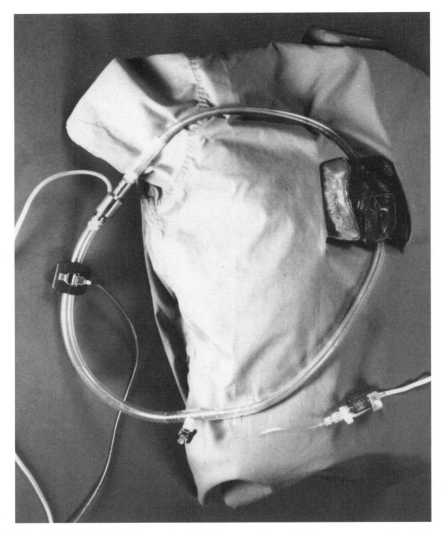

FIGURE 8. Model of United States Surgical Corporation axial flow pump system. The pump is connected to standard cannulae with inflow via either the left ventricle apex (shown) or left atrium and outflow to the ascending aorta.

pump is equipped with a bubble sensor that triggers immediate cessation of pumping should air be detected at the inflow cannula. A ventricular pressure transducer regulates ventricular unloading.

Experimental Results

In an ovine CABG model, the pump is capable of generating flow rates of 4 to 6 L/min at speeds ranging from 8000 to 13,000 rpm.[44] The device is capable of complete aortic pressure and flow wave capture in the β-blocked heart with subsequent profound reductions in myocardial oxygen demand and left ventricular external work. The safety net of axial flow left heart support provides maintenance of normal hemodynamics and access to all coronary territories in the β-blocked beating heart. No significant hemolysis or end organ damage has been observed after 3 hours of pump support. Recent studies in a primate model of left heart bypass using the USSC cannula pump have documented less complement activation, thrombin generation, and cytokine release when compared with standard CPB.[46]

Future Developments

Animal work on the USSC cannula pump has led to an IDE application. Limited human studies with the device are expected within the next 12 months. Its initial planned use will be in routine CABG patients as an alternative to CPB.

References

1. DeRose JJ Jr, Argenziano M, Umana JP, et al. Implantable left ventricular assist devices provide an excellent outpatient bridge to transplantation and recovery. *J Am Coll Cardiol* 1997;30:1773–1777.
2. DeRose JJ Jr, Argenziano M, Sun BC, et al. Implantable left ventricular assist devices: An evolving long-term cardiac replacement strategy. *Ann Surg* 1997;226:461–470.
3. Winowich S, Nastala CJ, Pristas JM, et al. Discharging patients who are undergoing mechanical circulatory support. *Ann Thorac Surg* 1996;61:478–479.
4. Hornick P, Taylor K. Pulsatile and nonpulsatile perfusion: The continuing controversy. *J Cardiothorac Vasc Anesth* 1997;11:310–315.
5. Hickey P, Bockley M, Philbin D. Pulsatile and nonpulsatile cardiopulmonary bypass: A review of a nonproductive controversy. *Ann Thorac Surg* 1983;36:720–737.
6. Angell-James J, de Burgh Daly M. Effects of graded pulsatile pressure on the reflex vasomotor responses elicited by changes of mean pressure in the perfused carotid sinus-aortic arch regions of the dog. *J Physiol* 1971;214:51–58.
7. Kohlsaedt K, Page I. The liberation of renin by perfusion of the kidneys following a reduction in pulse pressure. *J Exp Med* 1970;72:201–205.
8. Taylor KM, Bain WH, Russell M, et al. Peripheral vascular resistance and angiotensin II levels during pulsatile and nonpulsatile cardiopulmonary bypass. *Thorax* 1979;34:594–598.
9. Watkins DM, Peterson MB, Kong DL, et al. Thromboxane and prostacyclin changes during cardiopulmonary bypass with and without pulsatile flow. *J Thorac Cardiovasc Surg* 1982; 84:250–256.
10. Noris M, Morigi M, Donadelli R, et al. Nitric oxide synthesis by cultured endothelial cells is modulated by flow conditions. *Circ Res* 1995;76:536–543.
11. Taylor KM, Wright GS, Reid JM, et al. Comparative studies of pulsatile and non-pulsatile flow during cardiopulmonary bypass II: The effects of adrenal secretion of cortisol. *J Thorac Cardiovasc Surg* 1978;75:574–578.
12. Taylor KM, Wright GS, Bain WH, et al. Comparative studies of pulsatile and no-pulsatile flow during cardiopulmonary bypass III: Anterior pituitary response to thyrotrophin releasing hormone. *J Thorac Cardiovasc Surg* 1978;75:579–584.
13. Levine FH, Iverson S, Hetzer R, et al. Plasma vasopressin levels and urinary sodium excretion during cardiopulmonary bypass with and without pulsatile flow. *Ann Thorac Surg* 1981;32:63–67.
14. Mathie R, Desai J, Taylor K. The effect of normothermic cardiopulmonary bypass on hepatic blood flow in the dog. *Perfusion* 1986;1:245–253.

15. Moores W, Gago O, Morris J, et al. Serum and urinary amylase levels following pulsatile and continuous cardiopulmonary bypass. *J Thorac Cardiovasc Surg* 1977;74:73–76.
16. Gaer J, Shaw A, Wild R, et al. Effect of cardiopulmonary bypass on gastrointestinal perfusion and function. *Ann Thorac Surg* 1994;57:371–375.
17. Dapper F, Neppl H, Wozniak G, et al. Effects of pulsatile and nonpulsatile perfusion mode during extracorporeal circulation–a comparative clinical study. *J Thorac Cardiovasc Surg* 1992;40:345–351.
18. Wakisaka Y, Taenaka Y, Chikanari, et al. Long-term evaluation of a nonpulsatile mechanical circulatory support system. *Artif Organs* 1997;21:639–644.
19. Reddy RC, Goldstein AH, Pacella JJ, et al. End organ function with prolonged nonpulsatile circulatory support. *ASAIO J* 1995;41:M547-M551.
20. Allen GS, Murray KD, Olsen DB. The importance of pulsatile and nonpulsatile flow in the design of blood pumps. *Artif Organs* 1997;21:922–928.
21. Golding L, Murakami G, Harasaki H, et al. Chronic nonpulsatile flow. *ASAIO Trans* 1982;28:81–86.
22. Hindman BJ, Dexter F, Smith T, Cutkomp J. Pulsatile versus nonpulsatile flow. No difference in cerebral blood flow or metabolism during normothermic cardiopulmonary bypass in rabbits. *Anesthesiology* 1995;82:241–250.
23. Tominaga R, Smith WA, Massiello A, et al. Chronic nonpulsatile blood flow I. Cerebral autoregulation in chronic nonpulsatile biventricular bypass: Carotid blood flow response to hypercapnia. *J Thorac Cardiovasc Surg* 1994;108:907–912.
24. Sakaki M, Taenaka Y, Tatsumi E, et al. Influences of nonpulsatile pulmonary blood flow on pulmonary function. Evaluation of a chronic animal model. *J Thorac Cardiovasc Surg* 1994;108:495–502.
25. Tominaga R, Smith WA, Massiello A, et al. Chronic nonpulsatile blood flow III. Effects of pump flow rate on oxygen transport and utilization in chronic nonpulsatile biventricular bypass. *J Thorac Cardiovasc Surg* 1996;111:863–872.
26. Tominaga R, Smith WA, Massiello A, et al. Chronic nonpulsatile blood flow II. Hemodynamic responses to progressive exercise in calves with chronic nonpulsatile biventricular bypass. *J Thorac Cardiovasc Surg* 1996;111:857–862.
27. Sezai A, Shiono M, Orime Y, et al. Renal and cellular metabolism during left ventricular assisted circulation: Comparison study of pulsatile and nonpulsatile assists. *Artif Organs* 1997;21:830–835.
28. Jarvik R, Westaby S, Katsumata T, et al. LVAD power delivery: A percutaneous approach to avoid infection. *Ann Thorac Surg* 1998;65:470–473.
29. Westaby S, Katsumata T, Houel R, et al. Jarvik 2000 heart: Potential for bridge to myocyte recovery. *Circulation* 1998;98:1568–1574.
30. Pierce WS, Aaronson AE, Prophet GA, et al. Hemodynamic and metabolic studies during two types of left ventricular bypass. *Surg Forum* 1972;23:176–178.
31. Pennock JL, Pierce WS, Waldenhausen JA. Quantitative evaluation of left ventricular bypass in reducing myocardial ischemia. *Surgery* 1976;79:523–533.
32. Shiiya N, Zelinsky R, Deleuze PH, Loisance DY. Changes in hemodynamics and coronary blood flow during left ventricular assistance with the Hemopump. *Ann Thorac Surg* 1992;53:1074–1079.
33. DeRose JJ Jr, Umana JP, Madigan JD, et al. Mechanical unloading with a miniature in-line axial flow pump as an alternative to cardiopulmonary bypass. *ASAIO J* 1997;43:M421-M426.
34. Kaplon RJ, Oz MC, Kwiatowski PA, et al. Miniature axial flow pump for ventricular assistance in children and small adults. *J Thorac Cardiovasc Surg* 1996;111:13–18.
35. Macris MP, Parnis SM, Frazier OH, et al. Development of an implantable ventricular assist system. *Ann Thorac Surg* 1997;63:367–370.
36. Westaby S, Katsumata T, Evans R, et al. The Jarvik 2000 Oxford System: Increasing the scope of mechanical circulatory support. *J Thorac Cardiovasc Surg* 1997;114:467–474.
37. Parnis SM, Conger JL, Fuqua JM Jr, et al. Progress in the development of a transcutaneously powered axial flow blood pump ventricular assist system. *ASAIO J* 1997;43:M576-M580.
38. Thomas DC, Butler KC, Taylor LP, et al. Continued development of the Nimbus/University of Pittsburgh (UOP) axial flow left ventricular assist system. *ASAIO J* 1997;43:M564-M566.

39. Butler K, Thomas D, Antaki J, et al. Development of the Nimbus/Pittsburgh axial flow left ventricular assist system. *Artif Organs* 1997; 21:602–610.
40. Yamazaki K, Kormos RL, Litwak P, et al. Long term animal experiments with an intraventricular axial flow blood pump. *ASAIO J* 1997;43:M696-M700.
41. Macha M, Litwak P, Yamazaki K, et al. Survival for up to six months in calves supported with an implantable axial flow ventricular assist device. *ASAIO J* 1997;43:311–315.
42. Kawahito K, Damm G, Aber G, et al. Ex vivo phase 1 evaluation of the DeBakey/NASA axial flow ventricular assist device. *Artif Organs* 1996;20:47–52.
43. Kawahito K, Benkowski R, Otsubo S, et al. Ex vivo evaluation of the NASA/DeBakey axial flow ventricular assist device. Results of a 2 week screening test. *ASAIO J* 1996;42: M754-M757.
44. Kawahito K, Benkowski R, Otsubo S, et al. Improved flow straighteners reduce thrombus in the NASA/DeBakey axial flow ventricular assist device. *Artif Organs* 1997;21:339–343.
45. Sweeney MS, Frazier OH. Device-supported myocardial revascularization: Safe help for sick hearts. *Ann Thorac Surg* 1992;54:1065–1070.
46. Chen JM, Spanier TB, Choudhri AF, et al. Isolated left ventricular bypass produces less complement activation and inflammation than conventional cardiopulmonary bypass. *Circulation* 1998;98(17 suppl 1):I829.

Chapter 27

The DeBakey Ventricular Assist Device

George P. Noon, MD, Deborah Morley, PhD,
Suellen Irwin, RN, and Michael E. DeBakey, MD

Device Description and Design Rationale

The DeBakey VAD℠ is a miniaturized axial flow blood pump intended for use as mechanical support for patients with end-stage heart failure. The concept was developed in 1988 through a comprehensive research and development process that included input from Drs. Michael E. DeBakey and George P. Noon and engineers at the NASA Johnson Space Center. MicroMed Technology, Inc. (Houston, TX) received the license for the technology in June 1996 and has since been developing the device for commercial use. The designers' objective was to develop a ventricular assist device (VAD) system that was safe, effective, reliable, user-friendly, and affordable. The design of the axial flow pump targeted the reduction of hemolysis, thrombosis, and noise and heat generation. The goal for the entire system was also to allow patients to move about freely with a portable controller and battery.

Design controls consistent with the requirements outlined in the Food and Drug Administration Quality Systems Regulation and the European Active Implantable Medical Device Directive were used in the development process of the pump, controller, and clinical data acquisition system (CDAS). More than 50 pump design iterations were evaluated by NASA design engineers. MicroMed Technology, Inc. assembles the subsystems and distributes the final system.

Figure 1 depicts the DeBakey VAD human configuration. The system consists of three subsystems: a pump system (Figs. 2 and 3), a controller system (Fig. 4), and a CDAS (Fig. 5). The miniaturized blood pump, intended to provide mechanical assistance to the failing left ventricle, is an implantable titanium electromagnetically actuated axial flow pump. The miniaturized pump can provide flows in excess of 10 L/min. The pump is 1.2″ (30.5 mm) in diameter and 3.0″ (76.2 mm) in length and weighs 93 g. A titanium inflow cannula connects the pump to the ventricular apex and a Dacron℠ vascular graft (outflow conduit) connects the pump to the ascending

From Goldstein DJ and Oz MC (eds). *Cardiac Assist Devices.* Armonk, NY: Futura Publishing Co., Inc.; ©2000.

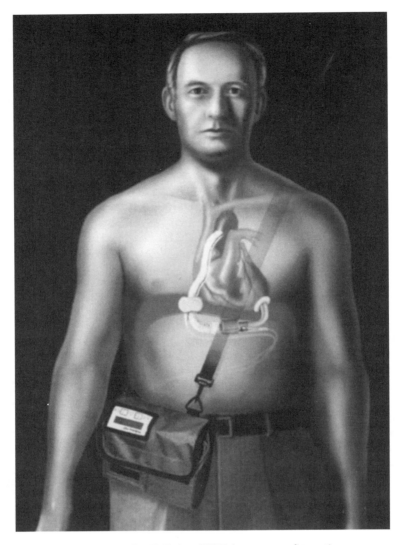

FIGURE 1. The DeBakey VAD human configuration.

aorta. Blood flow from the pump is measured by a flow probe placed around the outflow conduit. The wiring of the flow probe is bundled with that of the pump motor in a coated cable assembly. The cable assembly exits the skin from the abdominal wall superior to the iliac crest, and attaches to the VAD's external controller system. The controller (Fig. 4) provides energy to the device from the CDAS or from external batteries, causing the impeller to rotate and pump blood. The CDAS (Fig. 5) receives measurements of pump speed, flow, power and, current signals from the controller and displays that information so the user can monitor and adjust pump operation.

The VAD system is designed to be simple to use by both the patient and the clinician. Pump performance levels cannot be adjusted by the patient. All of the primary operating parameters can be viewed on the controller module's liquid crystal

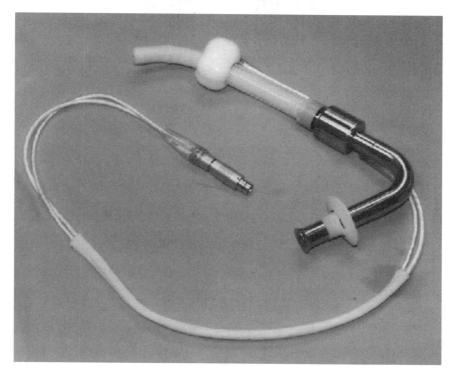

FIGURE 2. The DeBakey VAD pump system.

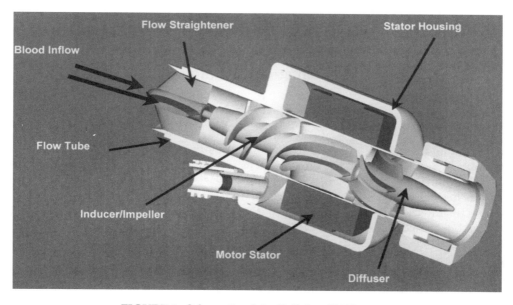

FIGURE 3. Schematic of the DeBakey VAD pump.

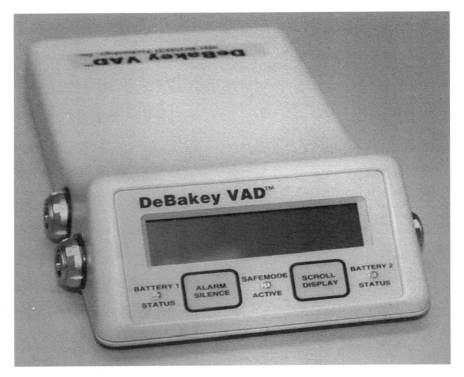

FIGURE 4. The DeBakey VAD controller.

display. The controller is designed to operate the pump. The CDAS is connected to the controller and stores pump-operating data, and displays pump and physiologic information. The CDAS also may be used to adjust the pump speed.

Implantation Techniques

Prior to the start of the operative procedure, the pump is immersed in saline, connected to the controller with battery power, and tested. An outflow graft is mounted and secured to the outflow end of the pump. A flow probe is placed on the outflow graft to measure pump flows after implant.

For pump implant, a median sternotomy incision is performed, extending several inches below the xyphoid process. An abdominal wall pocket is formed below the rectus muscle. The size and configuration of the pocket are determined by using the real or mock pump as a model. To provide access to the left ventricular apex, the pericardium is opened, the diaphragmatic attachment to the costal margin is divided, and both are extended laterally beyond the apex.

After institution of cardiopulmonary bypass, the left ventricular apex is elevated and the insertion site of the inflow cannula is selected. The apical fixation ring is sewn in place with at least eight interrupted 2-0 polypropylene mattress sutures with large Teflon felt pledgets. A trocar is connected to the pump drive line to

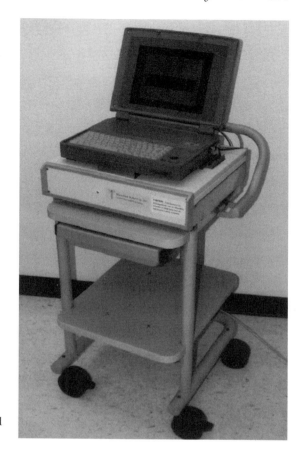

FIGURE 5. The DeBakey VAD clinical data acquisition system.

facilitate tunneling of the cable from the abdominal wall pocket across the midline to exit through the skin in a convenient position above the right iliac crest. The trocar is then removed and the drive line is connected to the controller.

In preparation for insertion of the pump inflow cannula, the left apex is elevated. The heart may remain beating, fibrillated, or arrested. Using an 11 blade, a full thickness cruciate incision is made inside the apical ring. The ventricular apex is manually compressed to prevent bleeding. A round bladed coring device is inserted into the left ventricle to extract a core of the left ventricular apex. To confirm precise apical coring and extraction, the apical tissue is removed from the coring device and carefully examined for completeness. Digital ventricular exploration is performed to evaluate the position of the core and to ensure absence of any potential obstruction to inflow. The pump outflow graft is clamped and the inflow cannula is inserted into the left ventricular apex. Proper placement of the inflow cannula inside the ventricle is imperative. The cannula opening must be clear of any ventricular tissue and must not be positioned in a way in which the free ventricular wall or septum could obstruct its opening. Using the previously placed polypropylene sutures, the suture ring on the inflow cannula is sewn to the apical fixation ring. The pump and left ventricle are de-aired by allowing the ventricle to fill with blood. The pump and outflow graft are elevated and filled with blood from the ventricle by releasing and reapplying the clamp on the outflow graft. To assure hemostasis, it may be necessary to further seal the ventricular sewing ring attachment by approximating the left ventricular apex and the sewing ring with a Teflon felt strip and continuous 2-0 polypropylene suture.

The DeBakey VAD is placed into the abdominal pocket and the length of the outflow graft is measured and trimmed. The graft should lie under the right sternal border without kinking or overstretching. A proximal, external graft protector is designed to prevent graft kinking. Care is taken to ensure that the flow probe is placed immediately proximal to the graft protector, as this helps in proper positioning of the outflow graft. A partial occlusion clamp is placed on the ascending aorta. A longitudinal aortotomy is made and the outflow graft is sewn to the lateral ascending aorta with 5–0 polypropylene. After the anastomosis is complete, an 18 gauge needle is placed in the outflow graft between the aortic anastomosis and graft clamp. With the temporary release of the aortic partial occlusion clamp, the distal aortic graft is filled with blood, and trapped air escapes through the 18 gauge needle. The aorta is reclamped. Remaining air in the system is released through the 18 gauge needle by unclamping the outflow graft and intermittently starting and stopping the pump. The aortic partial occluding clamp is then removed and continuous pumping is begun at 7500 rpm.

Pump flows are begun at 7500 rpm and adjusted to maintain a cardiac index of approximately 2.0 L/min/m². Hypovolemia and excessive pump speed are avoided to prevent ventricular collapse and diminished flows. By use of echocardiography, the location of the inflow cannula is viewed and the ventricles are assessed for volume, function, and presence of air. The inflow cannula must be free of obstruction. When placement of the cannula is noted to be satisfactory and flows are adequate, the patient is weaned from cardiopulmonary bypass and protamine is given to reverse heparin. After meticulous hemostasis, drains are placed in the mediastinum and the pump pocket and the incision is closed. The drive line exit site is approximated and the line secured in place with a suture.

After surgery, inotropic medications are continued to support the right ventricle. If the right ventricle fails in spite of medical management, a temporary right ventricular assist device is implemented. An intra-aortic balloon device may also be inserted for temporary pulsatile flow and/or hemodynamic support, if desired. Coagulopathies are treated and the patient is not placed on anticoagulant therapy until postoperative bleeding is minimal and coagulopathy is controlled, usually within 24 to 48 hours post implant.

Patients with continuous flow pumps may not have palpable pulses or blood pressures audible with a sphygmomanometer. Because the pulse is diminished, pulse oxymeters may not accurately measure peripheral oxygen saturation. Indwelling arterial catheters or Dopplers may be needed to evaluate blood flow and to measure blood pressure in heart failure patients with continuous flow devices.

Indications

The DeBakey VAD is currently indicated for use as a bridge to transplant in patients who are accepted by their institution's transplant committee prior to implantation. Future indications for the DeBakey VAD will be as a bridge to recovery and as a chronic implant. The small size of the VAD is advantageous in that it can be implanted in smaller patients than can the pulsatile VADs. Use of the DeBakey VAD extracorporeally in small children and infants may be a future application.

Limitations

Use of pulsatile versus nonpulsatile flow assist devices has been a controversial subject among scientists for years (see Chapter 26). Studies involving nonpulsatile extracorporeal circulation during cardiopulmonary bypass suggest that neuroendocrine mechanisms, which are triggered by baroreceptor discharge, are altered. These include changes in catecholamine release, activation of the renin-angiotensin system, increased secretion of vasopressin, and the production of local tissue vasoconstrictor agents.[1] Departure from normal blood flow physiology in animals has exhibited a degree of adaptability by reestablishing near normal physiology after initial postoperative increase in catecholamine levels.[2] The recent implantation and maintenance of the DeBakey VAD in humans now affords an opportunity to assess the neurovascular and neuroendocrine effects of a long-term reduced-pulsatile axial flow pump. Patients implanted with the device adapt physiologically to the reduced pulsatile flows; however, further studies will determine the long-term effects and any limitations of less pulsatile perfusion.

Another potential limitation of continuous flow devices is the potential for regurgitant flow in the event that the pump stops. Pump stoppage of the DeBakey VAD will allow regurgitant blood flow into the heart and possibly worsen the patient's heart failure. Because of this potential, a pump design with the ability to occlude the outflow graft, preventing regurgitation, is being considered.

At this time, the system lacks speed control with a controller algorithm. The current pump speed is fixed and can only be changed when the controller is attached to the CDAS. When not connected to the CDAS, a situation could occur in which a patient would benefit from a change in pump speed, and this would not be possible. A planned future generation of the DeBakey VAD will include a controller with an adjustable flow rate algorithm that will adapt pump flows to the patient's changing metabolic needs.

Preclinical Testing

Preclinical testing of the DeBakey VAD has been divided into several phases. Each phase has had a specific objective.

During the first phase of studies, a polycarbonate version of the pump was used. The purpose was to develop the pump design that was the least hemolytic and thrombogenic. Parametric bench testing of iterative pump designs identified the least hemolytic pump. Next, ex vivo tests of iterative pump designs were conducted to identify the pump that was least thrombogenic. For these tests, a pump was mounted in a saddle on a calf's back so that blood flowed through the device until thrombosis occurred or the experiment duration was met.[3–5] Using this paradigm, the pump design that could be used for up to 2 weeks without significant hemolysis or thrombosis was identified.

The next group of studies was in vivo,[6] ie, a titanium pump was intrathoracically implanted in 24 calves. The purpose was to ensure that the least hemolytic and thrombogenic design had been identified using titanium. The study also determined the safety of the DeBakey VAD for long-term support. The DeBakey VAD was shown to safely operate in animals for up to 145 days. Average pump outputs were maintained above 3.0 L/min with power consumption of 10 W or less. No significant hemolysis or end organ dysfunction occurred. Complications included one incidence of device-related infection and two incidences of pump thrombus. One pump thrombus incidence occurred after a malfunction in an early controller model. The second involved a small hub thrombus. These experiments also allowed the final design of the controller and the CDAS to be established.

Further in vivo studies were conducted to demonstrate safety of the entire system (pump, controller, CDAS) in support of European clinical trials. Six of the eight calves studied in this phase of preclinical testing survived 90 days post implant. One animal was sacrificed soon after surgery because its hypercontractile ventricle obstructed flow through the pump. The other animal was sacrificed for a pump stoppage on postoperative day 24. Explant analyses demonstrated a ring thrombus at the rear bearing. Pump output for the six surviving animals ranged from 3.3 to 5.4 L/min. Power consumption was 10 W or less. There were no incidences of end organ dysfunction, hemolysis, or infection. Although minor mechanical malfunctions such as a computer screen freezing and a cable disconnection did occur, each was readily resolved. Occasional resynchronization episodes were noted; however, in all cases the pump restarted according to design. The results supported safety of the entire system configuration and European clinical trials were begun in November 1998.

In vitro performance tests have been conducted with a mock circulation to define characteristics of pump function in response to normal and abnormal vascular conditions and ventricular performance. Studies completed to date[7,8] demonstrate that the DeBakey VAD can adequately unload the failing left ventricle, and does perform as expected when physiologic parameters such as preload or heart rate are varied.

Other studies are ongoing to determine whether bearing wear can be detected vibroacoustically. There are two types of studies being conducted: induced wear tests and endurance tests. The objective of induced wear tests is to quantify the relationship between artificially induced bearing wear, hemolysis, and the resulting vibroacoustic signature. No significant level of hemolysis has been observed at any level of artificially induced bearing wear, and no difference in hemolysis has been demonstrated between any artificially induced bearing wear step. The objective of the endurance tests is to examine endurance and the extent of bearing wear during continuous pump operation. As part of the endurance tests, 10 pumps have been operating continuously for 23 months (since May–June 1997). Two pumps have shown evidence of a minimal degree of wear; these pumps are still running.

Implantable components of the DeBakey VAD system have been subjected to both hemocompatibility and biocompatibility studies. The purpose of hemocompatibility studies was to identify blood-titanium interactions with the DeBakey VAD. These tests were performed with human blood in a mock circulation. Results demonstrate that the pump is not the source of thrombi or emboli and that it is otherwise hemocompatible. Biocompatibility tests that have been completed show the device to have no systemic toxicity, local toxicity, cytotoxicity, genotoxicity, pyrogenicity, physiochemical toxins, mutagenicity, and sensitization. The process by which implantable components are sterilized in ethylene oxide has been validated as well.

The controller and CDAS are manufactured for MicroMed Technology, Inc. by outside contractors. These firms have conducted independent testing to demonstrate that both components meet all standards required by the Active Implantable Medical Device Directive and applicable regulatory standards in the United States. Both components have been demonstrated to be electrically safe and to withstand environmental factors such as temperature and shock. Software validation has also been conducted; both the controller and the CDAS have been shown to comply with applicable standards.

DeBakey VAD Clinical Experience

The DeBakey VAD was introduced into clinical trials in November of 1998. To date, 10 (8 male, 2 female) patients have received the device. Five patients have been successfully transplanted. Support duration has ranged up to 115 days. Seven patients have been supported for more than 30 days, while four patients have been supported for more than 60 days. Figure 6 illustrates pump function for the first nine patients enrolled in the clinical trial.

During this early clinical trial, positive observations have been noted. The pump is placed just below the diaphragm in a small abdominal pocket (Figs. 7 and 8). The

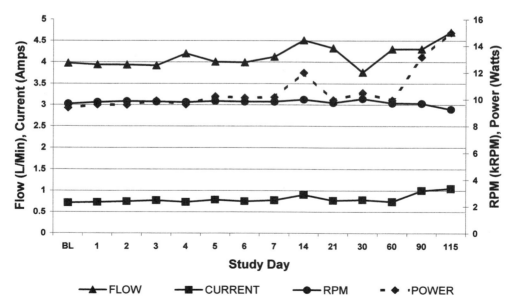

FIGURE 6. Trends for pump parameters for the first nine patients implanted with the DeBakey VAD.

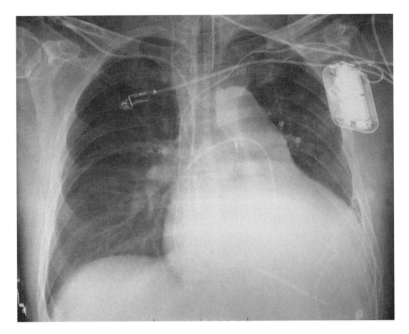

FIGURE 7. Pre-VAD implant chest x-ray of a patient with ischemic cardiomyopathy post myocardial infarction with intra-aortic balloon pump, endotracheal tube, and automatic implantable cardioverter defibrillator. The heart is enlarged.

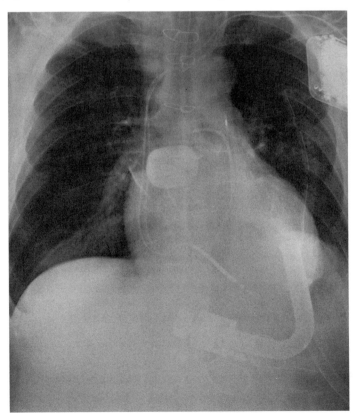

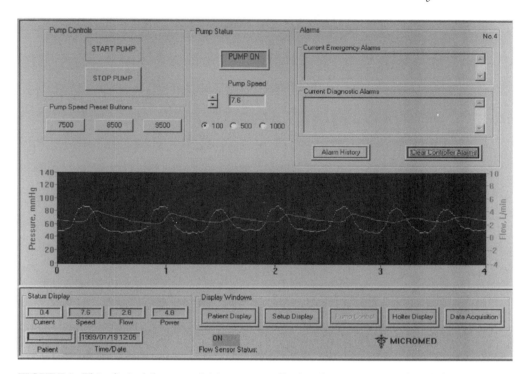

FIGURE 9. This clinical data acquisition system display demonstrates pulsatile flow between 1 and 5 L/min and a systolic pressure difference of 20 mm Hg with the aortic valve not opening.

dissection and pocket size are much less than required for the larger pulsatile pumps and result in less perioperative bleeding and potential for infection. De-airing is simple compared to pulsatile devices. The device is almost noiseless and patient awareness of the device is minimal. Although the pump is in a continuous flow mode, it does exhibit pulsatility depending on the strength of the heart's native contractility and the resulting delta P (Figs. 9 and 10). End organ function after implant has either shown improvement or remained stable at baseline for the patients supported on the DeBakey VAD. Patients have been able to perform normal low-level activity and have tolerated position changes without difficulty or evidence of postural hemodynamic changes. Select patients have taken supervised out-of-hospital excursions.

The DeBakey pump represents an exciting new generation of ventricular assist devices which have the potential to revolutionize our current algorithm for the surgical management of end-stage heart failure.

FIGURE 8. Chest x-ray showing the DeBakey VAD and flow probe in the immediate postoperative period. There is marked decrease in left ventricular size.

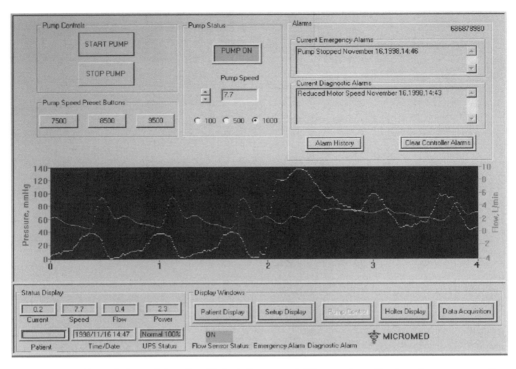

FIGURE 10. From left to right, the clinical data acquisition system display shows a negative pump flow with the pump stopped, a surge of positive blood flow with the pump started, and 0 to 6 L/min at 7600 rpm. There is a decrease in systolic diastolic pressure differential with pumping.

References

1. Hornick P, Taylor K. Pulsatile and nonpulsatile perfusion: The continuing controversy. *J Cardiothorac Vasc Anesth* 1997;11(3):310–315.
2. Allen GS, Murray KD, Olsen DB. The importance of pulsatile and nonpulsatile flow in design of blood pumps. *Artif Organs* 1997;21(8):922–928.
3. Damm G, Mizuguchi K, Aber G, et al. In vitro performance of the Baylor/NASA axial flow pump. *Artif Organs* 1993;17:609–613.
4. Mizuguchi K, Damm G, Bozeman RJ, et al. Development of the Baylor/NASA axial flow ventricular assist device: In vitro performance and systematic hemolysis test results. *Artif Organs* 1994;18:32–43.
5. Kawahito K, Damm G, Benkowski R, et al. Ex vivo phase 1 evaluation of the DeBakey/NASA axial flow ventricular assist device. *Artif Organs* 1996;20:47–52.
6. Fossum T, Morley D, Benkowski R, et al. Chronic survival of calves implanted with the DeBakey ventricular assist device. *Artif Organs* 1999;23:802–806.
7. Mitzuguchi K, Damm G, Benkowski R, et al. Development of an axial flow ventricular assist device: In vitro and in vivo evaluation. *Artif Organs* 1995;19:653–659.
8. Morley D, Benkowski R, Tayama E, et al. The DeBakey VAD®: Progress with in vivo studies. *Artif Organs* 1998;44:30.

Chapter 28

Epicardial Compression Mechanical Devices

John H. Artrip, MD and Daniel Burkhoff, MD, PhD

Introduction

Treatment of end-stage heart disease remains a major clinical challenge regardless of whether it is due to an acute myocardial insult or the consequence of decompensation in the setting of longstanding heart failure. Although a variety of ventricular assist devices are available, most of these devices require direct contact with the patient's blood; thus, thromboembolic events, anticoagulation- and hemolysis-related complications, and immune reactions are ever present problems. Accordingly, there has been renewed interest in the development of techniques to support the circulation by compressing the weakened heart from its epicardial surface or direct cardiac compression (DCC).

Insights into the effects of DCC on ventricular pump function have been gained from experience with biomechanical compression therapies and with newly developed mechanical compression devices. Biomechanical therapies such as dynamic cardiomyoplasty physically wrap the patient's skeletal muscle around the failing heart and electrically stimulate the muscle wrap to contract with the native heartbeat. Mechanical compression devices such as cuffs or cups fit around the heart and compress the weakened heart in synchrony with ventricular contraction. Although there are advantages and disadvantages specific to each form of therapy, the physiologic principles governing their mechanism of action are essentially the same.

Physiology of Epicardial Compression

Our understanding of the effects of DCC on ventricular mechanics stems from investigations using isolated canine hearts placed inside compression chambers whose pressure could be varied in synchrony with cardiac contraction.[1-4] Results of these studies showed that net ventricular pumping capacity can be augmented by

From Goldstein DJ and Oz MC (eds). *Cardiac Assist Devices*. Armonk, NY: Futura Publishing Co., Inc.; ©2000.

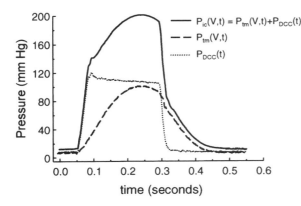

FIGURE 1. Left ventricular pressures obtained from an isolated canine heart undergoing synchronized epicardial compression under isovolumic ejection conditions. The pressure measured inside the ventricular cavity, Pic (V,t), is the sum of the transmural ventricular pressure, Ptm (V,t), plus the epicardial compression pressure, PDCC (t).

external pressure such that the forces applied to the heart's surface add to the ventricular pressure generated by the contracting myocardium. This is clearly demonstrated with studies performed under experimental conditions where the ventricular volume remains fixed (ie, isovolumic contractions) so that the strength of ventricular contraction is readily indexed by increases in ventricular pressure. Under these conditions, the pressure measured inside the ventricular cavity equals the sum of the pressure generated by the contracting myocardium (normally referred to as the transmural pressure) plus the pressure applied to the heart surface. This is illustrated in Figure 1 and can be expressed mathematically as:

$$\text{Pic } (V,t) = \text{Ptm } (V,t) + \text{PDCC } (t) \tag{1}$$

where Pic (V,t) is the intrachamber ventricular pressure, Ptm (V,t) is the transmural ventricular pressure, and PDCC (t) is the pressure generated by DCC. Applying this principle over a series of fixed ventricular volumes, it becomes apparent that DCC shifts the end-systolic pressure-volume relationship (ESPVR) upward by an amount related to the compression pressure (Fig. 2). With biomechanical wraps (ie, dynamic cardiomyoplasty), the skeletal muscle used for epicardial compression is subject to myofibril length-tension variation; for this reason, PDCC varies with ventricular size. As the ventricular size changes with filling volume, the length-tension relationship

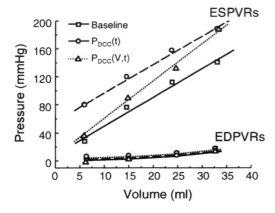

FIGURE 2. The effects of direct cardiac compression (DCC) on the end-systolic pressure-volume relationship (ESPVR) and end-diastolic pressure-volume relationship (EDPVR) of the left ventricle of an isolated canine heart under isovolumic ejecting conditions. With compression pressures that are independent of ventricular size, PDCC (t), the ESPVR is simply shifted upward with no change in the slope; however, with compression pressures that vary with the ventricular size, PDCC (V,t), the slope of the line is significantly increased with little change in the volume-axis intercept. The EDPVR is not affected by epicardial compression.

of the myofibrils of the muscular wrap changes, thus altering the amount of compression force delivered to the epicardium.[5] The ESPVR of a heart assisted with a skeletal muscle wrap is shown in Figure 2. The slope of the line (referred to as the end-systolic elastance [Ees]) is significantly increased with little change in the volume-axis intercept (Vo).[6,7] With mechanical compression devices, PDCC (t) is independent of ventricular size, so that the amount of compression pressure applied to the epicardial surface is the same regardless of the ventricular volume. Under these conditions, the ESPVR is simply shifted upward from the baseline by an amount equal to PDCC(t). The slope of the line is unchanged but the Vo value is decreased (Fig. 2).[4]

With the compression chamber used in the ex vivo canine heart experiment, the benefit for systolic function is achieved with no effect on ventricular diastolic function.[4] This is illustrated in Figure 2 by the similar end-diastolic pressure-volume relationship (EDPVR) tracings for the assisted and unassisted hearts. Unfortunately, biomechanical wraps and mechanical compression devices designed for use in vivo may have small effects on ventricular diastolic properties. Effects on diastolic properties have been inconsistently observed among various investigators but, when present, induce small leftward shifts of the EDPVR.[8,9] These shifts of the EDPVR are indicative of increased chamber stiffness that requires a higher filling pressure to obtain the same preload volume. Importantly, this effect was observed both with and without active compression, suggesting that the actual fixation of these wraps/devices to the heart accounts for this diastolic effect. Muscular wraps may also reduce the rate of diastolic pressure decay (negative dP/dt_{max}) and increase the time constant (tau) for ventricular relaxation, which has not been observed with mechanical compression devices.[9,10] This is likely due to the relatively slow relaxation period of skeletal muscle compared with cardiac muscle and the fact that the heart sits within the confines of the muscular wrap. The net effect of ventricular wraps and compression devices on the ventricular diastolic properties may lead to reduced ventricular preloads and potentially limit the degree of output augmentation obtained.[4,7,8]

Since DCC increases the ESPVR with little influence on the EDPVR, the overall effect is to increase pressure-volume area (PVA) confined between these two curves. This area reflects the external work of the heart and usually correlates with myocardial oxygen consumption (MVO_2). With mechanical compression from the epicardial surface, however, the PVA increases, but MVO_2 does not change.[3,4] This is shown in Figure 3 as a significant decrease in the slope of the MVO_2-PVA relationship with

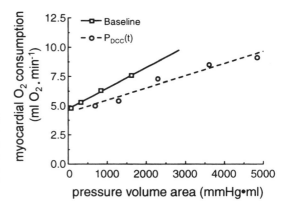

FIGURE 3. The effect of direct cardiac compression (DCC) on the relationship between myocardial oxygen consumption (MVO_2) and external work. DCC decreases the slope of the MVO_2-PVA relationship with little influence on the y intercept.

little influence on the y intercept. The slope changes of the MVO_2-PVA relationship observed with DCC do not reflect effects on myocardial properties, but rather the enhanced net pressure-generating capacity in the absence of an effect on intrinsic myocardial properties.

In contrast to isovolumic contractions, with physiologically ejecting conditions similar to those encountered in vivo, the increased pumping capacity of the ventricle with epicardial compression manifests not only as increases in end-systolic pressure, but also as increases in stroke volume.[4,8] However, preload volumes decrease as a consequence of the increase in ventricular ejection, and for this reason the degree of pressure and stroke volume augmentation anticipated by DCC is reduced to what would be expected if preload volumes remained constant. This is predicted from studies using isolated hearts ejecting against a computer-simulated physiologic afterload system,[4] and has been observed in vivo with studies using muscular wraps and compression devices.[7,8] Figure 4 shows pressure-volume tracings illustrating the preload shift that occurs with the increased pumping capacity of DCC. These observations can be explained with the use of modern theories of ventriculoarterial coupling,[11] and predict that the amount of stroke volume augmentation will be dependent upon the baseline myocardial contractile state, the baseline afterload resistance, and the degree of preload shift caused by PDCC (t).[4]

The inter-relationships between these parameters are further summarized in Figure 5, with the help of computerized modeling of the canine circulation. The dotted line in panel A shows how stroke volume varies as a function of contractile state at a fixed preload and a fixed afterload. The solid line at the top depicts how DCC would affect this relationship assuming that there was no change in preload. As preload decreases, however, this curve shifts downward, as shown by the dashed and dot-dashed solid lines. Graphs depicting the amount of stroke volume augmentation (expressed in absolute and relative terms, panels B and C, respectively) formally illustrate two fundamental aspects of the physiology of epicardial compression. First, the reduction in preload will blunt stroke volume augmentations and can even result in a diminution at higher baseline levels of contractility. Second, the amount of augmentation of effective ventricular contractile state afforded by DCC is a function of baseline contractile state. Substantial stroke volume augmentation is only achieved

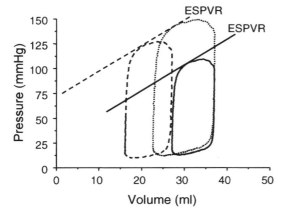

FIGURE 4. The effects of direct cardiac compression (DCC) on the left ventricle pressure-volume (PV) relationship of an isolated canine heart under computer-simulated physiologic ejecting conditions. With application of DCC, the end-systolic PV relationship is shifted upward from baseline (dashed versus solid line). Under conditions where neither preload volume nor afterload resistance changes, the new PV relationship increases with a significant increased stroke volume (dotted versus solid PV loop). However, preload volume is reduced during DCC and the PV loop shifts leftward (dashed PV loop), thus reducing the augmenting effects of DCC on stroke volume.

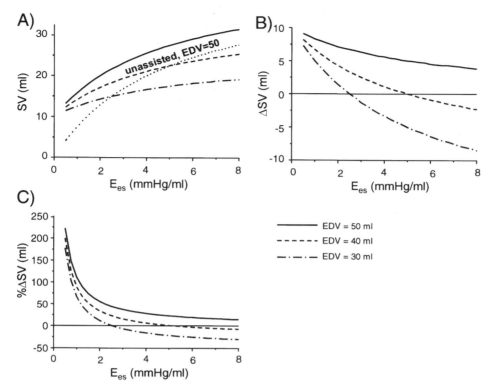

FIGURE 5. The effect of direct cardiac compression (DCC) on the relationship between stroke volume and ventricular contractility for three different preloads (EDV of 30, 40, and 50 mL) for a 24 kg adult male dog. Ventricular contractility is indexed as the end-systolic elastance (Ees) value, which is approximately 8 mm Hg/mL in a healthy adult male dog. The plots are depicted in (A) stroke volume versus Ees, (B) change in stroke volume (stroke volume = stroke volumeDCC—stroke volumebase) versus Ees, and (C) the percent increase in stroke volume (% [stroke volume = (stroke volumeDCC—stroke volumebase)/stroke volumebase) × 100] versus Ees. Stroke volumeDCC is stroke volume with DCC and stroke volumebase is the baseline stroke volume.

in a weak heart (40% normal). These principles have been verified in vivo with the use of a constant pressure epicardial compression device and a canine model of heart failure in which graded levels of heart failure were achieved by coronary artery microembolization.[8] The plot shown in Figure 6 is taken from the in vivo experiments and is analogous to the plot illustrated in panel B of Figure 5.

A full explanation of the physiology of DCC is still more complicated. DCC affects both ventricles equally, and only a single ventricular analysis has been discussed above. The intrinsic contractile strength and afterload resistance are lower for the right ventricle than the left ventricle. Thus, the effects of DCC on the right ventricle are proportionally greater.[4,8] Since under steady state conditions the stroke volume must be approximately the same for both ventricles, the effect of DCC on the right ventricle cannot translate into a larger stroke volume for the right ventricle than for the left ventricle. The degree of cardiac output augmentation will depend on the effects of DCC on the unequal pumping capacity and vascular resistance of

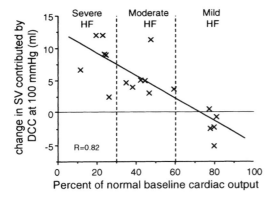

FIGURE 6. A plot of the change in the stroke volume produced by direct cardiac compression (DCC) versus the degree of heart failure indexed as the percent the normal baseline value. The correlation coefficient is 0.82.

the left ventricle and right ventricle, such that the ultimate degree of compression pressure to be used will be critically dependent on the effect of DCC on the right ventricle.[8] That is, increasing compression pressure to values above those required to completely empty the right ventricle will likely fail to further increase left ventricular outputs.

Biologic Compression Devices or Muscle Wraps

Skeletal Muscle as a Pump

Not surprisingly, early investigations into the effects of epicardial compression used skeletal muscle autografts to provide the supplemental pumping force. Skeletal muscles are capable of developing large forces, they do not require an external energy source, and they are not subject to immunologic rejection. In initial investigations, the left hemidiaphragm was wrapped around the distal thoracic aorta and contractions were stimulated via the intact phrenic nerve.[12] Diastolic augmentation of aortic blood pressure was achieved, but the effect was inconsistent and short-lived because of muscle fatigue. Skeletal muscles have a lower density of mitochondria per individual muscle cell than do cardiac myocytes. For this reason, skeletal muscles fatigue easily compared with cardiac muscle.

Skeletal muscles can adapt to their pattern of use and can be trained to perform with increased fatigue resistance.[13] Long-term, low-frequency electrical stimulation can transform fast type II skeletal muscle fibers into the slow type I fibers.[14–16] The fast-to-slow transformation improves the match between adenosine triphosphate production and utilization under continuous working conditions, thus making the muscle resistant to fatigue. With the muscle transformation, there is an associated loss of muscle mass, power, and contractile speed; however, it initially appeared that the remaining power would be more than required for ventricular assist.[17] Histologic and morphologic examinations have confirmed muscle transformation in both animal models and humans. However, it is evident that stimulation frequencies and patterns employed thus far have been unsuccessful in producing a transformation that results in muscle characteristics sufficient to aid muscular contraction over long periods.[18]

Surgical Technique

Carpentier and Chachques[19] reported the first successful cardiomyoplasty in 1985. The left latissimus dorsi muscle was transferred into the chest cavity to patch a large myocardial defect following resection of a cardiac tumor. Although more than 400 procedures have since been performed worldwide, the procedure has remained essentially unchanged. The procedure is illustrated in Figure 7. The patient is placed in the lateral decubitus position and a longitudinal flank incision is made extending from the axilla to iliac crest. The left latissimus dorsi muscle is freed from its tendinous insertions, and care is taken to preserve the neurovascular bundle. The anterior two thirds of the second or third rib is resected, allowing the latissimus dorsi muscle flap to be pulled into the thoracic cavity, and the proximal tendon is sutured to the periosteum of the second rib. A sternotomy or left thoracotomy is performed to expose the mediastinum. The pericardial sac is then opened and the latissimus dorsi muscle is wrapped around the heart to encompass both ventricular chambers. The wrap is secured to the pericardium posteriorly and the myocardium anteriorly. Myocardial pacing electrodes are placed intramuscularly in the proximal part of the latis-

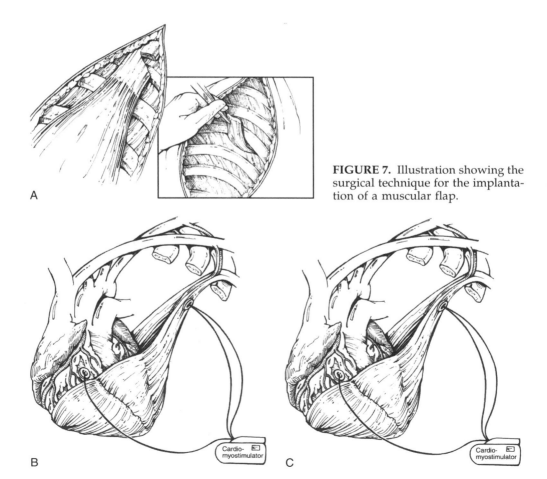

FIGURE 7. Illustration showing the surgical technique for the implantation of a muscular flap.

simus dorsi muscle, and sensing electrodes are sewn into the right ventricle. Both electrodes are connected to the cardiomyostimulator (Medtronic Inc., Minneapolis, MN), which is placed in a subrectus pocket in the abdominal wall. The cardiomyostimulator senses the R wave and stimulates the latissimus dorsi muscle wrap to contract with the native heartbeat. A delay period between 2 and 3 weeks prior to muscle stimulation enables the latissimus dorsi muscle to recover from loss of its blood supply and to develop adhesions between the epicardium and the muscle flap.[20-22] A 6-week muscle-conditioning period is begun in which the pulse frequency is gradually increased from 2 to 30 Hz.

Clinical Experience with Dynamic Cardiomyoplasty

Cardiomyoplasty as a treatment for end-stage heart disease has been performed at several centers across Europe and the Americas.[23-27] Patient selection for this therapy has been relatively confined to those suffering from severe heart failure (New York Heart Association [NYHA] functional Classes III to IV) and those who are not candidates for revascularization surgery or heart transplantation. Among the various study groups, including the American Cardiomyoplasty Study Group consisting of the eight centers in North and South America,[23] the patient population was predominantly male, average age ranging from 55 to 58 years, and the etiology of heart failure was mixed between idiopathic and ischemic cardiomyopathies. Concomitant procedures were performed in 29% to 44% of the patients in various study groups, and included ventricular aneurysm resection, tumor resection, valve replacement, and coronary artery bypass grafting. The reported rates for in-hospital mortality associated with cardiomyoplasty varied from 11% to 54% depending on the individual institutional experience with the procedure. The risk factors for in-hospital mortality were age, associated surgical procedures, biventricular heart failure, and preoperative requirement for hospitalization. Following cardiomyoplasty, the 1-year survival rates ranged from 65% to 71%, with the most common causes of death being heart failure and ventricular arrhythmias. Risk factors at the time of surgery that influenced 1-year survival were NYHA functional Class IV, biventricular heart failure, atrial fibrillation, and ejection fraction less than 15%. The inability of cardiomyoplasty to offer assistance to the failing heart during the immediate perioperative period was considered to account for the high early mortality rates. It has been suggested that patients who are to undergo this procedure should have enough residual ventricular function to support them throughout this period. This has practically limited selection criteria for cardiomyoplasty to NYHA functional Class III patients.

Symptomatic improvement was observed in patients who had cardiomyoplasty with reported significant decreases in NYHA functional class and increases in activity of daily living score. Improvements in ejection fractions were also observed among the various studies, and consistently correlated with symptomatic improvement. However, the increase in ejection fraction was rather modest, going from 23% to 26% to only 25% to 33%. More important indices of cardiac function such as cardiac index, capillary wedge pressure, exercise tolerance, or oxygen consumption have not been consistently improved with cardiomyoplasty. Thus, the improvement in patients' symptoms has been suggested to reflect a placebo effect, or even an overall improvement in medical management of these patients. Alternatively, it has been suggested that the procedure may attenuate the progression of left ventricle enlargement and limit further ventricular deterioration of the ejection fraction—the so-called girdling effect.[28-30] In support of this concept, similar levels of improvement from cardiomyoplasty, in terms of ejection fraction and ESPVRs, were observed with the cardiomyostimulator turned off, as well as with it turned on.[29]

Limitations

Despite the sound physiologic principles of epicardial compression, cardiomyoplasty has not been able to provide significant and consistent improvements in ventricular performance. Reduced ventricular preload volumes and suboptimal loading conditions of the skeletal muscle wrap can partially explain the lack of hemodynamic benefit. As discussed in an earlier section, preload volumes are reduced with epicardial compression, resulting in diminished stroke volume augmentation. Additionally, suboptimal loading conditions of the skeletal muscle over time may result in a reduced force-generating ability as the muscle undergoes fatty replacement. Histologic examination of the latissimus dorsi muscle following the cardiomyoplasty suggests that the grafted muscle undergoes extensive fibrosis and fatty replacement.[26,27] Another undesirable effect of cardiomyoplasty is the distorting influence of the muscle on the heart. With each assisted contraction, cardiomyoplasty produces marked rotation and displacement of the left ventricle[31] that may impede ventricular filling or even possibly outflow; however, this remains unproved.

Mechanical Compression Devices

Mechanical Pumping Force

Skeletal muscle wraps have been unable to provide an effective and reliable source of epicardial compression. The lengthy preconditioning period required and the high perioperative mortality rate of this procedure have virtually excluded NYHA Class IV heart failure patients, the group of patients that would benefit the most from ventricular assist. Additionally, the use of the cardiomyostimulator virtually precludes the use of pacemakers and implantable defibrillators in a patient population prone to conduction disturbances and ventricular arrhythmias. For these reasons, investigators have turned to mechanically driven epicardial compression devices, which are currently under development at several different institutions across the United States and Europe. The basic components of these devices consist of a compression-driving system, an electrocardiogram sensor/digital controller, and an epicardial cup or cuff. Adaptations to these individual components have been used to design devices rather specifically for cardiopulmonary resuscitation (CPR), acute ventricular support, and long-term ventricular support. Although no device is currently available for routine clinical use, there are several systems under development and evaluation.

CPR Devices

In 1965 George Anstadt[32] introduced an epicardial compression device that could administer efficient and sustained CPR. This device, known as the Anstadt cup (Fig. 8), is an elliptically shaped cup that fits over both right and left ventricular chambers. It has a semirigid outer shell and an inflatable inner diaphragm that delivers compression forces to the heart. Vacuum pressure (70 mm Hg) at the apex of the heart is used to attach the cup to the heart and to prevent migration of the device. Positive and negative pressure is generated within the inner diaphragm with the use of a pneumatic drive system that is able to deliver pulsed pressure. Because the inner diaphragm is tightly sealed to the epicardial surface, the device can provide diastolic decompression, as well as epicardial compression. Cycle rates are fixed but can be adjusted to provide the compressions at the desired rate. However, for technical reasons the device was not designed to deliver epicardial compressions synchronized with the native heartbeat. Although asynchronous ventricular assistance has been attempted, the increased frequency of rhythm disturbances and the potential for injurious effects to the myocardium have limited investigation of the utility of this device to the realm of CPR.

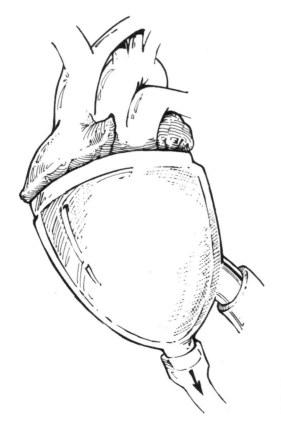

FIGURE 8. Illustration showing the Anstadt cup fitting around both ventricular chambers.

Devices Designed to Assist the Acutely Failing Heart

A ventricular support device designed to stabilize the acutely failing heart should be simple to apply in an unstable situation and freely adjustable to optimize ventricular outputs under a variety of clinical conditions. It should provide complete circulatory support in the event of cardiac arrest, and allow for easy removal following recovery of the failing heart. One system presently under development that meets these requirements is the CardioSupport System™ (Cardio Technologies, Inc., Pine Brook, NJ), which is illustrated in Figure 9. The device has a cuff-like structure that is placed around the outside of the heart between the atrioventricular groove and the apex. Negative pressure (200 mm Hg) applied to the apex of the heart is used to fix the device to the heart. The cuff's compression bladder circumscribes both ventricles around the base and is inflated synchronously with the heart's natural contraction when providing cardiac support. The inside of the vacuum seal has two finely meshed electrode bands which provide a reliable electrocardiographic source needed for timing the inflation and deflation of the compression system. The electrodes can also be used for defibrillation.

Upon inflation of the cuff, the ventricular walls are compressed, expelling the blood from the ventricles. Deflation of the cuff allows the ventricles to fill with blood, which is expelled during the next cuff inflation. The compression force is provided by an air compressor and is controlled with a computer console and electromechanical tether that regulates the amount, frequency, and duration of the compression

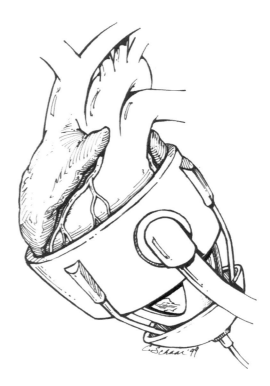

FIGURE 9. The CardioSupport System currently under development by Cardio Technologies, Inc. (The illustration was a generous gift from Bob Reinhardt, CTI Inc.)

pressure to be delivered to the epicardium. Individual parameters can be easily adjusted to optimize the ventricular assistance specific to the needs of the patient. In the CPR mode, the system inflates and deflates the cuff at a fixed rate that can be modified by the operator.

Devices Designed for Chronic Ventricular Support

Epicardial compression devices designed for chronic ventricular support should be both reliable and portable. The Heart Booster (ABIOMED, Inc., Danvers, MA), illustrated in Figure 10, is under development with design specifications suited for chronic ventricular support. The interface between the heart and the compression system is also a cuff-like apparatus that consists of several individual parallel compression tubes that are added serially to cover both ventricular chambers. These tubes form a band around the base of the heart and are held firmly to the epicardium with use of surgical adhesive. The device uses a hydraulic drive system that fills and empties the compression tubes with fluid during the respective half-cycles. These drive systems can be relatively small, they run on electricity, and they can operate on a rechargeable battery; hence, this type of device is well suited for chronic use.

Surgical Technique

Application of any of the three compression devices discussed is relatively simple and can be achieved through either a left thoracotomy or a median sternotomy.

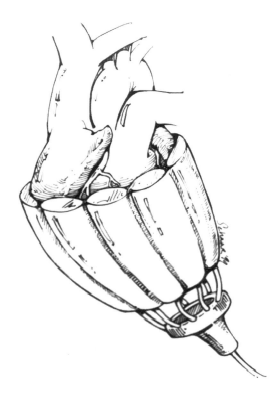

FIGURE 10. The Heart Booster currently under development by ABIOMED, Inc. (The illustration was a generous gift from Mike Milbocker, ABIOMED, Inc.)

Sizing of the Anstadt cup or the CardioSupport System is determined by visual inspection; however, estimates based on the size of the cardiac silhouette from chest x-ray or even measurement of the circumference of the heart at the base have proven helpful. The Anstadt cup and the CardioSupport System are sized by the inner diameter and are manufactured in increments of 5 to 10 mm. The inner diameter should be approximately the same diameter as the natural heart in order to ensure enough space to fit both ventricles adequately. The suction line and drive lines are brought out of the chest substernally or anterolaterally through an intercostal space, and care is taken to avoid kinking in either line. Before the chest is closed, compressions are initiated and, with the CardioSupport System and Heart Booster, synchronized with the native heartbeat by setting the onset of device compression pressure approximately equal to the onset of ventricular pressure increase. In the animal laboratory, this is accomplished with the use of a left ventricular pressure transducer; however, a pulmonary artery catheter pulled into the right ventricular chamber should provide a good approximation and is a feasible option clinically. The amount of compression pressure is slowly ramped upward until cardiac output is maximized. A left chest tube is placed and the chest is closed with the device actively assisting the heart.

Clinical Experience with Epicardial Compression Devices

To date, there have been no clinical studies using an epicardial compression device to assist the native ventricular contraction. The CardioSupport System and the Heart Booster are still under development, and only recently has the CardioSupport System been approved for phase I trials in Europe. Therefore, much of the clinical experience with epicardial compression comes from work done on the arrested heart using the Anstadt cup. The largest reported series of patients studied using this device comprised 12 patients.[33] The average age in the group was 48.2 ± 4.2 years, with a 5:7 female:male ratio. The average time from witnessed cardiac arrest to device application was 81 ± 9 minutes, although the time from skin incision to device application was reportedly less than 2 minutes. Systolic and diastolic blood pressures averaged 78 ± 4 and 41 ± 4 mm Hg, respectively, with a mean cardiac output of 3.14 ± 0.18 L/min obtained for periods ranging from 25 minutes to 18 hours (mean 228 ± 84 min). The Anstadt cup was compared to open-chest cardiac massage performed at similar compression rates and was more effective than open-chest cardiac massage at increasing arterial pressures (65% improvement) and cardiac output (190% improvement). Of the 12 patients reported on, 4 were successfully defibrillated; however, 2 died of heart failure within the first hour after resuscitation and 2 died from cardiac failure and respiratory insufficiency within 2 days from resuscitation. For one patient, the device provided adequate circulatory support to be bridged to emergent cardiopulmonary bypass, but the patient later died from a myocardial infarction. There were no complications associated with mechanical CPR; however, complications related to open-chest cardiac massage included a cardiac laceration during pericardiotomy and a ventricular rupture. Also of significance but not included in this study, was a report of successful circulatory support with the Anstadt cup for 56 hours with successful bridging to transplantation and the patient alive and well at 1-year follow-up.[34]

Potential Limitations

The potential injurious effects of direct mechanical compression on myocardium is a matter of concern with these or any other similar support mechanisms. Myocardial contusions, increased frequency of arrhythmias, and myocardial ischemia are the most obvious concerns. Early experience with the Anstadt cup demonstrated histologic evidence of nontransmural ecchymoses present on the endocardial surface of the right ventricle and pulmonary outflow tract when the device was used to deliver epicardial compression in dogs for periods between 6 and 24 hours.[35,36] When the duration of compression was increased to 3.5 to 20 months, histologic examination revealed a small scar in the same region. Importantly, these studies were performed with compressions asynchronous with the native heartbeat, making the likelihood for myocardial injury greater. A small amount of myocardial contusion and edema from direct mechanical compression may be unavoidable, but precautions such as fine adjustment of the synchronization of device contraction with ventricular contraction and avoidance of excessive compression will likely reduce these potential injurious effects. Since mechanical force can cause myocardial depolarization, DCC may increase the frequency of arrhythmias. Antiarrhythmic therapies such as lidocaine or bretylium and proper electrolyte management will be important to help control the frequency of arrhythmias. Unlike cardiomyoplasty, these devices do not represent contraindications to indwelling pacemakers or implantable defibrillators, which can be used if required. The potential for myocardial ischemia has also been considered a concern, especially since compression of the coronary arteries may theoretically impede blood flow. The majority of myocardial perfusion, however, occurs during diastole when the compression forces are reduced to zero, and with elevated arterial pressures from the device, myocardial perfusion may in fact improve.

Future Considerations

Although there has been a considerable amount of work done with epicardial compression, the potential of this mode of therapy as a therapy for patients with end-stage heart failure has yet to be realized. With the improvement in device design and with our understanding of the physiology of epicardial compression, however, such devices will provide an important future mode of left ventricular support. The most immediate application of these devices will be in the setting of acute heart failure, in which these devices will act to stabilize the heart for transplantation, permanent LVAD implantation, or even recovery of ventricular function. Recent studies have suggested that the heart can undergo reverse remodeling from prolonged ventricular unloading by conventional LVAD support[37] and that this is accompanied by histologic and molecular changes indicative of recovery of ventricular function. Conventional methods of ventricular support provide mechanical unloading; however, they do not assist with the actual muscular shortening as does epicardial compression. Assistance of myofibril shortening may offer theoretical advantages for ventricular recovery.

References

1. Kawaguchi O, Goto Y, Futaki, et al. Mechanical enhancement and myocardial oxygen saving by synchronized dynamic left ventricular compression. *J Thorac Cardiovasc Surg* 1992;103:573–581.
2. Kawaguchi O, Goto Y, Futaki S, et al. The effects of dynamic cardiac compression on ventricular mechanics and energetics. Role of ventricular size and contractility. *J Thorac Cardiovasc Surg* 1994;107:850–859.
3. Kawaguchi O, Goto Y, Ohgoshi Y, et al. Dynamic cardiac compression improves contractile efficiency of the heart. *J Thorac Cardiovasc Surg* 1997;113:923–931.
4. Artrip JH, Leventhal AR, Tsitlik JE, et al. Hemodynamic effects of direct bi-ventricular compression studied in isovolumic and ejecting isolated canine hearts. *Circulation* 1999; 99:2177–2184.
5. Spotnitz HM, Merker C, Malm JR. Applied physiology of the canine rectus abdominus: Force-length curves correlated with functional characteristics of a rectus powered ventricle. Potential for cardiac assistance. *Trans Am Soc Artif Intern Org* 1974;20B:747–755.
6. Aklog L, Murphy MP, Chen SB, et al. Right latissimus dorsi cardiomyoplasty improves left ventricular function by increasing peak systolic elastance (Emax). *Circulation* 1994;90: 112–118.
7. Cho PW, Levin HR, Curtis WE, et al. Pressure-volume analysis of changes in cardiac function in chronic cardiomyoplasty. *Ann Thorac Surg* 1993;56:38–45.
8. Artrip JH, Yi GH, Levin HR, et al. The physiologic and hemodynamic evaluation of non-uniform direct cardiac compression. *Circulation* 1999. In press.
9. Corin WJ, George DT, Sink JD, Santamore WP. Dynamic cardiomyoplasty acutely impairs left ventricular diastolic function. *J Thorac Cardiovasc Surg* 1992;104(6):1662–1671.
10. Salmons S, Jarvis JC. Cardiomyoplasty: The basic issues. *Card Chron* 1990;4:1–7.
11. Sunagawa K, Maughan L, Burkhoff D, Sagawa K. Left ventricular interaction with arterial load studied in isolated canine ventricle. *Am J Physiol* 1983;245:H773-H780.
12. Nakamura K, Glenn WL. Graft of the diaphragm as a substitute for myocardium. *J Surg Res* 1964;4+5–439.
13. Salmons S, Sreter FA. Significance of impulse activity in the transformation of skeletal muscle type. *Nature* 1976;263:30–34.
14. Salmons S, Vrbova G. The influence of activity on some contractile characteristics of mammalian fast and slow muscles. *J Physiol* 1969;201:535–549.
15. Sreter FA, Gergely J, Salmons S, Romanul F. Synthesis by fast muscle of myosin light chains characteristic of slow muscle in response to long term stimulation. *Nature* 1973; 241:17–20.
16. Clark BJ, Acker MA, McCully K, et al. In vivo 31P-NMR spectroscopy of chronically stimulated canine skeletal muscle. *Am J Physiol* 1988;254:C258-C266.
17. Salmons S, Jarvis JC. Cardiac assistance from skeletal muscle: A critical appraisal of various approaches. *Br Heart J* 1992;68:333–338.
18. Goldstein DJ, Costanzo MR, Rose EA. Novel cardiac replacement therapies. In Rose EA, Stevenson LW (eds): *Management of End Stage Heart Disease.* Philadelphia: Lippincott-Raven Publishers; 1998:255–261.
19. Carpentier A, Chachques JC. Myocardial substitution with a stimulated skeletal muscle: First successful clinical case. *Lancet* 1985;1:1267.
20. Mannion JD, Velchick M, Hammond RL, et al. Effects of collateral blood vessel ligation and electrical conditioning of blood flow in dog latissimus dorsi. *J Surg Res* 1989;47:332–340.
21. Chacques JC, Grandjean PA, Carpentier A. Patient management and clinical follow-up after cardiomyoplasty. *J Card Surg* 1991;6:89–99.
22. Chagas AC, Moreira LF, da Luz PL, et al. Stimulated preconditioned skeletal muscle cardiomyoplasty. An effective means of cardiac assist. *Circulation* 1989;80(5 Pt. 2):III202-III208.
23. Furnary AP, Jessup FM, Moreira LP. Multicenter trial of dynamic cardiomyoplasty for chronic heart failure. The American Cardiomyoplasty Group. *J Am Coll Cardiol* 1996;28(5): 1175–1180.
24. Carpentier A, Chachques JC, Acar C, et al. Dynamic cardiomyoplasty at seven years. *J Thorac Cardiovasc Surg* 1993;106(1):42–52.

25. Magovern JA, Magovern GJ Sr, Maher TD Jr, et al. Operation for congestive heart failure: Transplantation, coronary artery bypass, and cardiomyoplasty. *Ann Thorac Surg* 1993; 56(3):418–425.
26. Lucas CM, van der Veen FH, Cheriex EC, et al. Long term follow-up (12 to 35 weeks) after dynamic cardiomyoplasty. *J Am Coll Cardiol* 1993;22:758–767.
27. Moreira LFP, Bocchi EA, Stolf NAG, et al. Current expectation in dynamic cardiomyoplasty. *Ann Thorac Surg* 1993;55:299–303.
28. Capouya ER, Gerber RS, Drinkwater DC Jr, et al. Girdling effect of nonstimulated cardiomyoplasty on left ventricular function. *Ann Thorac Surg* 1993;56:867–871.
29. Kass DA, Baughman KL, Pak PH, et al. Reverse remodeling from cardiomyoplasty in human heart failure. External constraint versus active assist. *Circulation* 1995;91:2314–2318.
30. Patel HJ, Lankford EB, Polidori DJ, et al. Dynamic cardiomyoplasty: Its chronic and acute effects on the failing heart. *J Thorac Cardiovasc Surg* 1997;114(2):169–178.
31. Cho PW, Levin HR, Curtis WE, et al. New method for mechanistic studies of cardiomyoplasty: Three-dimensional MRI reconstructions. *Ann Thorac Surg* 1994;57:1605–1611.
32. Anstadt GL, Blakemore WS, Baue AE. A new instrument for prolonged mechanical massage. *Circulation* 1965;31(suppl. II):43. Abstract.
33. Anstadt MP, Bartlett RL, Malone JP, et al. Direct mechanical ventricular actuation for cardiac arrest in humans. A clinical feasibility trial. *Chest* 1991;100(1):86–92.
34. Lowe JE, Anstadt MP, Van Trigt P, et al. First successful bridge to cardiac transplantation using direct mechanical ventricular actuation. *Ann Thorac Surg* 1991;52:1237–1245.
35. Anstadt MP, Tedder SD, Vander Heide RS, et al. Cardiac pathology following resuscitative circulatory support: Direct mechanical ventricular actuation versus cardiopulmonary bypass. *ASAIO J* 1992;38:75–81.
36. Anstadt MP, Anstadt GL, Lowe JE. Direct mechanical ventricular actuation: A review. *Resuscitation* 1991;21:7–23.
37. Levin HR, Oz MC, Chen JM, et al. Reversal of chronic ventricular dilation in patients with end-stage cardiomyopathy by prolonged mechanical unloading. *Circulation* 1995;91(11): 2717–2720.

Chapter 29

The Pennsylvania State University Totally Implantable Left Ventricular Assist Device and Total Artificial Heart

Sanjay M. Mehta, MD and Walter E. Pae, Jr., MD

The success of mechanical circulatory support as a bridge to transplantation has renewed an interest in chronic circulatory support as an alternative means to treat patients with end-stage heart failure.[1,2] In fact, clinical trials are under way to evaluate "wearable" systems; over the last 30 years, investigators at the Pennsylvania State University (PSU), under the guidance of Dr. William Pierce, have worked toward the development of safe and reliable methods of sustained mechanical circulatory support. This work has culminated in the development of a completely implanted left ventricular assist device (LVAD) and a similarly implanted total artificial heart (TAH). This chapter provides a basic description of these systems, a summary of test data, a synopsis of indications for implantation of these systems, and a time table for planned ultimate clinical use.

The development of completely implantable mechanical circulatory assistance has evolved, in part, from the original pneumatically driven systems developed at PSU. The pneumatically driven TAH and LVAD were initially developed for extended circulatory assistance and for the resuscitation of patients in postcardiotomy cardiogenic shock.[3–5] These devices ultimately proved most useful as bridging tools for patients with end-stage heart failure who were awaiting cardiac transplantation.[6,7] The success of these systems at restoring normal perfusion has become apparent with extended clinical experience; they often reverse the sequelae associated with multisystem organ failure. Early experience with the PSU and Jarvik-7 (Symbion Inc., Salt Lake City, UT) TAHs proved that these devices could reliably resuscitate critically ill patients; however, the experience with both systems was hampered by problems with chronic mediastinal infections.[8–10] Subsequent experience with a variety of VAD systems has demonstrated the continued infectious risk associated with percutaneous external communication, even when these devices are used for short-

From Goldstein DJ and Oz MC (eds). *Cardiac Assist Devices.* Armonk, NY: Futura Publishing Co., Inc.; ©2000.

term support.[11-13] The externalized components of these systems are characterized by the inflow/outflow cannulae of the Thoratec (Thoratec Inc., Berkeley, CA) device, which evolved from the original PSU experience. Similar percutaneous communication exists with the blood tubing of the ABIOMED BVS 5000 (ABIOMED Cardiovascular Inc., Danvers, MA) device and centrifugal pumps, and though smaller in caliber, the externalized drive line of the pneumatic TCI HeartMate (Thermo Cardiosystems Inc., Woburn, MA). The electrically driven Novacor (Novacor Division, Baxter Healthcare Corporation, Oakland, CA) and electric TCI HeartMate pumps also require external venting, which mandates a percutaneous line. Great pains have been taken to minimize the risk of infection related to these lines by tunneling techniques and local line care, however, as with any break in the primary defense mechanism of the skin, the risk of infection persists. Furthermore, by definition the patient is always "coupled" to the device.

Device and line infections have at times proven devastating to patients awaiting cardiac transplantation. The ability to eradicate an active infection in an implanted foreign material continues to prove difficult and often mandates complete removal of the implanted device. Although chronic antibiotics have been used to suppress such infections in patients awaiting transplant, this approach has often resulted in virulent infections after transplant, and would likely find limited efficacy in patients receiving these devices as destination therapy. Additional lifestyle limitations can be imagined with devices that require a means of chronic external communication. Ultimately, a system designed for chronic mechanical circulatory support should allow return to a normal and comfortable existence for the recipient. This implies that the system should be quiet, reliable, free of vibration or noticeable motion, and should result in an acceptable level of hindrance of lifestyle, hygiene, or other day-to-day activities. In addition, there should be limited maintenance requirements. Concerns such as these have led us to develop a means of circulatory support that is completely implantable.

The Arrow Lionheart-2000 Completely Implanted LVAD

Rationale

Experience with temporary mechanical circulatory assistance has demonstrated that the majority of patients suffering end-stage heart disease can be supported with univentricular assistance.[7] Thus, the development of a chronically implanted LVAD should meet the demands of most patients who are otherwise deemed poor candidates for cardiac transplantation. The theoretic advantages of left ventricular support in comparison to a TAH are numerous. Implantation of the LVAD system is less complicated. The preperitoneal location of implantation minimizes the amount of foreign body within the mediastinum. Although left ventricular function is markedly impaired, there remains a potential back-up in the event of device failure. Finally, the less complicated design of ventricular assist pumps reduces the potential for mechanical failure with these devices.[14]

Device Description

The Arrow Lionheart-2000 LVAD (Arrow, Inc., Reading, PA) is composed of a heterotopically placed pump and its associated electronics hardware, as well as a variable volume compliance chamber, as depicted in Figure 1. The pump weighs 1.5 pounds and the complete set of components totals 3.2 pounds. The hardware comprising this system is implanted without the need for percutaneous communication.[15]

The pump comprises a titanium case that houses the motor, blood sac, and pusher-plate, as well as inlet and outlet mechanical heart valves (Fig. 2). A polyethylene form-based dipping process is used to construct the polyurethane blood sacs. This process results in a seam-free blood bag, which provides smooth blood contact surface for the pump. Delrin disk monostrut valves are used to assure unidirectional flow through the pump. A 27 mm valve is employed at the pump inlet and a 25 mm valve at the pump outlet, assuring durable, long-term valve reliability.

The pump is driven by a direct-current (DC) brushless motor, which drives a roller screw mechanism. A pusher-plate is attached at one end of the roller screw (Fig. 3). Linear motion of the roller screw is translated by the pusher-plate into reciprocating compression of the blood sac with concomitant pulsatile flow through the pump. The pusher-plate is not attached to the blood sac, so that during diastole

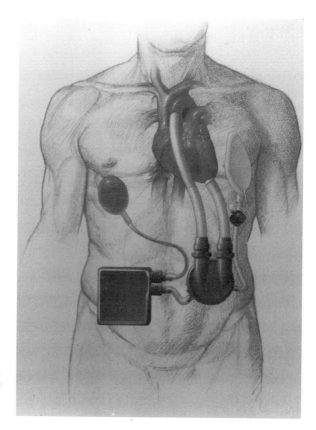

FIGURE 1. Schematic representation of Arrow Lionheart-2000 LVAD components as they appear in implanted positions.

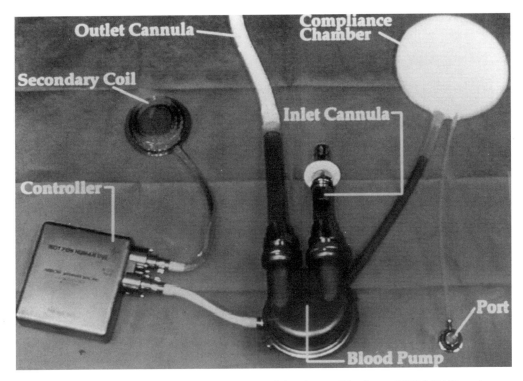

FIGURE 2. Labeled individual components of the Arrow Lionheart-2000-LVAD system.

the pump fills passively. The dynamic stroke volume of the pump is 64 mL, which allows a maximum sustained output of approximately 8 L/min. Motor position is monitored continuously by the pump controller via mounted Hall effect sensors.[15]

A gas-filled compliance chamber is attached to the motor housing to compensate for the gas-volume displacement produced by blood sac volume changes and diffusion gas losses across the blood sac, as shown in Figure 4.[16] The compliance chamber is placed in the left pleural cavity, and volume changes within the compliance system are monitored and adjusted via an attached subcutaneous infusion port placed over the left anterior chest wall. Volume changes within the system are accommodated by accessing the infusion port at approximately 3- to 4-week intervals.

The pump controller is implanted in the right lower quadrant and is responsible for power regulation of the external power supply, motor control, and monitoring, and houses rechargeable batteries which provide temporary power supply when the patient is disconnected from the external power supply. These batteries provide an emergent back-up for a malfunctioning external power supply and allow a minimum of 30 minutes of untethered activity with decoupling; they can be recharged to 85% of capacity within 5 hours. Telemetry is also provided, allowing intermittent monitoring of system data, and modification of controller software as dictated by clinical needs. The control system for the Lionheart-2000 relies on end-diastolic volume as a reflection of the patients pump needs, which are estimated by motor speed and voltage. Pumping characteristics are automatically adjusted by a software algorithm, which attempts to provide maximal filling of the pump with each stroke, by altering the pump speed.[15]

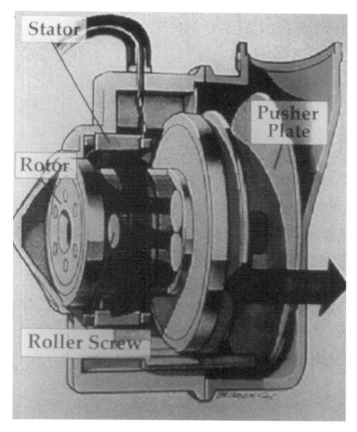

FIGURE 3. The roller screw and attached pusher-plates contained are shown in this cross-sectional diagram of the Arrow Lionheart-2000 LVAD.

Energy is supplied to the pump by means of a transcutaneous energy transmission system (TETS).[17] An external power pack consisting of rechargeable and replaceable cells provides DC power to a power transmitter, which converts this source to an alternating current supply, subsequently driving a wearable external primary power coil. This primary coil is secured on the skin overlying the secondary power coil, which is implanted and secured within the subcutaneous tissues of the right chest wall. Induction coupling provides a transcutaneous power source that is subsequently rectified to DC voltage, providing energy to the pump and controller (Fig. 5).

Finally, a physician's monitor has been developed to allow accurate telemetry communication with the controller to facilitate downloading of stored parameters and data, as well as modification of system software.

Technique of Implantation

The Lionheart-2000 LVAD requires dissection of the preperitoneal space, the left pleural space, and the subcutaneous tissues of the anterior chest wall for complete

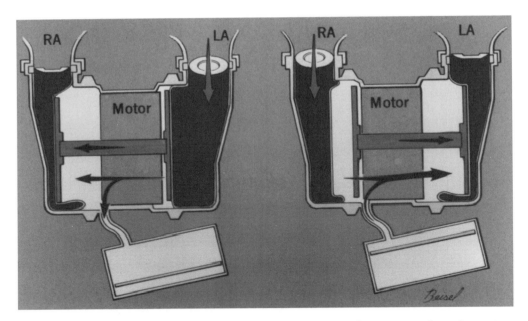

FIGURE 4. A simple representation of the compliance system demonstrates how the system compensates for gas volume changes within the motor housing. The diagram demonstrates the system as employed with the Pennsylvania State University total artificial heart in a manner comparable to that described for the left ventricular assist device.

implantation of its individual components. A traditional median sternotomy incision is continued to the level of the umbilicus. Prior to cannulation for cardiopulmonary bypass, the left rectus sheath is opened and a preperitoneal pocket is developed that will accommodate placement of the pump. Following institution of normothermic cardiopulmonary bypass , the diaphragm is opened for approximately 3 cm at the level of the ventricular apex to accommodate placement of the inflow cannula of the assist pump. A sewing ring is secured at the apex after apical coring with use of interrupted nonabsorbable sutures. The albumin-primed pump is place within the preperitoneal pocket and the inflow graft is brought up through the previously developed diaphragmatic rent at the level of the apex. The graft is subsequently secured to the previously placed apical sewing ring. A partial occlusion aortic cross-clamp is placed on the ascending aorta and an aortotomy is fashioned. An end-to-side anastomosis is created between the outflow graft and the aorta. The previously primed pump is de-aired via antegrade passive flow and is subsequently carefully secured to the outflow graft, which has been filled with a heparinized saline solution. Prior to heparinization a right lower quadrant transverse incision is used to fashion a second preperitoneal pocket for the electronics canister. The canister is inserted and a submuscular tunnel is developed for the cable between the pump and canister. An additional incision is made at the level of the sixth intercostal space over the anterior chest wall, and a subcutaneous pocket is developed to accommodate the secondary TETS coil. The electronic cable for the TETS system is subsequently tunneled to the electronics canister and attached to its designated connector. Finally, the left pleural space is entered to allow placement of the variable volume compliance chamber. The inlet/outlet tube of the compliance chamber is tunneled to the left

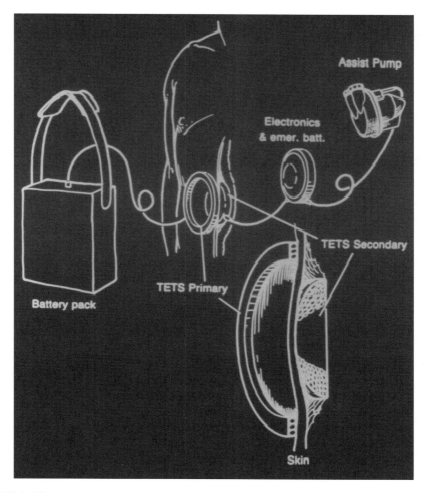

FIGURE 5. The transcutaneous energy transmission system (TETS) is shown schematically with its individual components including external power source, primary TETS coil, and secondary TETS coil.

upper quadrant and fastened and secured to the pump. A 2 cm incision over the lower anterior chest wall allows for the development of a subcutaneous pocket for the infusaport, the tubing of which is in turn tunneled between underlying ribs and secured to the compliance chamber.

When all of the components of the Lionheart-2000 have been attached and secured, a sterile primary TETS coil is utilized to supply power to the device, and flows are slowly increased via telemetry with concomitant weaning of cardiopulmonary bypass. Generally, preoperative inotropes are continued in the postoperative period, and weaned over the ensuing days as the patient's right heart function accommodates to left ventricular unloading. The patient's incisions are closed, over thoracostomy tubes, and closed suction drains are placed in the areas of preperitoneal dissection. Anticoagulation therapy is instituted within the first 24 hours postoperatively, when hemostasis is completely obtained as heralded by a consistent reduction in chest tube drainage. Heparin infusion without a bolus is initially instituted with a targeted thromboplastin time of 60 to 80 seconds. Upon extubation, the patient is begun on warfarin therapy, with oral anticoagulation goals mimicking those for implanted mechanical prosthetic heart valves.

Preclinical Experience

A reliable bovine model has been employed as a means of large animal testing mechanical circulatory assist devices at PSU for the last 30 years. Thus, in vivo testing of the Arrow Lionheart-2000 has proceeded similarly over the last 4 years.[12] Both acute and chronic studies have now been undertaken within National Institutes of Health (NIH) guidelines, and successful, safe, long-term support has been realized. A total of 21 devices have been implanted to date. End organ function has remained normal in all animal studies independent of the duration of support. Hemolysis, infection, and thromboembolic events have not been an issue, and the compliance chamber and TETS system have functioned flawlessly. These results have proven consistent with those described for pneumatic devices in previous studies. Additionally, an integrated in vitro testing facility, which allows continuous automated monitoring of these devices in simulated physiologic loops, is generating long-term durability data for the Lionheart-2000, with systems now functioning greater than 2 years.

Animal and mock circuit data have been completed for formal submission to the Food and Drug Administration toward approval for initial clinical testing, which will be realized within the next year.

The PSU/3M Health Care TAH

Rationale

A select population of patients suffering end-stage heart disease is unlikely to benefit from univentricular support. Conditions such as significant biventricular failure, large mural thrombus, refractory malignant arrhythmias, previous heart transplant, chronically elevated pulmonary hypertension, complex congenital heart disease, recent myocardial infarction, and significant valvular pathology or previous prosthetic valve replacement may preclude effective LVAD support. The absolute number of patients with end-stage congestive heart failure requiring a TAH is subject to speculation. However, this population is at least equal in number to the patients requiring concomitant right ventricular assistance in the bridge-to-transplant population, which is reported at 10% to 12%.[6] The TAH provides an effective alternative in this group of patients, as current system sizes would prohibit use of a completely implanted biventricular assistance system.

Concern regarding adequate circulatory support for this population of patients has led to the parallel development of a completely implantable TAH. The PSU and 3M Health Care Inc., (Minneapolis, MN) have worked, under contract support from the National Heart, Lung, and Blood Institute, toward the development of this TAH with the ultimate goal of realizing a clinically implantable system. Initially divided between three centers, this contract now has been narrowed to include this system, as well as the one under development at The Texas Heart Institute with the corporate partnership of ABIOMED Cardiovascular, Inc.

Device Description

The PSU/3M Health Care TAH is an electrically driven pump with no chronic percutaneous connections that is implanted in an orthotopic position, as depicted in Figure 6.[18,19] The pump consists of a titanium rigid casing, which encloses the blood sacs and energy converter. Each half of the pump is composed of a seamless blood sac that is constructed of polyurethane polymer. Blood flow is kept unidirectional by means of Delrin monostrut valves at the inlet (25 mm) and outlet (27 mm) connec-

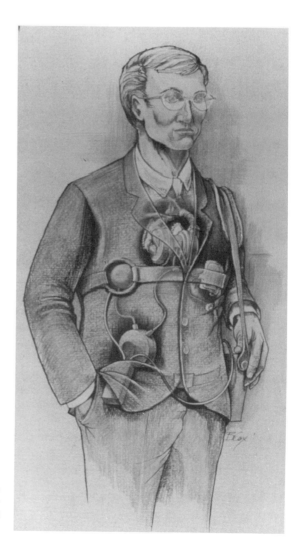

FIGURE 6. The Pennsylvania State University/3M Health Care Total Artificial Heart is shown schematically as it appears when implanted.

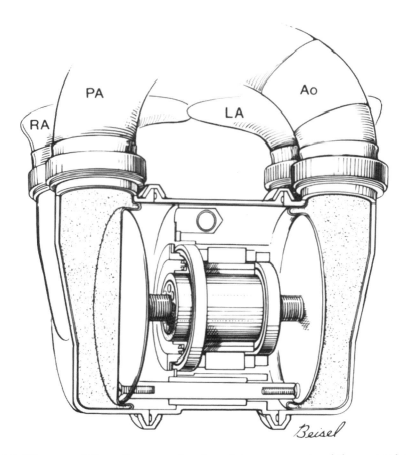

FIGURE 7. Diagram of the roller screw/pusher-plate components of the motor housing of the Pennsylvania State University/3M Health Care Total Artificial Heart.

tors for each pumping chamber. The energy converter is composed of a brushless DC electric motor, which actuates a roller screw with pusher-plates at either end (Fig. 7). Rotation of the roller screw translates into 1.9 cm of linear motion and results in alternate compression of the right- and left-sided blood sacs by the attached pusher-plates. The energy converter is housed between the blood sacs within the pump housing. Mechanical compression of the blood sacs by the pusher-plates against the rigid housing results in alternate emptying of the blood sacs. A direct connection of the blood sacs to the pusher-plates has been avoided to allow complete passive filling of the pump chambers during compression of the opposite side. The motor position is detected by a set of Hall effect sensors that are incorporated directly into the motor.[19] This system provides a relatively quiet device, with little associated vibration. Additionally, the total weight of the pump housing and its contents is approximately 1.1 pounds, resulting in a device that should be well tolerated by its recipient. Finally, a maximum cardiac output of 8 L/min with a stroke volume of 64 mL allows adequate perfusion under most physiologic conditions. Physiologic sensing is done through the left pump by use of estimated end-diastolic volume from motor speed and voltage, and thus provides information regarding the balance

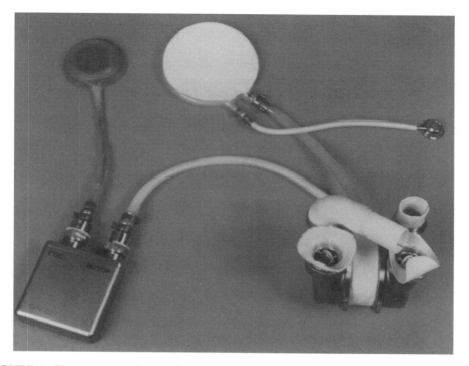

FIGURE 8. Shown as a unit are the motor housing, compliance chamber, transcutaneous energy transfer system unit, and electronics canister of the Pennsylvania State University/3M Health Care Total Artificial Heart.

between left- and right-sided pump outputs. This control process has previously been described by our group.[20]

The rigid housing has separate hermetically sealed connections, which provide attachment to the implanted electronics enclosure and the compliance chamber. The components of this system are shown in Figure 8. The titanium electronics canister is similar in dimension to an implanted automatic defibrillator and is designed to allow implantation in a preperitoneal position. Like the pump, its weight of less than 1 pound should be well tolerated by recipients. The enclosure houses the controller board, rechargeable batteries, and telemetry hardware. Telemetry allows intermittent diagnostic monitoring of the device as well as modulation of the controlling software. The nickel/cadmium batteries are quick-charging and provide an alternative power supply to allow intermittent short duration (up to 45 minutes) uncoupling from the external power source. Like the implanted LVAD, primary power is provided by transcutaneous energy transmission via induction coupling between an external power source with a wearable primary coil, and a subcutaneously implanted secondary coil (see Fig. 5). The system provides a means of monitoring internal battery charging so that the patient is aware of when he or she may safely remove the external power coil.[19]

A compliance chamber is coupled to the sealed motor housing. Although the alternating pumping associated with the TAH minimizes the internal pressure problems described above with the implanted LVAD system, the compliance system accommodates volume changes associated with gas diffusion across the blood sacs and changes in atmospheric conditions (see Fig. 4). The compliance chamber used is similar to that described above, and near-atmospheric pressure is maintained within the pump. Monitoring of system pressures and accommodation for system losses and varying atmospheric conditions is undertaken by accessing a subcutaneous infusion port incorporated into the system. Limited interval use and aggressive care of the infusion port during access should allow the reliance and longevity associated with infusion ports used clinically for chronic venous access.

Implantation Technique

Implantation of the PSU/3M Health Care TAH is undertaken via a median sternotomy. The recipient's heart is explanted with care to assure maintenance of adequate lengths of pulmonary artery and aorta, each which can be tailored at the time of anastomosis, and careful fashioning of atrial cuffs to minimize redundant tissue without compromising venous inflow. The Dacron® atrial cuffs of the pump are cut to match the retained recipient atria. These are subsequently sewn in place by running monofilament sutures with the left cuff preceding the right. The left and right outflow grafts are cut to prevent potential kinks and tension of the aortic and pulmonary artery anastomoses, and these in turn are fashioned with monofilament running suture lines. The albumin-primed pump is subsequently introduced into the chest and each of the connectors is fastened. Optimal installation is obtained when the order of connector coupling is left atrium, right atrium, aorta, and finally pulmonary artery. Careful de-airing of each of the pumping chambers is undertaken prior to initiation of TAH support and removal of the aortic cross-clamp.

The remaining hardware, including the preperitoneal electronics canister, secondary TETS coil, and compliance chamber with its perfusion port, are implanted in a fashion similar to the technique described at length for the Arrow Lion Heart-2000 LVAD. The patient is weaned from cardiopulmonary support with a compensatory increase in TAH flow until full support is realized. When stable TAH pumping and de-airing has been achieved, the patient is decannulated, and closed suction drains are placed prior to closure of all incisions. Anticoagulation therapy is instituted when chest tube drainage has subsided similar to the protocol described for the Lionheart-2000 LVAD.

Preclinical Experience

A large series of animal implantations were undertaken in calves, and were originally designed as long-duration implants that were terminated as the animals outgrew the devices.[18] The longest survivor in this group was supported for 388 days. A total of sixty-five 70 mL devices have now been implanted in calves without any means of percutaneous communication, and the last 49 have comprised the components planned for clinical implantation. Current studies have been tailored to contract specifications with pumps implanted for predefined 90-day study periods. Most recent studies have included assessment of hemodynamics of TAH support using invasive pressure monitoring as well as temperature probes to examine temperature changes associated with the different components of the device. The results of these characterization studies were recently published.[21] Finally, a long-term in vitro mock loop lab has been developed at our institution, where chronic durability studies are now under way, allowing continuous monitoring of multiple TAH loops for extended periods in a remote arrangement.

The PSU/3M Health Care TAH is being developed with the support of NIH contract N01-HV-38130. The continued device development characterized by phase I has been completed, and resulted in the current final device design. The second phase of the contract dedicated to preclinical animal and circuit testing is currently under way and expected to be completed within 1 year. Timely completion of the contract guidelines should assure clinical testing of a completely implanted TAH within the next 2 years.

Conclusions

The development of permanently implanted circulatory assist devices has evolved from a broad bridging experience and is extending the scope of therapy for this large population of patients with congestive heart failure, which continues to pose a significant public health problem. These devices should be ready for clinical implant studies within the ensuing 2 years. Future and ongoing studies are dedicated toward the development of pumps of differing sizes to increase the potential pool of support candidates, and to further the ongoing improvements in pump design and control software.

Acknowledgments   The authors wish to thank Dan Frank and Jim Thompson of Arrow International, Inc., and William Weiss, Gus Rosenberg, Alan Snyder, and George Felder of the Pennsylvania State University Division of Artificial Organs, for their thoughtful assistance with the preparation of this chapter.

References

1. Oz MC, Argenziano M, Catanese KA, et al. Bridge experience with long-term implantable left ventricular assist device. Are they an alternative to transplantation. *Circulation* 1997; 95:1844–1852.
2. Rose EA, Moskowitz AJ, Packer M, et al. The REMATCH trial: Rationale, design, and end points. Randomized evaluation of mechanical assistance for the treatment of congestive heart failure. *Ann Thorac Surg* 1999;67:723–730.
3. Zumbro GL, Kitchens WR, Shearer G, et al. Mechanical assistance for cardiogenic shock following cardiac surgery, myocardial infarction, and cardiac transplantation. *Ann Thorac Surg* 1987;44:11–13.
4. Pae WE Jr, Pierce WS. Temporary left ventricular assistance in acute myocardial infarction and cardiogenic shock: Rationale and criteria for utilization. *Chest* 1981;79:692–695.
5. Pierce WS, Parr GVS, Myers JL, et al. Ventricular-assist pumping in patients with cardiogenic shock. *N Engl J Med* 1981;305:1606–1610.
6. Pifarre R, Sullivan H, Montoya A, et al. Comparison of results after heart transplantation: Mechanically supported versus nonsupported patients. *J Heart Lung Transplant* 1992;11: 235–239.
7. Mehta SM, Aufiero TX, Pae WE Jr, et al. Combined registry for the clinical use of mechanical ventricular assist pumps and the total artificial heart in conjunction with heart transplantation: Sixth official report–1994. *J Heart Lung Transplant* 1995;14:585–593.

8. Griffith BP. Interim use of the Jarvik-7 artificial heart: Lessons learned at Presbyterian-University Hospital of Pittsburgh. *Ann Thorac Surg* 1989;47:158–166.
9. Joyce LD, Johnson KE, Toninato CJ, et al. Results of the first 100 patients who received Symbion total artificial hearts as a bridge to cardiac transplantation. *Circulation* 1989; 80(suppl III):III192-III201.
10. Cabrol C, Solis E, Muneretto C, et al. Orthotopic transplantation after implantation of a Jarvik 7 total artificial heart. *J Thorac Cardiovasc Surg* 1989;97:342–350.
11. Mehta SM, Aufiero TX, Pae WE Jr, et al. Results of mechanical ventricular assistance for postcardiotomy cardiogenic shock. *ASAIO J* 1996;42:211–218.
12. Herrmann M, Weyand M, Greshake B, et al. Left ventricular assist device infection is associated with increased mortality but is not a contraindication to transplantation. *Circulation* 1997;95:814–817.
13. McCarthy PM, Schmitt SK, Vargo RL, et al. Implantable LVAD infections: Implications for permanent use of the device. *Ann Thorac Surg* 1996;61:359–365.
14. Sapirstein JS, Pae WE Jr, Rosenberg G, et al. The development of permanent circulatory support systems. *Semin Thorac Cardiovasc Surg* 1994;6:188–194.
15. Weiss WJ, Rosenberg G, Snyder AJ, et al. A completely implanted left ventricular assist device: Chronic in vivo testing. *ASAIO J* 1993;39:M427-M432.
16. Lee S, Rosenberg G, Donachy JH, et al. The compliance problem: A major obstacle in the development of implantable blood pumps. *Artif Organs* 1984;8:82–90.
17. Weiss WJ, Rosenberg G, Snyder AJ, et al. In vivo performance of a transcutaneous energy transmission system with the Penn State motor driven ventricular assist device. *ASAIO Trans* 1989;35:284–288.
18. Snyder AJ, Rosenberg G, Weiss WJ, et al. In vivo testing of a completely implanted total artificial heart system. *ASAIO J* 1993;39:M177-M184.
19. Weiss WJ, Rosenberg G, Snyder AJ, et al. Recent improvements in a completely implanted total artificial heart. *ASAIO J* 1996;42:M342-M346.
20. Snyder AJ, Rosenberg G, Pierce WS. Noninvasive control of cardiac output for alternately ejecting dual-pusherplate pumps. *Artif Organs* 1992;16:189–194.
21. Rosenberg G, Snyder AJ, Weiss WJ, et al. Dynamic in vitro and in vivo performance of a permanent total artificial heart. *Artif Organs* 1998;22:87–94.

Chapter 30

The HeartSaver VAD:

A Fully Implantable Ventricular Assist Device for Long-Term Support

Tofy Mussivand, PhD, Paul J. Hendry, MD, Roy G. Masters, MD, and Wilbert J. Keon, MD

Introduction

The University of Ottawa Heart Institute began work on mechanical circulatory support in 1986 using the Jarvik 7–70 total artificial heart as a bridge to transplantation.[1,2] Since then, approximately 300 transplants have been performed and a variety of circulatory support devices have been used in 51 cases.[3–7] This experience resulted in the establishment of the Canadian Artificial Heart Program in 1988. The overall goal of the program was to develop an advanced ventricular assist device (VAD) capable of being implanted in the thoracic cavity, without the need for transcutaneous connections that would offer the recipient a near normal lifestyle with minimal limitations. The device developed through this program is now approaching clinical utilization and has been dubbed the HeartSaver VAD. This chapter presents an overview of the concept, development, and operation of this unique device, and discusses the current status of development and results of ongoing in vitro and in vivo experiments.

The Changing Paradigm

The HeartSaver VAD represents a major conceptual change from devices currently available for clinical use. With existing extracorporeal devices such as the

This work was supported by the Medical Research Council of Canada, the Natural Sciences and engineering Council of Canada, the University of Ottawa Heart Institute, Industry Canada, and WorldHeart Corporation.
From Goldstein DJ and Oz MC (eds). *Cardiac Assist Devices*. Armonk, NY: Futura Publishing Co., Inc.; ©2000.

Thoratec biVAD (Thoratec laboratories Corp., Berkeley, CA), the ABIOMED BVS 5000 (ABIOMED, Danvers, MA), and early versions of both the Thermo Cardiosystems (Woburn, MA) and Baxter/Novacor (Baxter Heathcare Corp., Oakland, CA) devices, the power supply and control systems are located in an external console. Even with the advent of the wearable systems by both Thermo Cardiosystems and Novacor, the device is controlled by an external control system that is carried by the patient. In contrast, the HeartSaver VAD's control system is located in the implanted component. This is analogous to the early days of the computer industry when the so-called "dumb terminals" were rapidly replaced by the desktop computer and the intelligence of the system was moved from the mainframe to the microcomputer and eventually onto the desktop of the computer user. This evolution is widely regarded as the key reason for the widespread use of computers.

The HeartSaver VAD is a totally implantable device that was developed for long-term use in the outpatient setting. The device has several key technological advances that render it particularly attractive for this application. These include: 1) the incorporation of the controller into the implanted unit; 2) the use of a transcutaneous energy transfer system and wireless technology; 3) the absence of percutaneous vents afforded by an integral volume displacement chamber; and 4) the use of a rechargeable implanted power source. In combination, these attributes allow the patient independent existence with the ability to partake in a wide variety of activities without the need for any external accessories, for periods of time determined by existing and future battery technologies. Hence, this device affords independence and a quality of life that is not achievable with current wearable devices. The limitations imposed by present battery technology will be reduced by imminent developments in this field.

Early prototypes of the device have been evaluated in vitro with systems running for more than 6 years without failure. A series of in vivo studies (n = 25) with durations of support of up to 30 days has successfully demonstrated several important aspects of the design. First, it is feasible as a totally implantable system without percutaneous connections. Second, it can be powered transcutaneously. Third, it can be remotely monitored and controlled with use of infrared data transmission. Finally, it can support the failing heart. Clinical studies are still pending.

System Description

The HeartSaver VAD system consists of both implantable components and external accessories.

Implantable Components

The intracorporeal components (Fig. 1) include the following: 1) the implanted VAD unit, which includes the blood chamber, the volume displacement chamber, the electrohydraulic axial flow pump, and the electronic controller; 2) the internal transcutaneous energy transfer and biotelemetry coil; 3) the internal battery pack; and 4) the inflow and outflow conduits with integrated tissue valves. These components are capable of providing the required blood pumping function without the

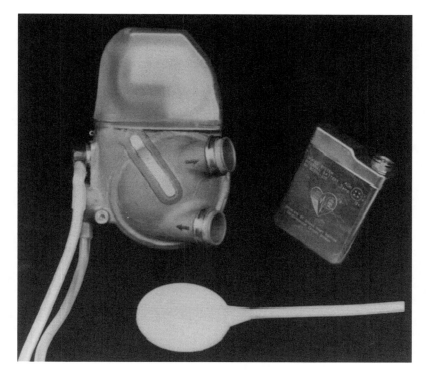

FIGURE 1. The implantable components of the HeartSaver VAD system.

need for the external components for periods determined by the energy storage capacity of the internal battery pack.

External Accessories

External accessories are shown in Figure 2. They include: 1) the remote biotelemetry monitor; 2) the external transcutaneous energy transfer and biotelemetry coil; and 3) the external battery pack. These components are worn by the patient and provide complete mobility. An additional external accessory is the clinical user interface (Fig. 3), which is used to control and monitor the device during implantation, to monitor device function in the early postoperative period in the intensive care unit and hospital wards, and for remote monitoring and control of the implanted device in the outpatient setting.

Intrathoracic VAD Placement

Advantages

The implanted VAD unit (Fig. 4) is the main blood pumping unit. It is designed specifically for implantation in the left hemithorax, and is connected to the heart via

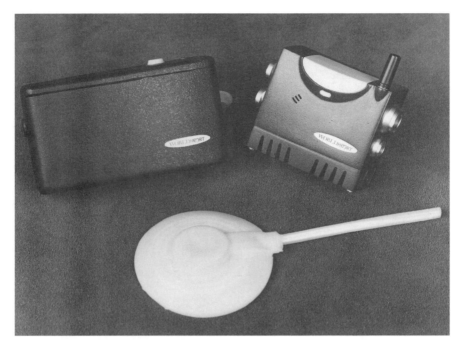

FIGURE 2. The external accessories of the HeartSaver VAD system. All external components are designed to be worn by the patient to provide complete mobility.

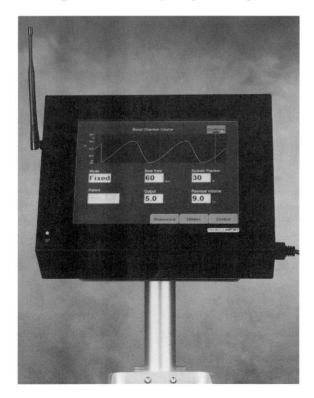

FIGURE 3. The clinical user interface designed for use in the operating room during device implantation, in the intensive care unit and ward postoperatively, and by the clinician to remotely monitor and control the device after patient discharge.

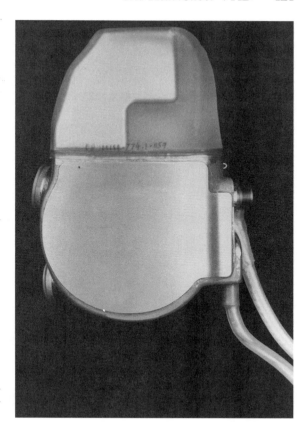

FIGURE 4. The implanted ventricular assist device unit designed for intrathoracic placement.

a left apical inflow cannula, and to the systemic circulation with an aortic outflow cannula (Fig. 5). An extracorporeal placement was not considered due to unsuitability for chronic use. Complications of intra-abdominal implantation can include erosion, bowel perforation or obstruction, diaphragmatic hernia, and wound dehiscence.[8] While some improvements have been observed with preperitoneal implantation, complications such as fascial dehiscence, infection, early satiety, and vomiting, as well as concern regarding pump erosion through the skin, have been reported.[9] In contrast, an intrathoracic placement offers several important benefits. First, the inflow and outflow cannulae can be made extremely short; this mitigates hydraulic losses and reduces potential cannula twisting, kinking, and adverse flow patterns, which can result in thrombosis and thromboembolic complications. Second, the intrathoracic implantation is less invasive, as it does not require extension of the wound into the abdomen or perforation of the diaphragm. Third, the rib cage provides an excellent anchoring base for the system to prevent device migration. Last, the need for percutaneous venting to atmospheric pressure can be eliminated by using an intrathoracic volume displacement chamber.

Anatomic Fit

To assess the optimal size and geometry for intrathoracic device insertion, fit studies in cadavers and intraoperative human fit trials were conducted.[10] These ef-

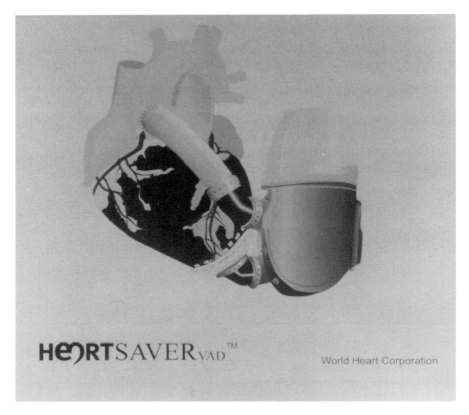

FIGURE 5. Connection of the developed device to the natural heart and systemic circulation.

forts along with detailed fluid dynamic analysis,[11–13] were used to derive the various anatomic dimensions and resulting geometric constraints of the intrathoracic implant site. Based on these constraints, preliminary device models were developed and used for follow-up fit studies.[14] A 600 mL model confirmed acceptable fit in patients as small as 64 kg. To ensure anatomic fit in a wider range of patient surface areas, efforts have been ongoing to further reduce the volume and weight of the implanted unit, and have resulted in the current device volume of approximately 530 mL.

To allow implantation in patients with smaller stature, an alternative device placement has been assessed in cadavers. This involves detachment of the diaphragm at its insertion into the anterior chest wall to establish a preperitoneal space. This space allows the lower portion of the device to fit into the left upper abdomen with the volume displacement chamber remaining in the left thorax. This positioning allows for the accommodation of different angulations of the cannulae to adapt to the variety of cardiac axes that may be present.

Operating Mechanism

The implanted VAD unit uses an electrohydraulic actuating mechanism. The VAD unit consists of a volume displacement chamber, a pumping chamber, and a blood chamber. The volume displacement and pumping chambers are separated by a bulkhead. The pumping and blood chambers are separated by a flexible polyurethane diaphragm. The unit incorporates an axial flow bidirectional brushless direct-current motor mounted on the bulkhead as an energy converter that pumps hydraulic fluid during systole from the volume displacement chamber into the pumping chamber. In turn, the hydraulic fluid actuates the flexible diaphragm, which then ejects blood from a flexible polyurethane sac. During diastole, the blood sac fills passively, thereby displacing the hydraulic fluid back to the volume displacement chamber via a custom one-way valve mounted on the bulkhead that operates automatically based on physiologic pressures. During passive filling, the energy converter operates at low rotational speed, which imparts negligible energy to the hydraulic fluid. If required, diastolic filling of the blood chamber may be augmented by operating the energy converter in an active filling mode.

Filling and ejection of blood are monitored using Hall effect sensors and a magnet embedded in the blood pumping diaphragm that allows the position of the latter to be dynamically determined during the pumping cycle by the internal electronic controller. These sensors detect both the full/fill and full/eject conditions of the blood sac, and thus allow for accurate control and optimization of the VAD operation. Additionally, electrical voltage and current levels, localized temperature fluctuations, diagnostic status of critical electronic components, and impeller position in the energy converter are continuously monitored to ensure proper system operation.

The VAD has four principal modes of operation. A single beat mode is used for de-airing purposes; a fixed beat rate; a full/fill–full/eject whereby a full stroke of the electrohydraulic mechanism occurs; and a default mode, which is used in emergencies. The latter has three safety levels that can be initiated in case of an emergency or electronic failure. First, there is a completely redundant, full function software code that will engage upon a primary software failure. Second, there is a default software mode of a fixed 60 bpm operation upon failure of the secondary software system. Finally, there is a hardware default mode of a fixed 60 bpm operation upon failure of the tertiary software system.

Elimination of Percutaneous Venting

To eliminate the need for percutaneous venting, a volume displacement chamber (VDC) was integrated into the implanted unit. The VDC allows for the displacement of the actuating hydraulic fluid during device diastole. It consists of an integrated hydraulic fluid chamber and a flexible diaphragm. The latter is in contact with the lung tissue, where the pressure is nearly atmospheric, thus eliminating the need for a percutaneous vent.

Thermal Management

The VDC also performs the secondary function of heat dissipation from the internal electronic module. The latter is mounted within the VDC and surrounded by hydraulic fluid, which allows excess heat generation to be transferred over the entire surface area of the implanted unit. Heat transfer to the body is accomplished across the flexible diaphragm and blood sac into the patient's blood system, across the VDC diaphragm to the lung tissue (and across the alveoli to the patient's inspired air), and across the housing to the surrounding tissue. By facilitating these large areas of heat transfer potential, local hot spots are eliminated and operating temperatures well within physiologic limits can be obtained, as demonstrated during in vivo studies.

Conduits and Valves

The conduits and valves are used to connect the device to the patient's circulatory system (Fig. 5). The inflow cannula conduit and valve assembly connect the inflow port of the VAD to the apex of the left ventricle via a rigid titanium conduit that is coated on the blood contacting surfaces with a biocompatible material. Similarly, the outflow conduit and valve assembly connect the outflow port of the VAD to the ascending aorta via a rigid titanium elbow coated with a biocompatible material on the blood contacting surface, and a flexible polyester velour graft that is sutured directly into the aorta. One porcine tissue valve is located in each inflow and outflow side of the assembly to ensure unidirectional flow through the device.

Elimination of Percutaneous Leads: The Transcutaneous Energy Transfer System and Biotelemetry System

Unfortunately, all circulatory support devices used to date require some form of percutaneous connection (pneumatic drive line, percutaneous power leads, monitoring cables, etc.) for powering, monitoring, and/or controlling the implanted device. To overcome the need for these lines, which have been implicated in the high rate of infectious complications seen with chronic use of these devices, a transcutaneous energy transfer and biotelemetry system was developed.[15–17] The transcutaneous energy transfer system (TETS)[18,19] consists of internal and external coils (Fig. 6) along with associated electronics located both within the implanted unit and in the remote biotelemetry monitor. The internal coil is implanted subcutaneously in the upper clavicle region and is connected to the implanted unit via a custom designed hermetic connector. The external coil is located extracorporeally directly over the top of the implanted coil and connected to the remote biotelemetry monitor worn by the patient via self-locking pin and socket connector.

The implanted unit is typically powered by an external power source (battery pack, wall socket, automobile cigarette lighter, etc.) and is periodically powered for short periods (approximately 1.5 hours) by the internal battery pack. The TETS uses the internal and external wire coils to form a transcutaneous air-core transformer. The transformer is used to transfer electrical energy across the skin and tissue barrier without the need for percutaneous connections. External power is delivered to electronics located in the remote biotelemetry monitor that use this power to drive an oscillator which energizes the external coil. This energy is then electromagnetically coupled across the skin and tissue barrier to the implanted internal coil. The induced voltage in the internal coil is then converted from an alternating current to a direct current. The output from this alternating current to direct-current conversion is used

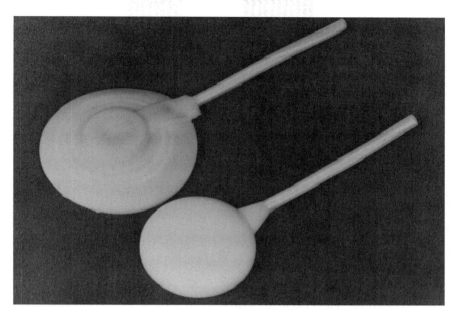

FIGURE 6. The internal and external coils of the transcutaneous energy transfer and biotelemetry system are used to power, monitor, and control the implanted ventricular assist device unit without the need for percutaneous connections.

to power the implanted unit as well as to recharge the internal battery pack. Autotuning circuitry has been implemented to reduce the effects from variations in-coil separation and coil misalignment. The autotuning circuitry tracks the transformer's natural resonant frequency and provides feedback control to the external coil oscillator.

The biotelemetry system uses infrared communication modules located at the center of each of the power transfer coils. Each of these modules contains multiple infrared transmitter and receiver components to provide operating redundancy and to minimize effects of coil misalignment. The infrared transmitters send direct digital (binary) data toward the receivers on the other side of the skin and tissue barrier. This signal passes across the skin and tissue layer and is picked up by the opposite infrared receiver. The infrared communication link accepts digital data streams at rates of up to 38,400 Baud and operates in a half-duplex mode to minimize signal feedback and cross-talk difficulties. Using this system, the operating status of the VAD unit is transferred to the remote biotelemetry monitor (Fig. 7) that is worn by the patient. The monitor provides device status displays and warning alarms to the patient and also offers the clinician the capability to perform remote device monitoring and control functions after patient discharge over standard telephone lines. Device operating status and various warning alarms are delivered to the patient using four distinct communication methods: 1) text messages via a liquid crystal display; 2) visual messages via light-emitting diodes; 3) audible messages via an acoustic generator (buzzer); and 4) a vibration alarm similar to those used on pagers.

These technologies play a key role in the total implantability of this device. Moreover, they should reduce device-related infections,[20–22] provide aesthetic acceptability, and eliminate the burden of continuous exit site wound care for these patients.

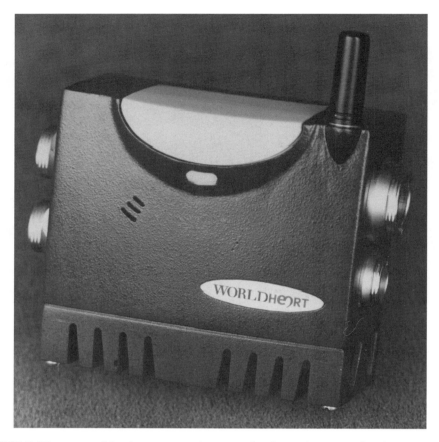

FIGURE 7. The remote biotelemetry monitor worn by the patient provides device operating status and warning messages via a liquid crystal display similar to a pager, as well as via audible and visual warning systems.

Clinical User Interface

The interface (Fig. 3) provides the clinician or clinical engineer the capability to perform advanced monitoring and to control functions. It is completely self-contained and touch-screen operated for ease of use. The unit is equipped with an integral back-up power supply that lasts for up to 1 hour. The interface software controls the data communication with the implanted device via the remote biotelemetry monitor, and presents clinical and engineering diagnostic information to the user, as well as allows the user to enter commands to modify operating parameters of the implanted device. The interface software runs on the Windows NT platform for increased stability. The software is presently password protected to ensure against unauthorized access, and additional security measures are under development to maintain higher level security controls. The interface can be operated in three distinct operating modes, each with separate password protection: 1) a control mode, which allows modification of clinical operating parameters intended for use during implantation and in the immediate postoperative period; 2) a monitoring mode, which presents various clinical operating parameters but prevents modification of these; it is intended for use in the ward prior to patient discharge and for remote monitoring of device function after patient discharge; and 3) a diagnostic mode, which is reserved for use by clinical engineering personnel.

The interface is capable of remotely monitoring and controlling the implanted unit via a telephone line or other public communications systems such as the Internet, satellite, or asynchronous transfer systems. This capability is a result of an integrated wireless (telephone) modem, which communicates with a dedicated home user interface unit connected to the telephone line at the patient's residence. The clinical user interface is also capable of interfacing to a hospital database for storage of patient data as back history and for post analysis.

Energy Storage

The HeartSaver VAD is designed to use two principal energy storage components, the internal and external battery packs. Initial energy storage efforts focused on the study of the impact of pulsed charge/discharge and normothermia on various cell chemistries. Based on these studies, further evaluation of nickel cadmium and lithium ion (Li/Ion) battery cells were conducted.[23–26] As a result of these studies and of the recent availability of high-quality Li/Ion battery cells, the latter were selected for the internal and external battery packs. They offer substantial improvements over other suitable chemistries in terms of energy density, recharge time, and cycle life. These attributes render these cells especially appropriate for this application, since the battery packs are either implanted and/or carried, making their overall volume and weight critical. In the case of the internal battery pack, cycle life is particularly critical because ambulatory surgery is required to replace the battery (much like generator replacements in pacemakers).

The internal battery pack is designed for subcutaneous implantation in the abdominal area and is rechargeable via the TETS and biotelemetry system. The internal battery pack serves as an interim power reserve when exchanging external batteries, in the case of emergencies, and to allow the patient to be disconnected from an external power source for limited periods of time to bathe, shower, and partake in various activities without the need for any external components whatsoever.

The pack consists of four "C" size, 4.1 V Li/Ion battery cells (Model R10198, Wilson Greatbatch, Clarence, NY), housed in a laser-welded titanium enclosure. The internal pack also contains electronics to maintain an accurate record of available battery capacity and to monitor each battery cell to ensure safe operation during charge and discharge, as well as to operate an integrated battery alarm that uses an acoustic generator to warn the patient of low charge conditions.

To provide an electrical connection from the internal battery pack to the implanted unit, a custom hermetic connector/feedthrough system was developed. This 8-pin connector system uses multiple sealing systems consisting of both o rings and an ionic barrier. The connector allows for easy linkage to the implanted unit during implantation and battery replacement when necessary (for patients receiving implants for greater than 2 to 3 years, the expected operating life of the internal battery pack).

The external battery pack is designed to be carried by the patient and is rechargeable with a stand-alone battery charger supplied to the patient. The external battery pack is connected to the biotelemetry monitor via a flying lead with a self-locking pin and socket connector. The external pack consists of two interconnected packages each containing 8 "D" size, 4.1 V Li/Ion battery cells (Model R10298, Wilson Greatbatch). Like the internal battery pack, the external unit also contains electronics to maintain accurate record of available battery capacity and to monitor each battery cell to ensure safe operation during charge and discharge.

In Vivo Studies

Two series of in vivo experiments were conducted (n = 25) using various prototype versions of the device in male Holstein calves.[27–29] The intent of all of the implants to date has been to supply input to the design process and aid in the development of an implantation procedure.

After insertion with inflow from the left ventricular apex and outflow to the descending aorta, the device was started in a fixed rate operating mode (50 bpm). Soon after functional operating status was confirmed by observation and stable hemodynamics were obtained, the device was switched to the full/fill–full/eject operating mode. After insertion of left and right chest tubes, the chest was closed and the animal was transferred to the recovery area. An automated data acquisition system was used to monitor and record the device and recipient parameters on an ongoing basis during the operative and postoperative phases.

During our experiments, the entire system including the TETS and biotelemetry system has been used to assess system design, total implantability, and overall device performance. The animals were supported for periods up to 5 days (mean 16.5 hours, range 1.5 hours to 5 days). The series demonstrated the feasibility of a totally implanted system using remote power transfer and wireless monitoring/control technologies, and provided input for the design optimization process. Figure 8 shows one of the calves from this series in the recovery pen; the external energy transfer and biotelemetry coil is seen on the flank of the animal, and it successfully provided continuous power and monitoring capabilities for the duration of these experiments.

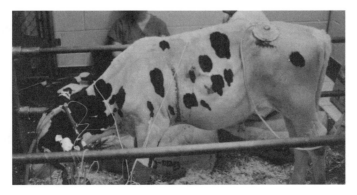

FIGURE 8. One of the calves from the in vivo evaluation in the recovery pen. The external energy transfer and biotelemetry coil can be seen on the left flank of the animal.

The second series of implants was conducted with a modified version of the device and focused on performance of the implanted unit; specifically, the inflow and outflow cannulae, assessment of the blood chamber fluid dynamics, device positioning in the calf model, and implant team preparation. The animals were supported for periods ranging from 1 hour to 30 days (mean duration 3.5 days).

With these advances demonstrated, we are pursuing clinical trials for long-term implantations.

Summary

Over the past 10 years, a totally implantable intrathoracic VAD has been developed which requires no percutaneous connections and which is expected to reduce the incidence of infection and to provide a better quality of life for future recipients. The device allows the patient independent existence and the possibility of partaking in a wide range of activities. The biotelemetry system allows for remote monitoring and control of operating parameters, thus eliminating the need for patients to visit the hospital for routine device assessment. This property is expected to provide patients with increased peace of mind after discharge from the hospital, as help is simply a phone call away. The intrathoracic implant site eliminates the need for external venting, and allows insertion via a simple median sternotomy. Each of these attributes enhances the potential of this device as long-term support for the treatment of end-stage heart disease.

Based on ongoing experimental studies, the HeartSaver VAD can function effectively as a totally implantable device. Formal evaluation of the preclinical device intended for clinical use is now beginning and clinical application in humans will follow, pending regulatory approval.

References

1. Keon WJ, Boyd WD, Walley V. Jarvik artificial heart for spontaneous left main coronary dissection. *Am Heart J* 1987;113:1538.
2. Keon WJ, Masters RG, Farrell EM, Koshal A. Use of the Jarvik total artificial heart as a bridge to transplantation. *Adv Cardiol* 1988;36:270–277.
3. Farrar DJ, Hill JD, Pennington DG, et al. Preoperative and postoperative comparison of patients with univentricular and biventricular support with the Thoratec ventricular assist device as a bridge to cardiac transplantation. *J Thorac Cardiovasc Surg* 1997;113:202–209.
4. Masters RG, Hendry PJ, Davies RA, et al. Cardiac transplantation after mechanical circulatory support: A Canadian perspective. *Ann Thorac Surg* 1996;61:1734–1739.
5. Arabia FA, Copeland JG, Smith RG, et al. International experience with the CardioWest total artificial heart as a bridge to heart transplantation. *Eur J Cardiothorac Surg* 1997;11: S5-S10.
6. Copeland JG, Pavie A, Duveau D, et al. Bridge to transplantation with the CardioWest total artificial heart: The international experience 1993 to 1995. *J Heart Lung Transplant* 1996;15:94–99.
7. Joyce LD, Johnson KE, Toninato CJ, et al. Results of the first 100 patients who received Symbion total artificial hearts as a bridge to cardiac transplantation. *Circulation* 1989;80: 192–201.
8. Phillips WS, Burton NA, Macmanus Q, Lefrak EA. Surgical complications in bridging to transplantation: The Thermo Cardiosystem LVAD. *Ann Thorac Surg* 1992;53:482–486.

9. McCarthy PM, Wang N, Vargo R. Preperitoneal insertion of the Heartmate 1000 IP implantable left ventricular assist device. *Ann Thorac Surg* 1994;57:634–638.
10. Mussivand T, Masters RG, Hendry PJ, et al. Critical anatomic dimensions for intrathoracic circulatory assist devices. *Artif Organs* 1992;16:281–285.
11. Mussivand T, Rajagopalan K, Robichaud R, et al. *Flow Visualization in an Artificial Heart Outflow Graft.* Proceedings of the 11th Canadian Symposium on Fluid Dynamics. Edmonton, Alberta, Canada: 1994.
12. Mussivand T, Rajagopalan K, Robichaud R, et al. Flow visualization in an artificial heart outflow graft. *ASAIO Abstracts* 1994;23:9.
13. Mussivand T, Navarro R, Chen F, et al. Flow visualization using diffuse and planar laser lighting. *Trans Am Soc Artif Intern Org* 1988;34:317–321.
14. Mussivand T. Lessons learned from the grandfather of artificial organs. *Artif Organs* 1998; 22:985–987.
15. Mussivand T, Hum A, Holmes KS. Remote energy transmission for powering artificial hearts and assist devices. In Akutsu T, Koyanagi H (eds): *Artificial Heart 6.* Tokyo: Springer-Verlag; 1988:344–347.
16. Mussivand T, Hum A, Holmes KS. Remote monitoring and control of artificial hearts and assist devices. In Akutsu T, Koyanagi H (eds): *Artificial Heart 6.* Tokyo: Springer-Verlag; 1988:370–374.
17. Mussivand T, Hum A, Diguer M, et al. A transcutaneous energy and information transfer system for implanted medical devices. *ASAIO J* 1995;41:M253-M258.
18. Miller JA, Belanger G, Mussivand T. Development of an automated transcutaneous energy transfer system. *ASAIO J* 1993;39:M706-M710.
19. Mussivand T, Miller JA, Santere PJ, et al. Transcutaneous energy transfer system performance evaluation. *Artif Organs* 1993;17:940–947.
20. Holman WL, Murrah CP, Ferguson ER, et al. Infections during extended circulatory support: University of Alabama at Birmingham experience 1989 to 1994. *Ann Thorac Surg* 1996;61:366–371.
21. McCarthy PM, Schmitt SK, Vargo RL, et al. Implantable LVAD infections: Implications for permanent use of the device. *Ann Thorac Surg* 1996;61:359–365.
22. Pennington DG. Extended support with permanent systems: Percutaneous versus totally implantable. *Ann Thorac Surg* 1996;61:403–406.
23. MacLean GK, Aiken PA, Duguay DG, et al. The effect of pulsatile power loads on nickel/cadmium battery cells for mechanical circulatory support devices. *ASAIO J* 1994;40:67–69.
24. MacLean GK, Aiken PA, Adams WA, Mussivand T. Evaluation of nickel/cadmium battery packs for mechanical circulatory support devices. *ASAIO J* 1993;39:M423-M426.
25. MacLean GK, Aiken PA, Adams WA, Mussivand T. Comparison of rechargeable lithium and nickel/cadmium battery cells for implantable circulatory support devices. *Artif Organs* 1994;18:331–334.
26. MacLean GK, Aiken PA, Adams WA, Mussivand T. Preliminary evaluation of rechargeable lithium ion cells for an implantable battery pack. *J Power Sources* 1995;56:69–74.
27. Hendry PJ, Master RG, Keaney M, et al. and the EVAD team. Evolution of an electrohydraulic ventricular assist device through in vivo testing. *ASAIO J* 1996;42:M350-M354.
28. Mussivand T, Hendry PJ, Masters RG, Keon WJ. Evaluation of a totally implantable intrathoracic ventricular assist device. *Cor Europaeum* 1997;6:110–114.
29. Mussivand T, Masters RG, Hendry PJ, Keon WJ. Totally implantable intrathoracic ventricular assist device. *Ann Thorac Surg* 1996;61:444–447.

Appendix:

Abbreviations

A-β_1-AAB = autoantibodies directed against the β_1-adrenoreceptor
ACE = angiotensin-converting enzyme
ACT = activated clotting time
ADP = adenosine diphosphate
AICD = activation-induced cell death
ALCAPA = anomalous origin of the left coronary artery from the pulmonary artery
ALVAD = abdominal left ventricular assist device
ANP = atrial natriuretic peptide
APC = antigen presenting cells
ASO = arterial switch operation
AVP = arginine vasopressin
biVAD = biventricular assist device
BSA = body surface area
CABG = coronary artery bypass graft
CDAS = clinical data acquisition system
cGMP = cyclic guanine monophosphate
CMA = centrifugal mechanical assist
CPB = cardiopulmonary bypass
CPR = cardiopulmonary resuscitation
CVVH = continuous venovenous hemofiltration
DC = direct current
DCC = direct cardiac compression
DNA = deoxyribonucleic acid
DRG = diagnosis-related group
DRT = device readiness testing
ECG = electrocardiogram
ECMO = extracorporeal membrane oxygenation
EDPVR = end-diastolic pressure-volume relationship
Ees = end-systolic elastance
ELSO = Extracorporeal Life Support Organization
ESPVR = end-systolic pressure-volume relationship
FADD = Fas-associated death domain protein
FDA = Food and Drug Administration
FLICE = caspase-8
FLIP = FADD-like interleukin-1β-converting enzyme

431

HIV-1 = human immunodeficiency virus type 1
HLA = human leukocyte antigen
IABP = intra-aortic balloon pump
ICU = intensive care unit
IDC = idiopathic dilated cardiomyopathy
IDE = investigational device exemption
IgG = immunoglobulin G
IgM = immunoglobulin M
IL-8 = interleukin-8
INR = international normalized ratio
IP = implantable pneumatic
IU = international unit
IVAS = Innovative Ventricular Assist System
IVIg = intravenous immunoglobulin
Li/Ion = lithium/ion
LOS = length of stay
LU = laboratory units
LVAD = left ventricular assist device
LVAS = left ventricular assist system
LVEF = left ventricular ejection fraction
LVIDd = left ventricular intracavity dimensions in diastole
MGH = Massachusetts General Hospital
MHC = major histocompatibility complex
MIP = macrophage inflammatory protein
mRNA = messenger ribonucleic acid
MVO_2 = myocardial oxygen demand
NFkB = nuclear factor kappa B
NHLBI = National Heart, Lung, and Blood Institute
NHLI = National Heart and Lung Institute
NIH = National Institutes of Health
NYHA = New York Heart Association
PABC = pulmonary artery balloon counterpulsation
PBMC = peripheral blood mononuclear cell
PDCC (t) = pressure generated by DCC
PEEP = positive end-expiratory pressure
PET = polyester
PFO = patent foramen ovule
Pic (V,t) = intrachamber ventricular pressure
Pi/PCr = phosphorous-to-phosphocreatine (ratio)
PRA = panel reactive antibodies
PSU = Pennsylvania State University
PTFE = polytetrafluoroethylene
Ptm (V,t) = transmural ventricular pressure
PTT = partial thromboplastin time
PVA = pressure-volume area
PVR = pulmonary vascular resistance
QALY = quality-adjusted life years
QoL = quality of life
Qs/Qt = transpulmonary shunt

RBC = red blood cell
REMATCH = Randomized Evaluation of Mechanical Assistance for the Treatment of Congestive Heart failure
R_{in} = pulmonary artery input resistance
rpm = revolutions per minute
RSCF = right-sided circulatory failure
RVAD = right ventricular assist device
RVSW = right ventricular stroke work
SI = stimulation index
SLE = systemic lupus erythematosus
SOLVD = Study of Left Ventricular Dysfunction
T_3 = tri-iodothyronine
TAH = total artificial heart
TCI = Thermo Cardiosystems, Inc.
TCR = T cell receptor
TEE = transesophageal echocardiography
TETS = transcutaneous energy transfer system
TGA = transposition of the great arteries
TNF-α = tissue necrosis factor-α
TPI = thrombodynamic potential index
UNOS = United Network of Organ Sharing
UOP = University of Pittsburgh
USSC = United States Surgical Corporation
V-A = venoarterial
VAD = ventricular assist device
VDC = volume displacement chamber
VE = vented electric
Vo = volume-axis intercept
VO_2 = oxygen consumption
V-V = venovenous

Index

Page numbers in italics indicate figures and tables.

ABIOMED BVS 5000, 235–250
  console, 237–239
  description, 235–239, *236*
  explanation techniques, 244
  implantation, 239–244, *239*
  indications for, 245–246, *245, 246*
  inflow cannulation, 240–244
    left-sided inflow, 241–244, *242, 243*
    right-sided inflow, 241
  limitations, 246–247
  outcome, 247–249
    institutional experience, 247
    Worldwide Registry, 247–249, *249*
  outflow cannulation, 239–240
    left-sided outflow, 240
    right-sided outflow, 240
  pump, 236–237, *238*
  transthoracic cannulae, 235–236, *237*
Aerobic training, left ventricular assist
  device recipient, 173–174
Anastomosis, outflow graft, Thermo
  Cardiosystems ventricular assist device,
  313–314
Anesthesia, 63–74
  cardiopulmonary bypass, separation
    from, 66–68
  heart failure, pathophysiology of,
    63–64
  intensive care unit, 71–72
  lining/induction, 65–66
  pharmacology, 64–65
  preoperative assessment, 65
  transesophageal echocardiography,
    68–71, *69, 70*
    during bypass, 70–71
    post bypass, 71
Aneurysm, ventricular, Thermo
  Cardiosystems ventricular assist device,
  317

Anomalous origin, left coronary artery,
  from pulmonary artery, pediatric
  patients, 49–51, *50, 52, 53, 54*
Antibodies, preformed, device selection
  and, 33
Anticoagulation, centrifugal pumps,
  222–224
Antithrombotic therapy, Novacor left
  ventricular assist system, 329
Aortic valve regurgitation, Thermo
  Cardiosystems ventricular assist device,
  317
Apical cuff, Thermo Cardiosystems
  ventricular assist device, 314–315, *314,
  315, 316*
Arginine vasopressin, 116–117
  deficiency, vasodilatory shock,
    114–115, *114, 115*
  with heart transplantation, 117, *117*
  hemodynamic effects of, 113–114, *113*
  mechanism of action of, 117–118
  for vasodilatory shock, 112–115
Arrhythmias, in left ventricular assist
  device recipients, 103–110
  electrophysiologic effects, device
    placement, 109
  postoperative management, 104–109,
    107
  preoperative, 103–104
Arrow Lionheart–2000 completely
  implanted left ventricular assist device,
  404–410
Artificial heart, CardioWest, 341–356
  clinical results, 354–355
  device description, 341–346, *342, 343,
    344*
  implantation technique, 346–352, *346,
    347, 348, 349, 350, 351, 352*
  indications for, 352–353, *353*
  limitations, 353–354

435

Autoimmunity, 200–201
Axial flow pumps, 359–374
    cardiopulmonary bypass, 359–360
    DeBakey/NASA axial flow
        ventricular assist system, 368–369
    Jarvik 2000 axial flow pump, 361–366
        description, 361–363, *363*
        experimental results, 364–365
        future developments, 365–366
        implantation, 363–364, *364*
    myocardial unloading, with axial flow
        support, 361, *362*
    Nimbus/UOP axial flow system,
        366–368
        description, 366–367, *366*, *367*
        experimental results, 367–368
        future developments, 368
        implantation, 367
    pulsatile, *vs.* nonpulsatile flow,
        359–361
    United States Surgical Corporation
        axial flow cannula pump, 369–371
    ventricular assist systems, 360–361

B cell hyper-reactivity, 199–200, 202–203
Balloon pump, intra-aortic, 291–306
    anticoagulation, during balloon
        pumping, 297
    complications of, 300–302
        balloon rupture, 301–302
        infectious complications, 302
        intra-abdominal complications, 301
        neurologic complications, 301
        vascular complications, 300–301
    development of, 291–292, *293*
    indications for, 294–295
    intraoperative placement, 295
    in pediatric patients, 302
    physiology of support, 292–294
    placement, 295–297
    postoperative placement, 295
    preoperative placement, 294–295
    removal of, 298–299
    results of, 299–300
    timing, 297–298, *298*
    weaning, 298–299
Berlin Heart device, 275–287
    blood pumps, *278*, 278–279
    cannulae, 277–278, *277*
    description, 276–282, *276*
    Deutsches Herzzentrum Berlin,
        283–284
    drive unit, 279–282, *280*, *281*, *282*
    implantation, 282–283
    pediatric assist, 284–286
Biologic compression devices, 392–395

Bleeding
    outpatient left ventricular assist
        therapy, 160–161
    perioperative factors, predisposing
        factors, 75–76, *76*
    perioperative management, 75–82
        consequences, 76–77
        incidence, 75–76, *76*
        management, 77–78
            hematologic, 77–78
            hemodynamics, 77
            humoral-pharmacologic, 78
        technical aspects, 78–79
    postoperative management, 79
    Thermo Cardiosystems ventricular
        assist device, 317
Blood type, device selection and, 33
Bridge to transplant device
    left ventricular assist devices, 7–10, *8*,
        9
    Novacor left ventricular assist system,
        330–333, *330*, *331*, *332*
    selection for, 32–33
    Texas Heart Institute, 7
Bypass
    cardiopulmonary, axial flow pumps,
        359–360
    transesophageal echocardiography
        anesthesia after, 71
        anesthesia during, 70–71

Cannula
    Berlin Heart device, 277–278, *277*
    fixation, centrifugal pumps, 221, *222*
    inflow passage, Thermo
        Cardiosystems ventricular assist
        device, 314–315, *314*, *315*, *316*
    selection, centrifugal pumps, 219–220,
        220
Cannulation, extracorporeal membrane
    oxygenation, 267–270
    circuit, 267
Cardiac arrest, extracorporeal membrane
    oxygenation, 265–266
Cardiogenic shock, extracorporeal
    membrane oxygenation, 265–266
Cardiomyoplasty, dynamic, clinical
    experience with, 394–395
Cardiopulmonary bypass
    axial flow pumps, 359–360
    separation from, anesthesia, 66–68
Centrifugal pump, 215–233. *See also under*
    type of device
    anticoagulation, management of,
        222–224
    bridge to transplantation, 227
    description of, 215–217, *216*, *217*

implantation techniques, 219–221
 cannula fixation, 221, *222*
 cannula selection, 219–220, *220*
 insertion technique, 219–220, *220*
 left heart bypass, 221
 right heart bypass, 221
 institutional experience with, 228–230,
  228, 229, 230, 230
 monitoring of, 224
 oxygenation, 225
 postcardiotomy ventricular failure,
  226–227
 post insertion, 221–224, *223*
 problems with, pediatric patients, 44
 surgery on thoracic aorta, 225–226,
  226
 ventricular assist device
  for pediatric patients, 49
  pediatric patients, 49
 in vitro comparison of, 217–218, *218*
 in vivo comparison of, 218–219
 weaning, 224–225
Columbia Presbyterian Outpatient
 Experience, 159–163, *160*
Community services, outpatient. *See*
 Outpatient
Coronary artery disease, Thermo
 Cardiosystems ventricular assist device,
 317
Cost
 left ventricular assist device, 183–192,
  187
  hospitalization, 184–186
  outpatient, 158–159, *159*, 187–188,
   188
  projections, 188–190, *190*
  rehospitalization, 187–188, *188*
 long-term support, pediatric patients,
  58
 outpatient, 158–159, *159*
Counterpulsation, balloon, pulmonary
 artery, 92
CPR devices, 396, *396*
Cuff, apical, Thermo Cardiosystems
 ventricular assist device, 314–315, *314,
 315, 316*

DeBakey/NASA axial flow ventricular
 assist system, 368–369
DeBakey ventricular assist device, 375–386
 clinical experience, 383–386, *383, 384,
  385, 386*
 description, 375–378, *376, 377, 378,
  379*
 design, 375–378, *376, 377, 278, 379*

implantation techniques, 378–380
 indications, 380–381
 limitations, 381
 preclinical testing, 381–383
Deficiency, vasopressin, vasodilatory
 shock, 114–115, *114, 115*
Device selection, 27–36
 community practice, 34–35
 current systems, 28–30
  implantable systems, 29–30
  paracorporeal, 28–29
 heart failure program, community
  practice, 35
 heart transplant program, practice
  with, 35
 patient-related issues, 33–34
  blood type, 33
  discharge, 34
  limitations, 34
  preformed antibodies, 33
  size, 33
  support, 33
 total artificial heart, 30–31
 type of support, 31–33
  bridge to recovery, 31–32
  bridge to transplantation, 32–33
Dilated cardiomyopathy, physiology,
 20–22, *21, 22, 23*
Discharge
 device selection and, 34
 patient, outpatient left ventricular
  assist therapy, 157–158
Donor heart dysfunction, pediatric
 patients, 55–56
Drive line tunnel, Thermo Cardiosystems
 ventricular assist device, 313, *313*
Dynamic cardiomyoplasty, clinical
 experience with, 394–395
Dyspnea, in heart failure, 140–141

ECMO. *See* Extracorporeal membrane
 oxygenation
Economic considerations, left ventricular
 assist device implantation, 183–192
 cost, 184–188, *186–187, 187*, 188–190,
  190
  rehospitalization, 187–188, *188*
 hospitalization, 184–186
 outpatient cost, 187–188, *188*
Education, postoperative, outpatient left
 ventricular assist therapy, 155
Electrophysiologic effects, left ventricular
 assist device placement, 109
Emergency resources, outpatient left
 ventricular assist therapy, 156–157
Energy storage, HeartSaver ventricular
 assist device, 427–428

Epicardial compression mechanical device, 387–402
  biologic compression devices, 392–395
  cardiomyoplasty, dynamic, clinical experience with, 394–395
  limitations, 395
  mechanical compression devices, 395–400
    acutely failing heart, *397*, 397–398
    chronic ventricular support, 398, *398*
    clinical experience, 399
    CPR devices, 396, *396*
    mechanical pumping force, 395
    potential limitations, 400
    surgical technique, 398–399
  muscle wraps, 392–395
  physiology, 387–392, *388, 389, 390, 391, 392*
  skeletal muscle, as pump, 392
  surgical technique, 393–394, *393*
Exercise capacity, measurement of, 137–138
Exercise performance, left ventricular assist device patients, 137–152
  arteriolar vasodilation, changes in, 138–139
  dyspnea, in heart failure, 140–141
  end-stage heart failure, 141–142
  exercise capacity, measurement of, 137–138
  exercise testing, to assess myocardial recovery, 147–149, *147, 148*
  in heart failure, pathophysiology of, 138–141
  maximal exercise capacity, 142–145, *142, 143, 144*
  metabolic abnormalities, 139–140
  serial assessment, exercise capacity, 146–147, *146*
  submaximal exercise capacity, 145–146, *146*
Exercise testing, to assess myocardial recovery, 147–149, *147, 148*
Extracorporeal devices, 213–287. *See also* Extracorporeal membrane oxygenation
  ABIOMED BVS 5000, 235–250
  Berlin Heart, 275–287
  centrifugal pumps, 215–233
  membrane oxygenation in adults, 263–274
  thoratec device, 251–262
Extracorporeal membrane oxygenation, 92–93, 263–274
  cannulation, 267–270
    cannulation, 267–270
    circuit, 267

    V-A mode, 267–269, *268*
    V-V mode, 269–270, *269*
  cardiac arrest/cardiogenic shock, 265–266
  complications, 271
  indications for, 264–267
  patient management, 270–271
  pediatric patients, 43–45, *45, 46*
  post-transplantation, left ventricular assist device, 266–267
  postcardiotomy cardiac support, 264–265
  postcardiotomy pulmonary support, 265
  primary respiratory failure, 266
  vs. ventricular assist device, pediatric patients, 56–58

Fail-safe rescues, outpatient left ventricular assist therapy, 156
Flexibility, rehabilitation, left ventricular assist device recipient, 174

Graft anastomosis, outflow, Thermo Cardiosystems ventricular assist device, 313–314
Great arteries, transposition of, pediatric patients, 51–55, *55*

Heart, artificial, CardioWest, 341–356
Heart failure
  dyspnea in, 140–141
  exercise performance, 138–141
  pathophysiology of, anesthesia and, 63–64
  program, community practice, device selection and, 35
Heart transplantation
  arginine vasopressin, 117, *117*
  program, practice with, device selection and, 35
HeartMate implantable VE left ventricular assist device, 9
HeartSaver ventricular assist device, 417–430
  advantages, 419–421, *421, 422*
  anatomic fit, 421–422
  clinical user interface, 426–427
  conduits, 424
  description, 418–419
  energy storage, 427–428
  external accessories, 419, *420*
  implantable components, 418–419, *419*
  intrathoracic ventricular assist device placement, 419–422
  operating mechanism, 422–428

percutaneous leads, elimination of, 424–426, *425*, *426*

percutaneous venting, elimination of, 423

thermal management, 423–424

valves, 424

in vivo studies, 428–429, *428*

Hematologic management, bleeding, perioperative, 77–78

Hemodialysis, immunobiology, 194

Hemodynamic interactions, physiology, 16–18

cardiac output, 16–17, *16*

pulmonary circulation, 17–18, *18*

Hemodynamics, perioperative management, 77

Historical perspective, left ventricular assist devices, 3–14, *7*

bridge to transplant, 7–10, *8*, *9*

DeBakey, intrathoracic circulatory device developed by, for left ventricular bypass, 4

HeartMate implantable VE left ventricular assist device, 9

landmark events in development, 11

long-term support, 10–11, *10*

modern era, mechanical circulatory support, 3–5, *4*, *5*

national programs, 5–6, *6*

Novacor implantable left ventricular assist device, 8

Texas Heart Institute, bridge-to-transplantation procedures at, 6–7, *7*

Thoratec extracorporeal ventricular assist device, 9

Home environment, outpatient left ventricular assist therapy, 156, *157*

Hospitalization cost, left ventricular assist device implantation, 184–186

Humoral-pharmacologic management, bleeding, perioperative, 78

Hypertension, pulmonary, reducing, 90–92, *90*, *91*

Hypotension, vasodilatory, incidence, predictors of, 116–117, *116*

Immune activation, systemic consequences of, 196–197, *197*, *198*

Immune deficiency, diseases of, 197–199

Immunobiology, 193–212

autoimmunity, 200–201

B cell hyper-reactivity, 199–200, 202–203

hemodialysis, 194

immune activation, systemic consequences of, 196–197, *197*, *198*

immune deficiency, diseases of, 197–199

immune system, effects on, 194–196

implanted biomaterials, human immunologic responses to, 194

macrophages, deposition of, on left ventricular assist device surface, 194–195, *195*

monocyte T-cell interactions, left ventricular assist device surface, 195–196

monocytes, deposition of, on left ventricular assist device surface, 194–195, *195*

T cell cytokine profile, 199

T cell defects, 202–203

Implantable systems, device selection, 29–30

Implanted biomaterials, human immunologic responses to, 194

Infection

device-related, outpatient left ventricular assist therapy, 161–162

non-device-related, outpatient left ventricular assist therapy, 161

outpatient left ventricular assist therapy, 161–162, 161–163

Inflow cannula passage, Thermo Cardiosystems ventricular assist device, 314–315, *314*, *315*, *316*

Inpatient rehabilitation unit, rehabilitation, left ventricular assist device recipient, 171–172

Intensive care unit, anesthesia, 71–72

Intracorporeal devices, 288–356

CardioWest total artificial heart, 341–356

intra-aortic balloon pump, 291–306

Novacor left ventricular assist system, 323–340

Thermo Cardiosystems ventricular assist devices, 307–322

Intra-aortic balloon pump, 291–306

anticoagulation, during balloon pumping, 297

complications of, 300–302

balloon rupture, 301–302

infectious complications, 302

intra-abdominal complications, 301

neurologic complications, 301

vascular complications, 300–301

development of, 291–292, *293*

indications for, 294–295

intraoperative placement, 295

in pediatric patients, 302

physiology of support, 292–294

placement, 295–297

Intra-aortic balloon pump (*cont.*)
    postoperative placement, 295
    preoperative placement, 294–295
    removal of, 298–299
    results of, 299–300
    timing, 297–298, *298*
    weaning, 298–299
Intrinsic muscle changes, 139–140
Ischemia, physiology, 20

Jarvik 2000 axial flow pump, 361–366
    description, 361–363, *363*
    experimental results, 364–365
    future developments, 365–366
    implantation, 363–364, *364*

Landmark events, in development of left
    ventricular assist devices, 11
Left coronary artery, anomalous origin,
    from pulmonary artery, pediatric
    patients, 49–51, *50, 52-53, 54*
Left heart bypass, centrifugal pumps, 221
Left ventricular assist device
    exercise performance in patients with,
        137–152
    historical perspective, 3–14, 6
        bridge to transplant, 7–10, *8, 9*
        DeBakey, intrathoracic circulatory
            device developed by, for left
            ventricular bypass, 4
        HeartMate implantable VE left
            ventricular assist device, 9
        landmark events in development,
            11
        long-term support, 10–11, *10*
        modern era, mechanical circulatory
            support, 3–5, *4, 5*
        national programs, 5–6, *6*
        Novacor implantable left
            ventricular assist device, 8
        Texas Heart Institute, bridge-to-
            transplantation procedures at,
            6–7, *7*
        Thoratec extracorporeal ventricular
            assist device, 9
    immunobiology, 193–212
    implantation, economic
        considerations, 183–192
    placement, vasodilatory hypotension
        after, 111–120
        arginine vasopressin, 116–117
            with heart transplantation, 117,
                117
            hemodynamic effects of, 113–114,
                113
            for vasodilatory shock, 112–115

vasodilatory hypotension,
    incidence, predictors of, 116–117,
        116
vasodilatory shock, etiology,
    117–118
vasopressin deficiency, vasodilatory
    shock, 114–115, *114, 115*
quality of life issues, 177–182
recipient
    arrhythmias in, 103–110
        electrophysiologic effects, device
            placement, 109
        postoperative management,
            104–109, *107*
        preoperative, 103–104
    rehabilitation, 167–176
    support, left ventricular recovery
        during, 121–136
        beta-adrenoceptor, autoantibodies
            directed against, 123–124, *123*
        device explanation, 125–126
            timing of, 128–129
        follow-up, after device removal, 126
        implantation, perioperative
            management, 122
        left ventricular assist device
            implantation, cardiac
            performance following, 124
        medical therapy, 122–123
        predictive parameter, for weaning,
            130
        pump adjustment, following
            improvement, 124–125
        weaning from mechanical cardiac
            support, 121–122
Left ventricular recovery during left
    ventricular assist device support,
    121–136
    beta-adrenoceptor, autoantibodies
        directed against, 123–124, *123*
    device explanation, 125–126
        timing of, 128–129
    follow-up, after device removal, 126
    implantation, perioperative
        management, 122
    left ventricular assist device
        implantation, cardiac performance
        following, 124
    medical therapy, 122–123
    predictive parameter, for weaning,
        130
    pump adjustment, following
        improvement, 124–125
    weaning from mechanical cardiac
        support, 121–122

Long-term support
    left ventricular assist devices, 10–11,
        10
    pediatric patients, 58
LVAD. *See* Left ventricular assist device

Macrophages, deposition of, on left
    ventricular assist device surface,
    194–195, *195*
Malfunction, outpatient left ventricular
    assist therapy, 162–163
Maximal exercise capacity, exercise
    performance, left ventricular assist
    device patients, 142–145, *142, 143,
    144*
Mechanical support. *See also under* type of
    device
        overview, left ventricular assist
            devices, 3–5, *4, 5*
        weaning patient from, pediatric
            patients, 45–47
Metabolic abnormalities, exercise
    performance, left ventricular assist
    device patients, 139–140
Monocyte
    deposition of, on left ventricular assist
        device surface, 194–195, *195*
    T-cell interactions, left ventricular
        assist device surface, 195–196
Muscle, skeletal, as pump, 392
Myocardial unloading, with axial flow
    support, axial flow pumps, 361, *362*

National programs, left ventricular assist
    devices, 5–6, *6*
Neurologic events, outpatient left
    ventricular assist therapy, 161
Nimbus/UOP axial flow system, 366–368
    description, 366–367, *366, 367*
    experimental results, 367–368
    future developments, 368
    implantation, 367
Nitric oxide, effect on mean arterial
    pressure, 91
Nitrogen, effect on mean arterial pressure,
    91
Non-device-related infections, outpatient
    left ventricular assist therapy, 161
Nonpulsatile flow, *vs.* pulsatile flow, axial
    flow pumps, 359–361
Novacor left ventricular assist system, 8,
    323–340
        American bridge-to-transplant
            experience, 330–333, *330, 331, 331,
            332*

antithrombotic therapy, 329
destination therapy, 337
European bridge-to-recovery
    experience, 335–337, *336*
global experience, 333–335, *333, 334,
    335, 336*
implant technique, 328
outpatient support, 329–330
patient selection, 327–328
perioperative management, 328–329
quality of life, 337–338, *337*
results, 330–338
system evolution, 323–327, *324–326*

Outflow graft anastomosis, Thermo
    Cardiosystems ventricular assist device,
    313–314
Outpatient adverse clinical events,
    outpatient left ventricular assist therapy,
    160–163
Outpatient costs
    left ventricular assist device
        implantation, 187–188, *188*
    outpatient left ventricular assist
        therapy, 158–159, *159*
Outpatient left ventricular assist therapy,
    153–165, *154*
    bleeding, 160–161
    Columbia Presbyterian Outpatient
        Experience, 159–163, *160*
    community services, 157
    device malfunction, 162–163
    device-related infections, 161–162
    emergency resources, 156–157
    fail-safe rescues, 156
    home environment, 156, *157*
    infections, 161–163
    initiation of outpatient therapy, 155
    neurologic events, 161
    non-device-related infections, 161
    outpatient adverse clinical events,
        160–163
    outpatient costs, 158–159, *159*
    outpatient program, creating, 154–157
    patient discharge, 157–158
        general release protocol, 157–158
    postoperative education, 155
    preoperative patient education, 155
    program structure, 154
Outpatient management, left ventricular
    assist device recipient, 172–175
Oxygenation
    centrifugal pumps, 225
    extracorporeal membrane, 92–93,
        263–274

Oxygenation (*cont.*)
    cannulation, 267–270
        cannulation, 267–270
        circuit, 267
        V-A mode, 267–269, *268*
        V-V mode, 269–270, *269*
    cardiac arrest/cardiogenic shock,
        265–266
    complications, 271
    indications for, 264–267
    patient management, 270–271
    post-transplantation, left ventricular
        assist device, 266–267
    postcardiotomy cardiac support,
        264–265
    postcardiotomy pulmonary
        support, 265
    primary respiratory failure, 266

Paracorporeal systems, device selection,
    28–29
Patient discharge, outpatient left
    ventricular assist therapy, 157–158
    general release protocol, 157–158
Patient education, preoperative, outpatient
    left ventricular assist therapy, 155
Patient evaluation, rehabilitation, left
    ventricular assist device recipient,
    168–169
Pediatric patients, 37–62
    Berlin Heart device, 284–286
    centrifugal pump ventricular assist
        device, 44, 49
    donor heart dysfunction, 55–56
    extracorporeal membrane oxygenation
        strategy, 43–45, *45, 46*
    indications, 38–39
    intra-aortic balloon pump, 302
    left coronary artery, anomalous
        origin, from pulmonary artery,
        49–51, *50, 52, 53, 54*
    long-term support, 58
        cost, 58
    Royal Children's Hospital, 47–49
    transposition of great arteries, 51–55,
        55
    ventricular assist device, 39–43, *40, 44*
        vs. extracorporeal membrane
        oxygenation, 56–58
    weaning patient from mechanical
        support, 45–47
Pennsylvania State University
    3M health care total artificial heart,
        410–415
    total artificial heart, 403–416
    totally implantable left ventricular
        assist device, 403–416

Percutaneous leads, elimination of,
    heartSaver ventricular assist device,
    424–426, *425, 426*
Pharmacology, anesthesia, 64–65
Physiology, ventricular assistance, 15–26
    dilated cardiomyopathy, 20–22, *21,*
        22, 23
    hemodynamic interactions, 16–18
        cardiac output, 16–17, *16*
        pulmonary circulation, 17–18, *18*
        venous return, 16–17, *16*
    ischemia, 20
    mechanical anatomic interactions,
        18–20, *19*
    right ventricular function, in left
        ventricular assist device recipients,
        22–24
Postcardiotomy cardiac support,
    extracorporeal membrane oxygenation,
    264–265
Postcardiotomy pulmonary support,
    extracorporeal membrane oxygenation,
    265
Postcardiotomy ventricular failure,
    centrifugal pumps, 226–227
Postoperative education, outpatient left
    ventricular assist therapy, 155
Postoperative management, bleeding, 79
Preformed antibodies, device selection
    and, 33
Preoperative assessment, anesthesia, 65
Preoperative patient education, 155
    outpatient left ventricular assist
        therapy, 155
Preperitoneal pocket, Thermo
    Cardiosystems ventricular assist device,
    310–313, *312*
Primary respiratory failure, extracorporeal
    membrane oxygenation, 266
Protocol, release, patient discharge,
    157–158
Pulmonary artery balloon
    counterpulsation, 92
Pulmonary hypertension, reducing, 90–92,
    90, 91
Pulsatile, *vs.* nonpulsatile flow, axial flow
    pumps, 359–361

Quality of life
    left ventricular assist devices, 177–182
    Novacor left ventricular assist system,
        337–338, *337*

Regurgitation, aortic valve, Thermo
    Cardiosystems ventricular assist device,
    317

Rehabilitation, left ventricular assist device recipient, 167–176
    outpatient management, 172–175
        aerobic training, 173–174
        flexibility, 174
        strengthening, 175
    patient evaluation, 168–169
    treatment, 169–172
        inpatient rehabilitation unit, 171–172
        intensive care unit, 169, *170*
        regular floor care, 169–171, *171, 172, 173, 174*
        step-down unit, 169–171, *171, 172, 173, 174*
Rehospitalization costs, left ventricular assist device implantation, 187–188, *188*
Release protocol
    general, outpatient left ventricular assist therapy, 157–158
    patient discharge, 157–158
Respiratory failure, primary, extracorporeal membrane oxygenation, 266
Right heart bypass, centrifugal pumps, 221
Right-sided circulatory failure, 83–101
    diagnosis, 86–88, *86, 87, 88*
    hypertension, pulmonary, reducing, 90–92, *90, 91*
    medical therapy, 88–89, *89*
    nitric oxide, effect on mean arterial pressure, 91
    nitrogen, effect on mean arterial pressure, 91
    pathophysiology, 84–85, *84*
    perioperative contributions, 85–86, *85*
    preoperative contributions, 85–86, *85*
    surgical therapy, 92–98
    treatment, 88–98
Right-to-left venoarterial shunting, 93–94
Right ventricular assist devices, 94–98, *95, 97, 98*
Right ventricular function, in left ventricular assist device recipients, 22–24
Royal Children's Hospital, pediatric patients, 47–49

Serial assessment, left ventricular assist device patients, exercise capacity, 146–147, *146*
Shock
    cardiogenic, extracorporeal membrane oxygenation, 265–266
    vasodilatory, etiology, 117–118
Size, device selection and, 33

Skeletal muscle, as pump, 392
Step-down unit
    left ventricular assist device recipient, 169–171, *171, 172, 173, 174*
    rehabilitation, left ventricular assist device recipient, 169–171, *171, 172, 173, 174*
Submaximal exercise capacity, exercise performance, left ventricular assist device patients, 145–146, *146*
Support, device selection and, 33

T cell
    cytokine profile, immunobiology, 199
    defects, immunobiology, 202–203
Texas Heart Institute program, left ventricular assist devices, 6–7, *7*
Thermal management, HeartSaver ventricular assist device, 423–424
Thermo Cardiosystems ventricular assist device, 307–322
    aortic valve regurgitation, 317
    apical cuff, 314–315, *314, 315, 316*
    bleeding, 317
    contraindications, 318–319, *318*
    coronary artery disease, 317
    criteria selection, 318–319, *318*
    de-aring protocol, 315–316
    description, 308–309, *309, 310, 311, 312*
    drive line tunnel, 313, *313*
    historical perspective, 307–308, *308*
    implantable technique, 309–318
    inflow cannula passage, 314–315, *314, 315, 316*
    institutional experience, 319–320, *319, 320*
    limitations, 318–319, *318*
    outflow graft anastomosis, 313–314
    preperitoneal pocket, 310–313, *312*
    ventricular aneurysm, 317
    Worldwide Registry, 319–320, *319, 320*
Thoracic aorta, surgery on, centrifugal pumps, 225–226, *226*
Thoratec device, 251–262
    description, 251–253, *252, 254*
    implantation technique, 253–256, *255*
    indications, 256
    limitations, 257–258
    for pulmonary circulatory support, 257–258
    transplantation, bridging to, 258–260
Thoratec extracorporeal ventricular assist device, 9

Total artificial heart
  CardioWest, 341–356
    clinical results, 354–355
    device description, 341–346, *342,
      343, 344*
    implantation technique, 346–352,
      346, 347, 348, 349, 350, 351, 352
    indications for, 352–353, *353*
    limitations, 353–354
  device selection, 30–31
Transesophageal echocardiography,
  anesthesia, 68–71, *69, 70*
  during bypass, 70–71
  post bypass, 71
Transplantation
  bridge to
    centrifugal pumps, 227
    device selection, 32–33
    left ventricular assist, 7–10, *8, 9*
    Novacor left ventricular assist
      system, 330–333, *330, 331, 332*
    Texas Heart Institute, 7
    Thoratec device, 258–260
  extracorporeal membrane oxygenation
    after, 266–267
  program, device selection, practice
    with, 35
  vasodilatory hypotension, after left
    ventricular assist device placement,
    arginine vasopressin, 117, *117*
Transposition of great arteries, pediatric
  patients, 51–55, *55*
Transthoracic cannulae, ABIOMED BVS
  5000, 235–236, *237*
Treatment, rehabilitation, left ventricular
  assist device recipient, 169, *170*
Type of support, device selection, 31–33
  bridge to recovery, 31–32
  bridge to transplantation, 32–33

United States Surgical Corporation, axial
  flow cannula pump, 369–371

VAD. *See* Ventricular assist device
Vasodilatory hypotension
  after left ventricular assist device
    placement, 111–120
  arginine vasopressin, 116–117
    with heart transplantation, 117,
      117
    hemodynamic effects of, 113–114,
      113
    for vasodilatory shock, 112–115
  vasodilatory hypotension,
    incidence, predictors of, 116–117,
      116

vasodilatory shock, etiology,
  117–118
vasopressin deficiency, vasodilatory
  shock, 114, 115, *114, 115*
incidence, predictors of, 116–117, *116*
Vasodilatory shock, etiology, 117–118
Vasopressin, arginine, 116–117
  deficiency, vasodilatory shock, 114,
    115, *114–115*
  with heart transplantation, 117, *117*
  hemodynamic effects of, 113–114, *113*
  mechanism of action of, 117–118
  for vasodilatory shock, 112–115
Venoarterial shunting, right-to-left, 93–94
Ventricular aneurysm, Thermo
  Cardiosystems ventricular assist device,
  317
Ventricular assist device
  vs. extracorporeal membrane
    oxygenation, pediatric patients,
    56–58
  Thermo Cardiosystems, 307–322
    aortic valve regurgitation, 317
    apical cuff, 314–315, *314, 315, 316*
    bleeding, 317
    coronary artery disease, 317
    criteria selection, 318–319, *318*
    de-aring protocol, 315–316
    description, 308–309, *309, 310, 311,
      312*
    drive line tunnel, 313, *313*
    historical perspective, 307–308, *308*
    implantable technique, 309–318
    institutional experience, 319–320,
      319, 320
    outflow graft anastomosis, 313–314
    preperitoneal pocket, 310–313, *312*
    ventricular aneurysm, 317
Ventricular assist device strategy, pediatric
  patients, 39–43, *40, 44*
Ventricular assist devices, 94–98, *95, 97, 98*
Ventricular failure, postcardiotomy,
  centrifugal pumps, 226–227

Weaning
  from centrifugal pumps, 224–225
  from intra-aortic balloon pump,
    298–299
  from mechanical support, 121–122
    pediatric patients, 45–47
    predictive parameter, 130
Worldwide Registry
  ABIOMED BVS 5000, 247–249, *249*
  Thermo Cardiosystems ventricular
    assist device, 319–320, *319, 320*